NORMAN HAIRE
AND THE STUDY OF SEX

Diana Wyndham

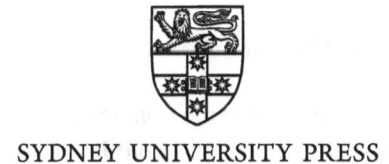

SYDNEY UNIVERSITY PRESS

Published 2012 by SYDNEY UNIVERSITY PRESS
sydney.edu.au/sup

© Diana Wyndham 2012
© Sydney University Press 2012
2013 printing

Reproduction and Communication for other purposes

Except as permitted under the Act, no part of this edition may be reproduced, stored in a retrieval system, or communicated in any form or by any means without prior written permission. All requests for reproduction or communication should be made to Sydney University Press at the address below:

Sydney University Press, Fisher Library F03
University of Sydney NSW 2006 AUSTRALIA
Email: sup.info@sydney.edu.au

National Library of Australia Cataloguing-in-Publication entry
Author: Wyndham, Diana.
Title: Norman Haire and the study of sex / Diana Wyndham. Foreword by Michael Kirby.
ISBN: 9781743320068 (pbk.)
Notes: Includes bibliographical references and index.
Subjects: Haire, Norman, 1892-1952.
    Sex educators--Biography.
    Sexologists--Biography.
    Sex.
    Birth control--History.
    Contraception--History.
    Contraceptive devices.
    Reproductive rights--History.
    Family planning--History.
Other Authors/Contributors:
    Kirby, M. D. (Michael Donald), 1939-
Dewey Number: 304.666

Cover design by Dushan Mrva-Montoya

Unless otherwise stated, all images are from the Norman Haire collection from the Rare Books and Special Collections Library at the University of Sydney.

Contents

Figures		4
Acknowledgements		7
Foreword by The Hon. Michael Kirby AC, CMG		9
1.	Introduction: Norman Haire – a man of valour	15
2.	Early years	21
3.	Zions the Scapegoat	49
4.	Haire the Phoenix	67
5.	Making his mark	107
6.	Moving up in the world	135
7.	Organising the 1929 congress	169
8.	The darkening years	193
9.	Escalating troubles	223
10.	Mounting gloom on most fronts	265
11.	Haire's homecoming	299
12.	Dr Wykeham Terriss writes for *Woman*	323
13.	The ABC population debate	343
14.	Final years	361
15.	Conclusion	397
Abbreviations		429
References		431
Index		469

Figures

Cover. Caricature of Haire by EX [Edmond Xavier] Kapp, 1929
2.1. Henry Zions (Norman's father) — 22
2.2. Clara Zions (Norman's mother) — 24
2.3. Norman Zions aged four — 27
2.4. 'Yours sincerely, Norman Zions, 1909' — 30
2.5. Henry Havelock Ellis, the 'Darwin of Sex' — 34
2.6. Sydney University Commemoration Day, May 1912 — 39
2.7. Four Zions siblings in 1916 — 42
2.8. Norman Zions as a medical graduate, 1915 — 43
2.9. Captain Norman Zions, 1915 — 46
3.1. Dr Norman Zions at Newcastle Hospital — 50
4.1. Countess of Hungary's £200 loan cheque to Haire — 73
4.2. Magnus Hirschfeld — 79
4.3. Eugene Steinach — 89
4.4. Haire pessary — 101
5.1. Diana Wyndham and Ralf Dose visiting the Magnus Hirschfeld Memorial in Berlin — 110
5.2. Sketch of Norman Haire by Chris Watt, July 1925 — 124
6.1. Clara Zions — 140
6.2. Flyer for Haire's Cromer Welfare and Sunlight Centre — 147
6.3. Mural at the Cromer Welfare and SunlightCentre — 150
6.4. 127 Harley Street London — 152
6.5. Haire's vast Chinese bed — 154
6.6. Norman beside his Rolls Royce — 156

6.7. Haire acts in Ivor Montagu's film *Bluebottles*	166
7.1. Wigmore Hall, London	173
7.2. Haire in rational dress at Ethel Mannin's 'cottage'	188
8.1. Haire, Hirschfeld and Giese at a WLSR congress	204
8.2. 1930 WLSR congress	205
8.3. The last WLSR congress in Brno, 1932	218
8.4. Haire with his camera in the Brno congress	220
9.1. WB Yeats before the 'rejuvenation' operation	246
9.2. Ethel Mannin, 1925. Photograph by EO Hoppé	247
9.3. Haire's friend 'Paddy' O'Connor with his car	251
10.1. Post card of Nettleden Lodge	271
10.2. Visitors' map of Nettleden Lodge	273
10.3. Norman Haire by P Tennyson Cole	277
10.4. Conchita Supervia and Ivor Newton	278
10.5. Conchita Supervia's grave	280
11.1. 7 Elizabeth Street	303
11.2. Hengrove Hall, 193 Macquarie Street	306
11.3. 1940s greeting from Norman to his brother Bert	307
11.4. Dr Lotte Fink in 1942	311
12.1. Publicity photograph of Haire	324
12.2. An article Haire wrote as Wykeham Terriss	326
13.1. Cartoon of Norman Haire and Dame Enid Lyons	348
13.2. The ABC's 'Population unlimited?' debate	350
15.1. Cartoon by George Molnar, 1952	403
15.2. Norman Haire and his partner, Willem van de Hagt	422
15.3. Haire's greeting card	426

Acknowledgements

I first wish to thank Sydney University's Faculty of Medicine for awarding me a Norman Haire Fellowship in 1998. My interest in Haire began even earlier and my many years' research for this biography involved travel, locating primary resources, interviewing Haire's colleagues, friends and relations and assembling the information. Two benefits flow from this. When I started, Sydney University Press (SUP) was dormant but now it is thriving and it is appropriate, sixty years after Haire's death, for them to publish a tribute to such an illustrious Sydney University graduate and generous benefactor. Secondly, my work has been enriched by many people whose help I greatly appreciate. Unfortunately, some of them have since died: Meg Brink, John Cargher, Dr Ian Cope, Dr Stella Cornelius, Ethelwyn Dawson Wallace, Averil Fink, Dr Frank Forster, Dr Ben Haneman, Jacquie Hart, Sir Rupert Charles Hart-Davis, Ron Horan, Patrick O'Connor, Professor John Passmore, Elizabeth Riddell, Betty Swabsky, Les Tanner, Dr Peter Tyler, Margaret Whitlam and my friend Dorothy Simons who provided encouragement and translated large amounts of German and French.

I received additional help with translations from Kep Enderby (Esperanto), Carmel Marjenberg (old shorthand), Agata Mrva-Montoya (Polish), Peter Walmsley (Latin) and Hugh and Josefina Wyndham (Spanish). Others provided expert advice: Professor RF Foster about Yeats' poetry, Dr Irvine Loudon about historical obstetrics, Dr Chandak Sengoopta about glands and hormones, Professor Gillian Shenfield about pharmacology and Ralf Dose who shared with me his encyclopaedic knowledge of Magnus Hirschfeld and the World League for Sexual Reform.

I appreciate the warm support I received from Haire's relatives: Norman Cohen in Israel, Gloria Savill and her son John Savill in Queensland, Gillian Shenfield in Sydney and Selwyn Torrance in

Philadelphia. I was assisted by the librarians and archivists whose institutions are listed in the bibliography and, while it is impossible to thank everyone, I acknowledge the assistance I received from Canon Stuart Babbage, Josephine Bastian, Dr Gaston Bauer, Dr Alison Beard, Professor Nancy Beere, Neil Boness, Stephanie Brody, David Bradshaw, Dr Pat Buckridge, Dr Graeme Budd, Paul Brunton, Dr Patrick Buckridge, Richard Casey, Professor Robert Clancy, Iain Clark, Peter Coleman, Dr Ivan Crozier, Alyson Dalby, Dr Marie de Lepervanche, Ken Dickson, Edwina Doe, John El-Badawi, Dr Yolanda Eraso, Professor Raymond E Fancher, Jean Faulks, Beat Frischknecht, Jonathan Gathorne-Hardy, Dr Una Gault, Dr Judith Godden, Professor Phyllis Grosskurth, Dr Lesley A Hall, Professor David J Handleman, Gwen Hause, Barbara Horton, Professor Anthea Hyslop, Dr Robert M Kaplan, Professor John Kelly, Francis King, Dr Michael King, Michael Kirby AC CMG, Phillip Knightley, Dr Paul Lancaster, Dr Lachlan Lang, Dr C W S LaSalle, Dr Ruth A Fink Latukefu, Dame Hermoine Lee, Professor Stephen Leeder, Antionette le Marchant, Ros McDonald, Professor John Mack, Renata Mancini, Miriam Margolyes, Professor Carmel Maguire, Lisa McGregor, Jan Monson, Kees Moeliker, Katie Molnar, Dr Nicole Moore, Professor Kevin Morgan, Dr Peter Morton, Dr Agata Mrva-Montoya, Dushan Mrva-Montoya, Susan Murray-Smith, Bronwyn O'Reilly, Brayden Phillips, Julie Price, Dr Jan Roberts, Liz Rouse, Dr D'Arcy Ryan, Lee Sands, Betty Sheehan, Dr Stefania Siedlecky, Dr Gary Simes, Jean Simpson, Nigel Sinnott, Dr Graeme Skinner, Paul Snijders, John Spence, Dr Margaret Spencer, Lois Sweet, Dr John Thearle, Dr Di Tibbits, Melissa von Bergner, Margaret Vos, Judy Wedderburn, Professor Jeffrey Weeks, Dr Ann Williams and most of all John Wyndham.

Foreword

The Hon. Michael Kirby AC, CMG*

On a parallel course

As I began reading this fascinating biography by Diana Wyndham, I became a little unsettled by the uncanny similarity between several aspects in the life of the hero of this book (for hero he is) and elements in my own life.

We were both born in Sydney. We both grew up in the suburbs during a time of prudish sexual morality, when sexual matters were private and 'not to be spoken of' by Christian or Jewish people. Religious opinions informed perceptions of morality and directly influenced politicians, officials, judges, police and other instruments of governmental authority. Laws, regulations and censorship were implemented to uphold religious norms and to curtail sexual freedom. Anyone who questioned these features of Australian society was either evil, or demented or, at best, eccentric.

Norman Haire attended Fort Street School, as I later would. He took a leading role in Play Day, which was the school's alternative to sport and cadets. It made him, and many after, such as Barwick, Wran and myself, devotees of acting. Haire graduated from Sydney University, as I did, choosing medicine after his parents thwarted his acting ambitions.

At an early stage Norman Haire realised that he was homosexual, as I would later do. But such were the criminal laws and social stigma of the time that he could not mention these taboo subjects because of the then prevailing rule of 'Don't ask. Don't tell'. Undoubtedly, this discovery contributed to his fascination with the whole subject of sexual expression.

Norman Haire went to London in 1919 and soon launched his crusade to save the world from sexual misery just as sexology

---

* Justice of the High Court of Australia (1996–2009).

was emerging as a discipline with wide-ranging concerns about contraception, sterilisation, abortion and the rights of people oppressed by religious control. He contacted leading figures in the fields of contraception, women's rights, eugenics and homosexuality. Very soon he was writing books, giving lectures and participating in committees and conferences. In addition, he worked as an honorary doctor in birth control clinics for poor women and established a flourishing gynaecological practice in Harley Street, London. He liked to confront people with his unsettling opinions about sex, in an attempt to shake them out of adherence to religious opinions, which he blamed for imposing misery, guilt, unwanted conception, impotence and suicidal depression because of a lack of sexual fulfilment.

Haire was, as Diana Wyndham's biography shows, a quick witted and talented public performer with an attractive voice who tirelessly challenged the prevailing 'sex negating culture.' Many people were shocked by his powerful and persuasive arguments which, he said, reflected his rationalist, humanist approach to sexual equality. As a result his supporters cheered; but his opponents tried to silence him.

Haire had no doubts about his decision to champion sexual reform but as he approached his premature death in 1952, it is inevitable that a man of such intelligence would have asked whether there was any evidence that his varied activities had altered the puritanical, sex negating, pleasure-hostile society into which he had been born.

An Australian hero

Norman Haire was born as Norman Zions, in Sydney in 1892, into a world plagued by sexual dysfunction, hypocrisy and anxiety. Even masturbation was regarded not only as a religious sin but also as a serious medical problem. This was the prevailing attitude that had endured for hundreds of years. In the reign of Queen Victoria, even up to the year of Haire's birth as the 11th, and last, child of modestly prosperous parents, the sexual order of things had remained largely unquestioned, in the British Empire at least. This would last well into the 20th century.

In the 19th century, Galton and Darwin re-examined the views about the evolution of the human species. So it was inevitable that rational proponents of their writings would question the prevailing rules on personal sexual morality. The intellectual liberation that followed Darwin's sensational hypothesis gave birth to scientific research and much scrutiny of human sexuality. The easier moral climate of Germany and the Austro-Hungarian Empire was conducive to research by Richard Krafft-Ebing, Sigmund Freud and Magnus Hirschfeld, the last of whom used empirical methodology in his research into homosexuality. In England, Havelock Ellis had started work on his epic *Studies in the psychology of sex*. Norman Haire arrived in London during these heady times. He was to contribute to this progress and to collaborate with female champions of women's reproductive rights including Marie Stopes, Margaret Sanger and Dora Russell.

Haire came to play a significant role in this international movement, as described in Diana Wyndham's book. Indeed, he played a catalytic role in the growth of a new global science of sexuality. In a sense, he was, with others, laying the grounds for the remarkable work of taxonomy performed by Dr Alfred Kinsey at Indiana University in Bloomington, in the United States of America in the 1940s and 1950s.

As this book reveals, Kinsey and Haire formed a bond of mutual admiration. Haire's work, and allied British and European studies, encouraged Kinsey in his examination of sexual variations in the lives of Americans. Like Haire, Kinsey, the quiet zoologist and expert in gall wasps, warmed to the role of popularising the new knowledge about human sexuality. With the aid of radio broadcasts and mass distribution newspapers and magazines, the moment for change had arrived. The attempt of religious orthodoxy to stamp out the fascinating information failed, thanks to gifted communicators such as Kinsey and Haire. Yet without modern media, they would have been unable to tap the interest and support of men and women in the suburbs whom Kinsey and Haire instinctively understood. Kinsey's research undoubtedly stimulated the moves in Britain to re-examine the criminal laws on homosexuality and prostitution. That led, in turn, to the repeal of the laws in Britain that criminalised homosexuals. A great global movement had begun.

Haire contributed to this movement both in the practical advice that he gave to patients and in the theoretical and descriptive underpinnings he provided in the well-expressed, simple and popular works that he wrote at a time when such writings were rare. Haire's medical qualification and experience gave him the cachet which made his writings acceptable in both scientific literature and popular outlets. They gave a green light to his engagement with popular media.

It would be an exaggeration to suggest that Norman Haire's efforts were central to the critical research of Alfred Kinsey and his followers and Diana Wyndham does not go so far. Nevertheless, he was, as her biography shows, an extremely well-known figure in the field of sexology during the 1920s to 1940s. To this extent, he prepared the way, not only in the movement for women's reproductive rights but also in helping to loosen the oppressive barriers to the study of sexual health and satisfaction, including those faced by homosexuals, like Haire himself.

Dilemmas and progress

This book reveals a dilemma. Should we condemn Haire as an intellectual coward who used the stalking horse of female sexuality and contraception while remaining pitifully silent about the sexual oppression that affected him personally? Does his silence on this account show his essential defects as a scientist? Whilst views may differ over the answers to these questions, those offered by Diana Wyndham in the closing chapter of this book are convincing to me.

As one whose own puberty was emerging at about the time of Haire's death, I can affirm the tremendous power of oppression that was imposed upon homosexuals, especially males, who were then subject to criminal sanctions in most English speaking countries. One by one, the rational steps towards scientific reality and civic equality are being taken in western countries today. The grip of the old patriarchal pact between religion and politics is being broken. Norman Haire played an honourable part in bringing about the conditions in which this could happen. He was, as Diana Wyndham has suggested, a life-affirming man, an enlarger of human happiness whose colourful personality was well suited to challenging the straighteners, censors, wowsers and oppressors.

Foreword

This book is long overdue. It was to Sydney University that Haire willed the bulk of his estate in a bequest huge by the standards of the time. He thereby demonstrated his affection for his original homeland and place of learning. It is splendid that 60 years after his death, Sydney University Press should now publish this biography.

Happily, it turns out to be more than an institutional work of dutiful gratitude. It brings to life a colourful, witty and larger than life character who was well in advance of his time. He exhibited courage, imagination and persistence. How surprised, and pleased, he would be if he had lived to see that his dream has come closer to fulfilment. That human sexuality would be given the respect it deserves for the importance it holds in the lives of virtually everyone. And that honesty is on the way to replacing hypocrisy, transparency in the place of secrets and dialogue in the place of silence.

Michael Kirby

1 October 2012

1

Introduction: Norman Haire – a man of valour

Queen Victoria had nine children, despite her reservations (delicately expressed in French) about the inconvenience and hardship of having a large family.[1] Large families were the norm during her reign and the high birthrates in Britain and the Commonwealth went in tandem with high mortality rates of mothers and babies. Paradoxically, while Victorian artists and writers were preoccupied with death, it was indelicate, even taboo, to discuss the 'facts of life' even though unchecked childbearing so often caused death. One such unplanned and unwanted baby was born in Sydney on 21 January 1892, his parents' 11th and final child who, for the first 27 years of his life, was called Norman Zions. He left Australia in undeserved disgrace in 1919, changed his name to Norman Haire and began a new career in London.

My interest in him spans more than three decades. Following a feminist takeover of the Family Planning Association of New South Wales, I was employed to establish the library in 1975 and having acquired some of the books he had written decades before was struck by his sensible, lucid writing which still retained its relevance. In 1987 Stefania Siedlecky and I were members of the FPA Board and won a Bicentennial grant to write *Populate and perish: a history of Australian women's fight for birth control*. We discussed the shrinking of Australian families between 1870 and 1930 despite the unreliability of most contraceptive methods and the lack of clinics. It was driven by social and economic factors and in response the New South Wales government called a Royal Commission in 1904 to investigate the declining birthrate. As a result, baby health centres and a £5 baby bonus were

---

1 Queen Victoria asked her uncle Leopold, King of the Belgians, on 5 January 1841 if he really wanted her to be the *Mamma d'une nombreuse famille*.

introduced to try and reverse the trend. In 1921 the newly established Commonwealth Department of Health provided additional measures to help stamp out venereal diseases (VD), produce healthy families and increase the population; in 1925 and 1944 the federal government held enquiries into the threats posed by VD, a falling birthrate and a high maternal and infant mortality rate. People were starting to see that it was no use having a high birthrate if the babies did not survive. However, many politicians, clergy and doctors remained strongly opposed to birth control because they believed that Australia needed to 'populate or perish'; contraceptives were hard to obtain and abortion was illegal. Even in the 1960s many doctors refused to prescribe the Pill because they claimed it would encourage promiscuity and there was no federal government support for family planning until 1972.

Haire featured briefly in our book and, as he advocated birth control and eugenics, my next step was to examine the Australian eugenics movement in my history PhD thesis. Haire took centre stage in 1998 when I won a Norman Haire Fellowship from the University of Sydney's Faculty of Medicine. I was determined to finish the biography that a Melbourne gynaecologist began in 1978 after winning a Haire fellowship but then abandoned, saying the family had disowned Haire as a black sheep, a publisher wasn't interested, people became chilly on hearing his name and one woman had even consulted her solicitor. I read many more such stories and found there was no basis for them; at first the myths irritated me and then I became determined to do what I could to set the record straight.

I was pleasantly surprised to find that Haire's colleagues and relatives were very interested in my research and generously provided me with stories and photographs. The family had once been part of the Jewish community in Plock in Poland which used to be one of the biggest in Europe; they are very proud of Norman and there is no basis for the black sheep claim. Norman Cohen, an elderly relative who lives in Israel, is particularly proud of his illustrious namesake: he was named in Haire's honour by his mother Ettie Shrank who was the same age as her cousin Norman. As a young married woman living in Britain's north in the early 1930s, Ettie made annual trips to Harley Street to consult him about birth control and afterwards he would take her to lunch. As an old woman she livened up when his name was mentioned and she always stressed what a perfect gentleman he was. In Queensland, Norman's niece Gloria Savill has fond memories of him and said her father Bert was Norman's favourite brother (he called him Bertie) and they kept in touch by letter right up until he died. Professor Gillian Shenfield, a relative who lives in Sydney, also spoke about Ettie Shrank (her strong-willed grandmother and Norman Cohen's mother), one of the Scottish branch of the family who as a teenager climbed out of her bedroom window to take part in an amateur dramatics performance. Ettie liked sharing his company and told Gillian stories (always prefaced by the warning 'don't tell your mother') and said her sex life had improved greatly once he helped her to obtain contraception. Ettie was widely read, knowledgeable about music, passionate about the theatre and she would have been proud to say 'my cousin Norman Haire the distinguished gynaecologist in London', although she would not have said he practised birth control and gave sex advice because that was not spoken about in polite society.

I immersed myself in books and articles by and about Haire and tried to form a picture of his life. Gradually I began thinking that Haire would like this or laugh at that, and without these warm feelings about this passionate man I would never have devoted so many years to this project. His relatives were helpful and so were people who responded to my RSVP request in the *Sydney Morning Herald*. I started to give conference papers about Haire and this stimulated people to provide me with anecdotes and the names of people who had known him in the 1940s, and with this help I contacted Margaret and Gough Whitlam who as students had met him through the Sydney University Dramatic Society, Jan Monson who as a teenager had typed his letters, Una Gault who went to one of his psychology lectures, Stefania Siedlecky who as a young doctor attended his obstetrics lecture and Stella Cornelius who with her husband consulted him as patients. I spent a morning with the poet Elizabeth Riddell who spoke fondly about their collaboration when he wrote a sexual advice column in the women's magazine she edited. In Sydney I visited the site of the house where he was born in

Paddington, and collected reviews and programs of his acting and recital performances, which began while he was still at school. I photographed the apartments where he lived in the 1940s and Hengrove Hall in Macquarie Street where he worked. In Britain I took photographs of his Harley Street residence and workplace, attended a Wigmore Hall concert (the venue of a spectacularly successful congress he and Dora Russell organised in 1929), visited the Tudor gatehouse he owned as a retreat in Hertfordshire and saw the beautiful sculpted grave of one of his patients. Since he attracted the attention of British and Australian security services in the 1940s I was able to scour security service files as well as the archives of such icons as Dora Russell, Havelock Ellis, Marie Stopes, Norman Himes and Margaret Sanger which include Haire's reports and his correspondence. It is fortunate that so many of these papers survive because Haire's executors deliberately burnt his papers on the grounds that they contained correspondence from a number of distinguished persons which might have caused embarrassment in the wrong hands. Much of the information has also survived because he was a famous lecturer and author who was also a copious letter writer and mixed with famous and influential people, many of whom recorded their impressions about him.

Other pioneers have been recognised: the openly homosexual Magnus Hirschfeld became a hero to the gay movement, Margaret Sanger and Marie Stopes became feminist icons, and the importance of Sigmund Freud, Havelock Ellis and Alfred Kinsey is widely acknowledged. However, Norman Haire, who had to conceal his homosexuality, has been overlooked or maligned. Haire revered Havelock Ellis and admired his ability to be 'sincere without being crude' and to 'tell all that is essential to tell' while leaving many things 'to be read clearly enough by intelligent readers, between the lines'. Haire shared this gift. James Capshew and other researchers at Indiana University Bloomington examined Alfred Kinsey's life 'as a scientist and a person' while taking care not to 'add fuel to the persisting fire that surrounds him and his legacy'. Their study included an analysis of Jonathan Gathorne-Hardy's biography of Kinsey which corrected the errors made by another biographer who focused on the man's flaws

Introduction

and missed the point: Vincent van Gogh's room was untidy and Frank Lloyd Wright had debts and his roofs leaked but their failings do not diminish their contributions to art and architecture. Similarly, Haire's critics mistook his ebullience for self-aggrandisement and criticised his aesthetic house décor and his gourmand's eating habits while ignoring his achievements in making birth control available and his work to reform laws relating to abortion and sexuality.

Supporters admired his zeal but his detractors hated him for it and tried to undermine his work by spreading lies or disparaging his achievements. It is time to rebut the rumours and recognise this tenacious, humane, witty, innovative and brave man's contribution to birth control, sexology and human rights history.

2

Early years

Norman's grandfather, Louis Levy Zajac, married twice and had 'at least' three sons: Simon who was born about 1829, Solomon in about 1834 and Henry, Norman's father, in 1841.[1] Confusingly, Simon changed his surname twice; Solomon became Solomon Abrahams and Henry changed his name to Zions. Polish Jews had to do this to survive – death was the alternative to name-changing or emigration when Poland was ruled by Russia which decreed that everyone in their empire had to serve in the Russian army. The requirements were harshest for Polish Jews, who from the age of 12 became army conscripts for 25 years and very few survived.[2] Fortunately, Simon, Solomon and Henry escaped to Britain. Simon settled in London where he was a tailor and married at least twice; he and his first wife had a daughter and, after his wife's death, Simon remarried and emigrated to Australia with the two sons of his second marriage and, like Henry, adopted the Zions surname.

Norman's uncle, Solomon Abrahams, settled in Duntocher (near Glasgow) and started a money-changing business for immigrants and a furniture factory. This branch of the family grew wealthy and established a large dynasty after Abrahams converted the town's old cotton mill into a furniture factory known as the 'Jew's Mill'. Employment in cotton mills had ceased in the 1860s when the American Civil War put an end to Britain's cotton trade with the United States, so the factory gave welcome work to 100 people and provided them with housing and a synagogue. When any poor Polish or Russian Jewish families arrived in Britain, other members of his family would send the refugees to

---

1 Most of the information comes from a genealogy of the Zajac/Zions family, compiled by Selwyn Torrance in Philadelphia and supplemented by other relatives. His grandmother began this family history.

2 Details are from The Simon Wiesenthal Center, quoting from the 1972 edition of the *Encyclopaedia Judaica*.

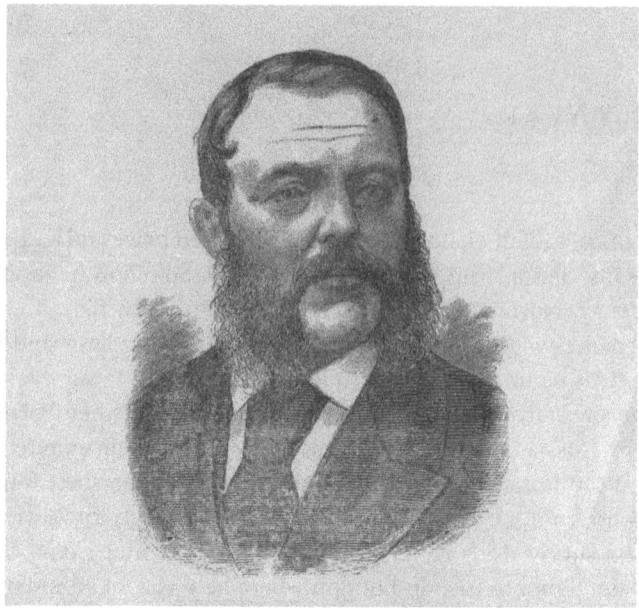

Figure 2.1. Henry Zions (Norman's father), a candidate in the NSW elections in 1880.

Duntocher where Abrahams housed and fed them until they could re-embark, usually for America.

If he is to be believed, Henry was only a child when he and his brothers fled from Poland. Henry spent seven years in England and then travelled to New Zealand where he remained for over 12 months, and came to Sydney in 1860, which he then made his home.

Henry gave these details in a flyer when he was a candidate for the districts of Hastings and Manning in the New South Wales 1880 general election.[3] From 1871 to 1873 he was involved in mining but this venture failed. In 1872 he owned and farmed Waterview Park at Fairfield in

---

3 The 1880 candidates were listed in *The Maitland Mercury & Hunter General Advertiser* on 23 October, 6 and 13 November. On 30 November it reported that Messrs Young and Andrews had been elected for the seat of Hastings and Manning. Messrs Zions and Richard forfeited their £40 deposit.

Sydney's west where he had stood for the seat of Central Cumberland but he was narrowly defeated because of the 'false misrepresentations' by his opponents. Henry gave one address in Lake Innes, Port Macquarie, on the mid north coast of New South Wales and the other at 409 George Street in central Sydney. He attributed his success in life to his 'energy and straight forwardness' and said he was a steady advocate for colonial industries and the advancement of the working man and had spent over £100,000 to further this cause, including the erection of many buildings 'some of which are an ornament to this city'.

After establishing himself in Australia, Henry made a leisurely tour of the neighbouring colonies, travelled overland to Europe and, after a year in England, married Clara Cohen on 18 November 1874 at Mile End (now Stepney) in London's East End. He was 33 and his bride was 22; Henry was listed as a 'gentleman' on the British marriage certificate while in contrast his down-to-earth Australian death certificate classified him as a 'tailor'. The Zions sailed to Australia and were living at 76 Elizabeth Street, Sydney, when their first child was born in 1875.

The couple suffered two major setbacks: on 7 May 1883 the *Brisbane Courier* reported a gas explosion which had shattered their house, slightly injuring Zions and his assistant, cracking the plaster and smashing the doors, windows, and furniture. This was followed by a major fire in the Zions Buildings at 613–617 George Street on Sydney's Brickfield Hill. The *Sydney Morning Herald* reported on 16 December 1885 that the blaze began on the second floor, gutting both the second and third floors. City and suburban fire brigades evacuated several people who had been sleeping there and saved the buildings, but a large stock of goods which Zions had stored in an upstairs room were badly damaged. Zions' tailoring establishment, on the ground floor of 613, and Mr Kaiser's dining rooms at 615, suffered water damage. The damage was 'between £2000 and £3000' but the buildings and stock were insured.

When Norman was born in 1892 his parents were living at 255 Oxford Street, Paddington, near the town hall and fire station. This birth came 16 years after their first child was born and three years after

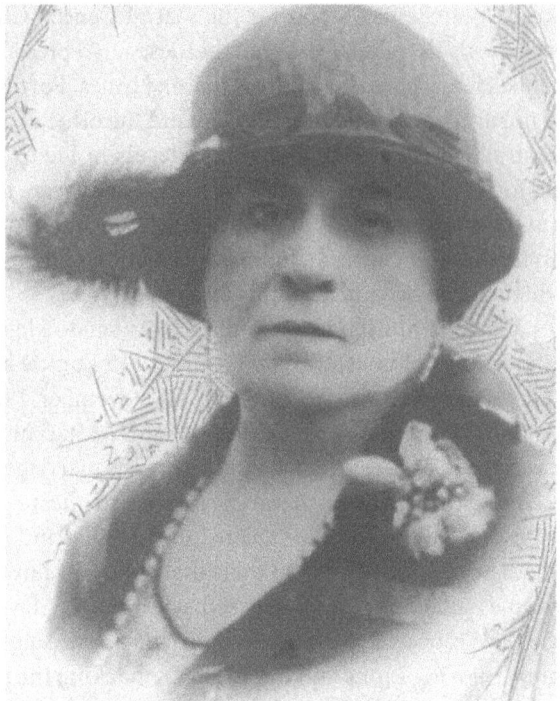

Figure 2.2. Clara Zions (Norman's mother) aged about 40.

their infant daughter Minnie died. Norman grew up in 'Morepo', their Paddington home, and his parents lived there for the rest of their lives.[4]

Like Alfred Kinsey, Norman was a weak, sickly child who was frequently bullied at school and lived in terror of his authoritarian father. He was also manipulated by his mother, and both parents influenced his career choice. Years later Norman said he was 'a French letter baby resulting from a pin-hole burst' when his father was 51 and his mother was 40.[5]

---

4 In the 1870s, 89 percent of Sydney's Jewish population lived in central Sydney and, by 1901, 78 percent had moved to the nearby suburbs of Paddington, Surry Hills, Darlinghurst, Glebe and Newtown (Rutland 2005, 37, quoting Charles Price). The Zions family had made this upmarket move by 1875.

5 Clara Zions was born in 1852 so she would have been 40 when Norman was born in 1892, not 37, the age given on Norman's birth certificate.

He described her desperate attempts at abortion when she nearly poisoned herself with huge overdoses of purgative pills if she had missed a period. His early life was largely spent running to and from the neighbouring chemist's shop to buy boxes of a certain brand of pill, which his mother swallowed, a whole box at a time. It was only later that he realised why she took them. Her health, which had already been shattered by having 11 babies in 16 years, was further damaged by this desperate attempt to control her fertility. In another account, he said a *relative's* mother 'took B's pills a whole box at a time'. The B stood for Beecham's Pills – laxatives made of aloe, ginger and soap which were advertised as being worth a guinea a box, the same price as a back street abortion, and were widely used as abortifacients in the 1890s.[6]

In this decade Australia was hit by a financial crisis so Norman's father, 'after years of leisure' was forced to work. They had servants, food, warm clothes, sunlight and fresh air but his mother was usually pregnant or breast feeding. His parents' heavy responsibilities made them bad-tempered and although his mother was 'devoted' (excessively so), his father made Norman's life 'as unhappy as possible'. There was little money for visits to doctors or dentists, so the children had poor teeth and Norman did not wear glasses until he was 11, even though he had needed them at least five years before that. However, he was aware that the plight of households with unemployment or drunkenness was far worse and later he quoted statistics which showed more sadness, sickness and higher mortality rates in very large families.

Norman's older siblings had attended expensive schools but after the financial crisis had to find jobs. The younger children were sent to state schools which were free. He explained in *Some more medical views on birth control* that as he lived in Sydney, where state schools were

---

[6] Volume II of the 1904 *Royal Commission on the decline of the birth-rate* (paragraph 1671) quoted a Newtown chemist and druggist who, when asked if women asked him for abortion pills, agreed they did but said he gave them purgatives because if he refused they would buy a box of Beecham's Pills which had the same effect. The second volume dealt with methods of contraception and abortion; Neville Hicks realised this suppressed volume existed after reading Norman Himes' 1936 *Medical history of contraception* and found a copy in America's National Library of Medicine.

better than the expensive private ones, this was not a disadvantage. He acknowledged that it was only because he was the youngest that he was able to make the most of his intelligence, unlike his siblings who were denied the opportunities to make the most of theirs through having to go out to work younger.[7] It was not until he became an adolescent that the family's financial circumstances gradually improved and, because there were no younger children to be provided for, they could afford to send him to university.

Curiously, in his 1934 bestseller *How to be happy though human*, Beran Wolfe turned this story on its head with the claim that Dr Norman Haire, as the youngest of eleven children, was denied the educational advantages of his elder brothers and sisters because his father suddenly became impoverished and, because of this, devoted his life to the amelioration of the condition of unwanted children by becoming the champion of birth control. This myth might have been inspiring, if one didn't wonder how poor Norman Zions became rich Dr Haire, but this fiction has a function, as Canadian historian Angus McLaren explained in 1995 when he debunked similar 'sexual stories': Stopes was not the married virgin she pretended to be in *Married love*; Sanger was not propelled by the death of a New York mother to launch her birth control campaign; and Kinsey was collecting data on sexuality long before his university asked him to but these stories, myths and parables were needed to make sense of the changes of modern life. While Norman's emotional deprivation was a factor, he scotched the myth about his life's work being motivated by physical deprivation. He also scuppered stories about large happy families, writing in 1943 that his irritable parents used to send the three youngest children to bed at 6 o'clock to get them out of the way and, as it was too early to sleep, four-year-old Norman, nine-year-old Annie and ten-year-old Bert played games; inevitably sexual games became a regular and considerable part in the evening routine.

---

7 This was not quite true because at least one of his siblings – 'Morris Zions, Chemist, Sea Lake' (a small town in north-west Victoria) – had a professional qualification which he listed in the death notice he wrote for his 'beloved father' Henry Zions of Paddington in *The Argus* on 8 January 1920.

EARLY YEARS

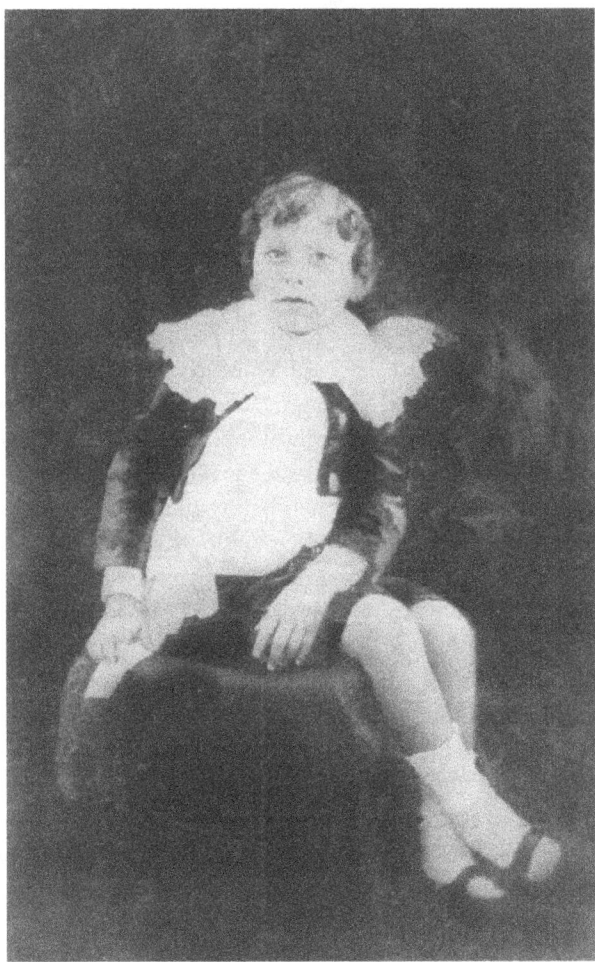

Figure 2.3. Norman Zions aged four.

Norman's school life began badly in 1896: on his first day at Paddington Public School the teacher, a 'soured spinster', threatened to 'put him up the chimney' for talking in class and he feared she really would kill him. He ran back home refusing to return. For the next few years he attended a 'dame school' in the home of an untrained young woman who was better suited to looking after small children. Then he returned to his first school which now had a wiser teacher who 'did not terrorise her pupils unnecessarily'. He was bright and intelligent, mostly well behaved, near the top of the class and said his teachers treated him well and promoted him rapidly. The result was that this small, younger, short-sighted, delicate and timid student was often bullied. When he was 12, three much older boys made his life so miserable that he again refused to go school and his misery intensified after Bert ran away to sea to get away from their domineering mother. The first time his mother found him and brought him back, but Bert tried again and escaped to Queensland where he achieved his dream of becoming a farmer.

Norman now had to sleep alone and the creaks and noises in the old house terrorised him. He imagined the noise of water dripping from an outside drain pipe was a burglar tapping to loosen the putty round the glass in a dining room window. He would hold his breath and listen for the sound of the window catch being lifted as the burglar entered. In his mind's eye he could see him creeping stealthily across the room, opening the dining room door and creeping up to the fourth stair of the flight leading up to his room. Paralysed with terror, holding his breath and his mouth too dry to scream, he would wait for a head to appear round the door. If he had taken a candle and matches to bed he would light the candle and the worst would be over but he would sometimes run screaming into his parents' room and sleep there for the rest of the night. Finally, they arranged for another member of the family to sleep in his room because the night terrors only struck when he was alone.

He spent the next 18 months at the nearby Darlinghurst Public School until he was fortunate enough to be admitted to Sydney's Fort Street Model School[8] in 1907 when it was on Observatory Hill, AJ Kilgour was the headmaster, and the school was at its best. Norman would have suffered in an authoritarian school which valued sport and compliance but he blossomed at Fort Street because the school valued culture and encouraged creativity. Kilgour formed the school's literary

---

8 The building was designed in 1815 as a military hospital, then it was acquired by the government in 1849 and the school opened in 1851. This government school provided Australia's first teacher training. The buildings now house Sydney's National Trust Centre (Barcan 1965).

and debating society in 1905 with a syllabus and weekly two-hour meetings with debates and lectures alternating.[9] From 1906 Norman began to hone these skills in after-school technical college elocution classes run by Miss Rose and, in exchange, her star pupil agreed to give recital performances which advertised the excellence of her teaching. These details come from an article George Munster wrote for the *Sydney Morning Herald* in 1983, compiling most of it from Haire's own papers, particularly the (now lost) diary of his life from 14 to 21.[10] Most of the entries referred to his public appearances which began in December 1906 when he won a silver medal at the Ashfield Eisteddfod. Norman became the stage manager of Fort Street's dramatic society in March 1908.

The school's newspaper, *The Fortian*, discussed the boys' speeches and debates, although it gave no details of Norman's first lecture on conscription which the headmaster praised.[11] Another article discussed the newspaper parodies which were tactfully criticised by George Mackaness,[12] a gifted English teacher the boys called 'Creeping Jesus' because his rubber-heeled shoes enabled him to surprise wrongdoers. In the 12 May 1908 issue of *The Fortian* he asked why the craze had

---

9   Bruce Mitchell, in his *ADB* entry for Alexander James Kilgour, said 'he became a legend in his lifetime for the scholastic excellence of Fort Street and for his dedication to discipline and hard work'. The school's archivist Ronald Horan said that unfortunately, although they were a most important element of school life, none of the literary and debating society's records were kept.

10 Munster noted that Norman listed all his recitals, but said little about his private life other than to mention being 'in love for a week' when he was 18 but described it as a 'calfy' infatuation.

11 In 1903 Australia passed a *Defence Act* allowing home service conscription in wartime and in 1909 the government approved of compulsory military training for men aged from 12 to 26. In 1916 and 1917 the Jewish community strongly supported the two referenda in which Prime Minister Billy Hughes tried to implement conscription.

12 Mackaness was an educationist, author and bibliophile who began teaching at Fort Street in 1903 and became the English master and deputy headmaster in 1912. He developed a new teaching approach and pioneered the Play Day Movement in NSW: Fort Street became noted for its annual days in which every class acted scenes from Shakespeare or other writers.

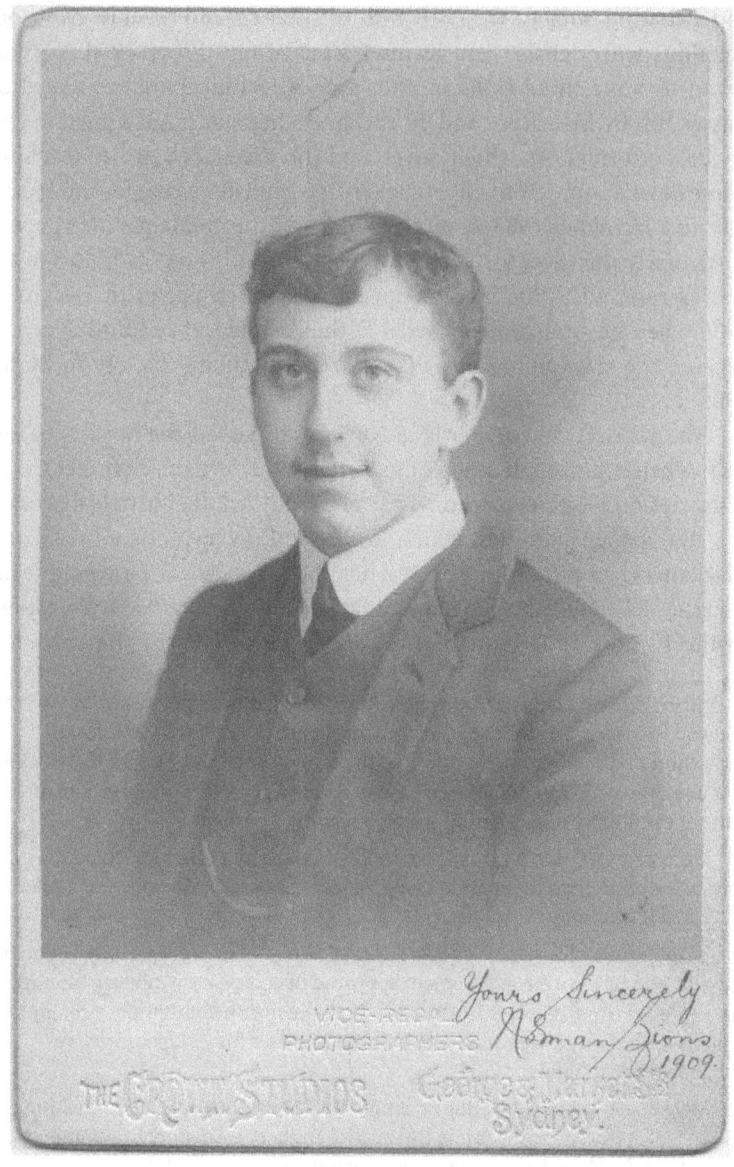

Figure 2.4. 'Yours sincerely, Norman Zions, 1909'.

taken such a hold on the members of the society and suggested they should find more original ways to display their genius. Secondly, he mentioned 'a tendency to buffoonery' in some of their advertisements, 'a form of literature requiring very little intellect to write' and, although some were witty, most were rather pointless. Thirdly, he commented on the editor's habit of summarising previous debates which were 'generally well written' but 'might be omitted occasionally'. Fourthly, many papers were so long there was no time for discussion 'which was surely the most profitable part of the exercise; he was pleased that papers were now limited to eight pages but hoped the quality would improve. Fifthly, he wanted to see many more separate articles, 'either grave or gay'. Sixthly, he did not want them to take these remarks as 'carping criticism' but felt it was his duty to point out genuine defects and hoped in future to see more original material such as an original diary, or illustrated sketches, or an imitation of some literary work.

The boys heeded his advice and the next issue of *The Fortian*, in its account of the 'Society's Afternoon with the Novelists', included a discussion of Norman's 'lecturette' on Marie Corelli, who was once the most widely read author in Britain and whose melodramatic style, oratorical skills and huge sales probably impressed Norman. *The Fortian* usually included monthly updates about Norman; in July 1908 he won two first prizes at the Wollongong Eisteddfod for a Shakespearian oration and a humorous recital and in August he became editor of the debating society's journal. In September Mackaness praised perhaps one of the finest issues of the journal for its articles and an elocution editorial (Norman's specialty) which showed 'deep thought, originality, and a large amount of learning'.

Mackaness wrote in October, 'Zions acted up to his reputation. The histrionic art is making great progress in the school: It is not beyond the improbable to dream of another David Garrick'. This teacher was a discerning man so Norman must have had great acting skill to have been equated with this famous 18th-century actor who was renowned for his comic and tragic performances. Norman continued to debate and act until the last months of his final year at school but, despite these distractions, he matriculated in 1909 with First Class Honours in

English, Second Class Honours in French; Bs for Latin and Algebra and Cs for German, Geometry and Trigonometry. Given his later passion for Germany and his fluency in the language his poor marks in this subject are surprising. In 1910 he came third in the Shakespearian section and second in the humorous section at the Commonwealth Eisteddfod.

Norman noted that none of Fort Street's teachers said a single word about any aspect of sex, with the result that he had a 'liberal education, of a smutty and furtive character', from his schoolmates in the classroom and the playground. Some of the boys supplemented theory by practice and 'masturbation in class was not uncommon, sometimes secret, less frequently with exposure under the desk'. During World War II, Norman's schoolboy reminiscences were of great interest to officials in the Australian Department of Security Services and, in one of the many files in Norman Haire's dossier, there are lines scrawled down the margin beside the reference to the boys' 'undercover' work. Some boys had made sexual advances to other classmates and one boy offered to pay for sex with sweets, theatre tickets or the promise of sex with his own sister, who, as a result, had had multiple sexual partners before she was 12. Norman was intellectually curious but physically unadventurous so he didn't participate although he did have a rich inner sexual life and had 'lived largely in the realm of fantasy from the age of five when Bert taught him to masturbate', insisting that 'every drop of semen was worth two ounces of blood'. At school, diagrams of asexual bodies were used in physiology classes and the teachers' textbook did not mention reproduction, defecation or micturition but Norman blamed the system, not the magnificent teachers; if any trespassed in 'this forbidden field', his motives would have been suspected and it would have led to disaster.

The security service also marked this sentence: 'How much they knew of what went on under the desks and in the playground, and in our lives away from school, I do not know. But officially we were children, and officially children were asexual. So sex was totally ignored'. Students gossiped but teachers were silent when a 16-year-old boy was forced to marry a girl he'd made pregnant and Norman gave some other tragic consequences of this ignorance. One boy caught gonorrhoea from a servant and another tried to castrate himself in an attempt to stop masturbating. Many young lives were warped by this neglect and by their parents' warnings against indulging in irregular sexual conduct because, as Barbara Tuchman wrote so eloquently, 'In struggles to oppose the strongest human instinct the idea of equating sex with sin has left the greatest train of trouble'.

As an adult Norman referred to the attempted suicide of a close friend who was 'a very religious boy' of 18, during their last year at school because of the extreme conflict between his very powerful sexual urge and the restrictive sexual norms of his upbringing. He took an overdose of a sedative drug, and swam out to sea at Coogee, but the tide washed him back to shore where the doctors managed to revive him. Even so, his friend was determined to die and enlisted as soon as World War I broke out and was killed in France. It is likely that this friend was the debating society's secretary Eric Leask who was 24 when he died on 20 July 1916 in the Battle of Fleurbaix (also called the Battle of Fromelles). Leask's name is on the rolls of honour at his school and in the archives of the Australian War Memorial which include this tribute:

> Young Leask, a Divinity Student was one of the best that were with me; quiet and unassuming, he exercised a power of good over those serving under him, to whom his conduct was a pattern. I had already recommended him for a commission which he had earned.

He died in a British-led, poorly planned 27-hour battle, memorialised by the Cobbers statue,[13] below which is a plaque stating the British suffered 1567 casualties, the Australians a devastating 5333.

Close friendship between the introverted Eric and the extroverted Norman might at first seem unlikely but Norman hid his timidity behind a shield of bravado in debates and on stage. He would later explain to Havelock Ellis that he was occasionally aggressive in an attempt to compensate for a sense of inferiority. As an 18-year-old he had discovered Havelock Ellis' five-volume *Studies in the psychology of*

---

13 The Cobbers statue is in Fromelles' Australian Memorial Park. The sculptor is Peter Corlett of Melbourne. Leask is buried in Plot I. K. 81 of the Rue-Petillon Military Cemetery, Fleurbaix, Pas-de-Calais, France.

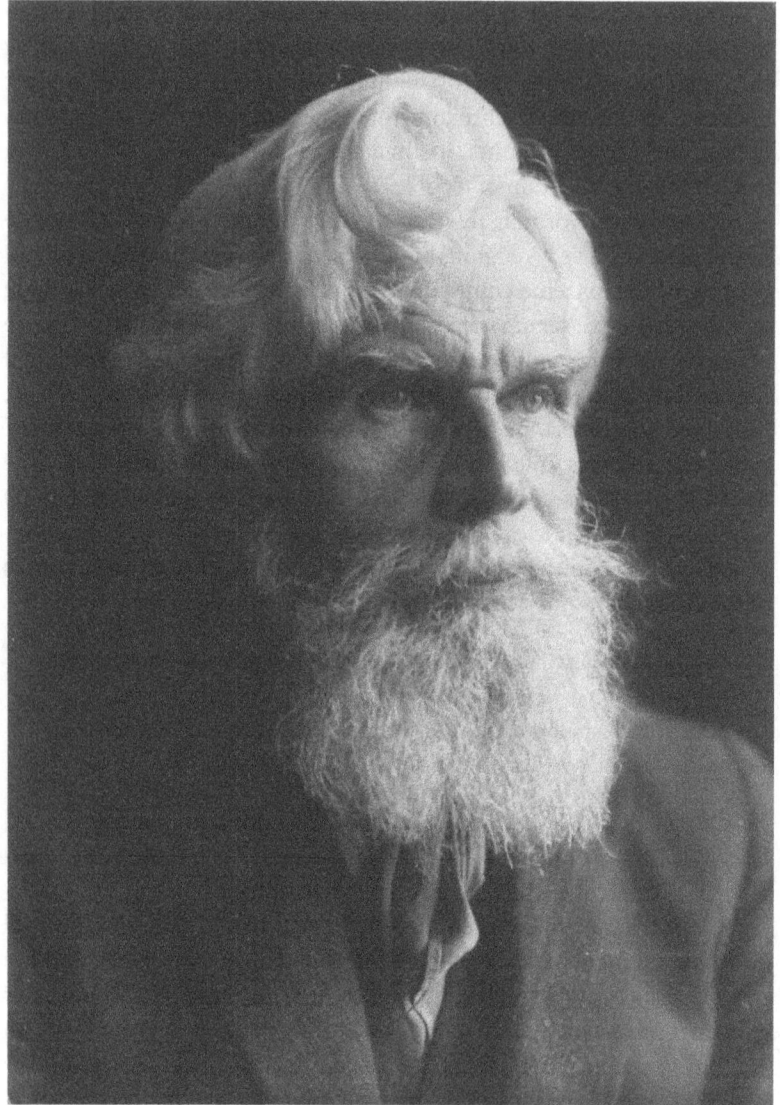

Figure 2.5. Henry Havelock Ellis, the 'Darwin of Sex'.

sex in Sydney's public library and, as a result of his avid reading, suffered a 'bad attack of mental indigestion'. He soon recovered and started to have a better understanding of himself and others. The 'relief' sparked an epiphany: he would devote his life to the study sex so that he could also help others. He felt it was the only way to repay the debt he owed the 'Darwin of Sex' who was to become his mentor.[14]

Norman's determination to do this developed as a result of his troubled childhood and his sexual anxieties, the same stimuli that had motivated Havelock Ellis. In 1908 Henry James explored the reality of a writer's 'impulses' which he said 'were like those of the navigator, the chemist, the biologist, scarce more than alert recognitions. He comes upon the interesting thing as Columbus came upon the isle of San Salvador, because he had moved in the right direction for it'. Norman recognised that sexual anxiety was the catalyst for his 'interesting thing' and he later observed some curious parallels: Havelock Ellis had trained as a teacher at Norman's old school (Fort Street), matriculated to his university (Sydney), and spent many hours in the same public library in Sydney trying to determine *his* life's work.

Havelock Ellis was a sickly 16-year-old in 1875 when he arrived in Sydney aboard his father's ship and, as the next port was Calcutta, the ship's doctor convinced the father to leave the boy in Sydney in the hope that the climate would improve his health. Fortunately, he was a resilient youth and, after some inept attempts to teach, Havelock Ellis, or HE as he was known,[15] enrolled in a teacher-training course and wrote in his diary that the three months of training 'were not unpleasantly spent' although he also said they were 'acutely distressing'. He wandered all day about the classrooms at Fort Street, following the prescribed routine with his fellow students. When the casual course of his training at Fort Street was over, he had to give a test lesson to a class and pass an informal examination by a Scotsman called Forbes, who asked him a few questions and gave him an easy passage in Latin to translate. The

---

14 Haire (1951, 4).

15 Few people called Havelock Ellis by his first name, Henry, and he and others often abridged his surname to 'HE' (also short for His Eminence or His Excellency) which is ironic because he hated to be lionised.

master 'improved the situation – it was midsummer – by eating an orange'. This is an evocative but erroneous image because oranges ripen in winter.

After 'one or two interviews with the headmaster', Ellis was appointed at the half-time schools at Sparkes Creek and Junction Creek (near Scone) with instructions to 'go there immediately'. In this rural setting he 'would stretch out in relaxation on a hard bench' and meditate after the pupils had gone home. He always 'thought best horizontally'[16] and was rewarded with a Eureka moment: 'he would study medicine and search for artistic and scientific truth'. As a teenager Ellis had spent three rather boring months at Fort Street as a trainee teacher but the 15-year-old Norman relished three very productive years there as a student.

Norman had two 'burning' ambitions when he left school: to save the world from sexual grief and to become an actor – already he was a very successful amateur and had made up his mind to be a professional. After he matriculated in November he had taken his sheaf of press cuttings to a theatrical manager and asked for a job. He was promised a job with Matheson Lang's theatre company in a performance which was opening in Sydney the following May. Meanwhile he worked as a clerk in a grain warehouse and, although the manager wanted him to stay, he left after only a month to take a more interesting and better paid job coaching the manager's son in his university subjects; although he had only just left school, his cheek and confidence landed him the job.

At home his thespian ambitions sparked a melodrama: his father threatened to throw him out of the house and 'never darken his doors again' if he didn't become a medical student and his tearful mother knelt down to beg him to study medicine because it was so much safer than the stage, which was so uncertain and so immoral. She wanted to tie him down as a doctor with a nice practice in Sydney, *near her* because, if he became an actor, he would travel and she might lose him. To keep the peace and please her, Norman registered as a medical student.

---

16 Ronald Horan, the school's archivist, was quoting from Havelock Ellis' diary and the same words appear in *My life: Havelock Ellis* (1939, 115–17).

Four days later a telegram arrived: 'Oscar Asche opening in *Count Hannibal*.[17] Small part for you. Come at once'.

The Australian-born Asche had been successful in London and, during his 1909–10 Australian tour, he saw Norman playing Mercutio (Romeo's lively and cynical friend) in *Romeo and Juliet* and offered to take him back to London and help further his progress. Norman replied in anguish that if he threw up his medical studies there would be a hell of a row – his father would be furious and his mother would have to bear it all. He imagined his father would say to his wife 'your son' – he always called Norman 'your son' when he wanted to be withering and only called Norman by his first name if he was pleased with him and that wasn't very often. '"Your son", he would say. "A fine beauty! Goes and spends my money at the University and then throws it all up the first week to go gallivanting on the stage"'. Much as Norman longed to go on the stage, he couldn't in these circumstances. So he wept and told the theatrical manager what had happened, and continued as a medical student.

Norman loathed physics and found botany terribly dull, although chemistry was easier and zoology was interesting until he had to dissect cockroaches, which he found peculiarly disgusting and loathsome. The dissecting room was a challenge because he had never seen a human corpse before and seeing 32 pickled and partly dissected bodies made him vomit. He couldn't attend any more lectures that day and refused to eat meat for a fortnight.

Ironically, after Norman had refused an acting job he now repeatedly begged the theatrical agent for work and the reply was always 'graduate first' and then he'd get his chance. Norman spent five nights a week rehearsing or acting with amateur companies or reciting at concerts and he made quite a respectable amount of pocket money from concert fees. He used to harrow audiences with *The signal-man's story* about a child on the railway track and the man's choice whether to save his son or doom a crowded express train. Of course he did his duty and the child

---

17 Asche's first Australian tour began in Melbourne on 17 July 1909 and lasted 18 months, ending in Perth. His repertoire included his own dramatisation of Stanley Wyman's novel *Count Hannibal*.

was saved too. He would make them weep with *Lasca down by the Rio Grande*, a cowboy's lament for his Mexican sweetheart who died while saving him in a stampede or convulse them with *The matinee hat*, a slapstick comedy. Audiences were much less sophisticated in those days, he was 'quite a good reciter' and it was a popular form of entertainment.

In June 1911 'Mr Norman Zions elocutionist' gave two performances in a YMCA hall: he recited a maudlin bush ballad (*His Gippsland girl*) and acted in the gossipy *Mrs Brown at the play*.[18] His acting puzzled one reviewer in the *Sydney Morning Herald* on 17 March 1913: 'Mr Norman Lions [sic], much too handsome and athletic for Whitelocks, the forlorn and faithful Fool in love with Yolande, delivered his lines with feeling'.[19]

Norman became more interested in medicine once he started to see patients; initially he was nauseated by sights in the casualty department but he gradually gained confidence and was relieved that he did not faint at his first major operation. He had good rapport with the patients and thought of them as people not cases, but he said he was not very good at history-taking because he was more interested in *them* than in their diseases. He walked the hospital by day and trod the boards by night, repeating his role in *Mrs Brown at the play* on 8 May 1914 and he recited *The green eyes of the yellow god* at a fundraising night in the Blue Mountains for the conservative Women's League. In July he appeared as the Rev. William Smythe in the long moralistic play *The servant in the house*[20] and four months later he took on the roles of stage manager and actor in Mary McIntire Pacheco's farce *Tom, Dick and Harry*.

Ivan Crozier is an Australian historian who wrote two hostile articles about Haire in 2001 and 2003 while he was a Post-Doctoral Research Fellow at London's Wellcome Trust Centre for the History of Medicine.

---

18 The poet Will Ogilvie was a Scot who worked in the Australian bush from 1889 to 1901 (Miller 1956, 364). *Mrs Brown at the play* was written by George Rose (as 'Arthur Sketchley'). He was an English entertainer who toured Australia and wrote 32 Mrs Brown novels.

19 Norman's onstage agility was remarkable in view of his dislike of organised sport and his muscular rheumatism which, over the previous six months, Pathology Professor DA Welsh had successfully treated with 'a vaccine'.

20 Written in 1908 by Charles Rann Kennedy, an Anglo-American dramatist.

EARLY YEARS

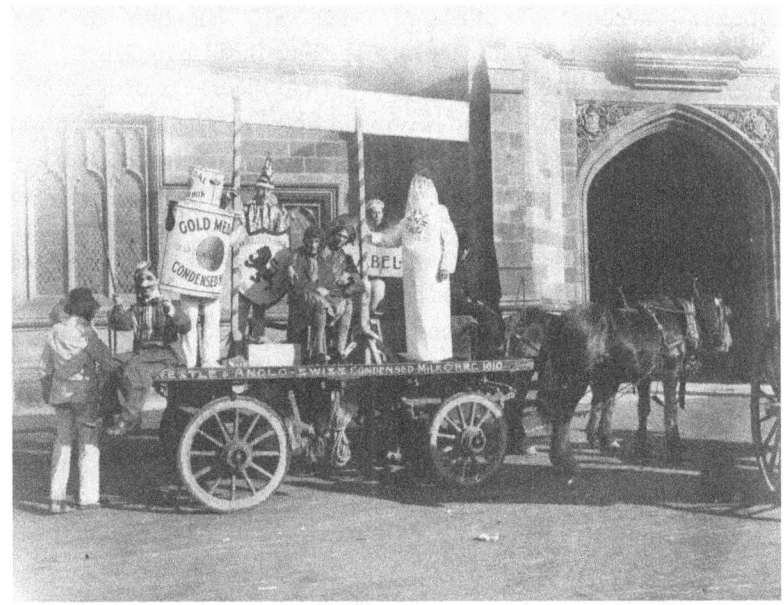

Figure 2.6. Sydney University medical students performing on Commemoration Day, May 1912.

In the first he wrote dismissively that Haire 'apparently acted with zeal in an amateur dramatic production at Sydney University as a loaf of bread, and later as a robber in Ivor Montagu's 1929 film, *Bluebottles*. Crozier grossly underestimated Haire's acting talent and made mistakes in the examples he chose: the film appeared in 1928 and Norman was *not* a loaf of bread or anything else in the May 1914 University of Sydney Commemoration Day skit in which, according to reports in *The Daily Telegraph* on 25 May and *The Daily Mail*, students dressed in white with hollowed loafs for hats, held placard slogans such as 'We bake between strikes' and one tried to smash a government loaf with a hammer, in a reference to Sydney's bread trouble that year.

Norman had featured in the university's May 1912 procession as one of six students on a horsedrawn dray with the words 'Nestlé &

Anglo-Swiss Condensed Milk Co. M.H.C. 1610'[21] along the edge and above them a banner with the words 'The Blue Bird Up to Date'.[22]

Bobbie Silberthau portrayed Nestlé's Gold Medal Condensed Milk, Norman Zions was Sugar and the others were 'Mytyl and Tytyl', Bread and Light with two non-medical 'interlopers' standing behind the dray. Zions and Silberthau had met in their school's debating society and the group of third-year medical students needed to take care to keep their balance; if Zions *had* acted with zeal, he would have frightened the horses and it is the *only* time he performed with his head in a bag. A 1912 slump in the condensed milk market coincided with the opening of Nestlé's butter and cheese factory in Kempsey on the mid north coast of New South Wales. This may have prompted the students' protest or it could have been in response to frictions between the factory owners and nearby farmers including the Zions family.

Welsh miners had bought their literature, song and music tradition with them during the gold rush and Norman won many prizes at the Ballarat Eisteddfod in 1914, claiming 'I was the best male amateur reciter in Australia' and the eisteddfod program and newspaper reports confirm this.[23] During the six-day festival he competed in every section open to him and on Monday 5 October, in an extraordinary marathon of stamina, skill, versatility and memory, he won three first prizes, two seconds and a third, giving performances in the morning at 10.30 and 11.30, in the afternoon at 2.00 and 3.30 and then again in the evening at 8.15 and 9.30. He began with an extract from Tennyson's sentimental poem *Enoch Arden*, followed by an impromptu reading. In the afternoon he spoke with simplicity and force in Abraham Lincoln's *Gettysburg*

---

21 In 1911, Nestlé built the world's largest condensed milk plant in Dennington, Victoria. The market crashed in 1912 because huge stocks of it made the price drop and forced plants to shut. [Online] Available: en.academic.ru/dic.nsf/enwiki/241312 [Accessed 8 October 2012].

22 Henri Nestlé launched the logo in 1868 as a pun on his name in German which meant little nest. It became the 'blue birds in a nest' trademark.

23 Peter Bowler (2005) sent me the 1914 program, newspaper clippings of the results and a publicity brochure – in 1998 the Grand National Eisteddfod of Australasia attracted over 7800 entries and an audience of 25,000.

address and *Shiel's reply to Lord Lyndhurst*,[24] rounding off with a speech by Mark Antony and playing both characters in a humorous interchange between David Copperfield and a waiter. The judges agreed that his voice was excellent, well modulated, clear and forceful; his emotional pauses were done well, that he had fine power and intensity and gave excellent performances with fine, powerful gestures. One said that he was too argumentative and not appealing enough as Lincoln and another thought his voice was too good for the waiter. World War I still seemed remote to Australia during this eisteddfod where excitement mounted as Mr Norman Zions and Miss Louie Dunn were close favourites but finally on 10 October 1914 *The Argus* announced that Norman was the winner.

A month later Australia was feeling the war's impact and Zions played the part of the premier in *Mrs Pretty and the Premier* at a fundraiser for those killed and wounded on the HMAS *Sydney* and to celebrate the Australian navy's first triumph. This was just ten days after the *Sydney* had sunk the German cruiser *Emden* on 9 November 1914 and, in the rush, the printer left a blank space in the program for the playwright's name – he was Arthur H Adams and the comedy was one of the *Three plays for the Australian stage* he wrote that year. After he had graduated, Norman continued to act in Sydney University Dramatic Society plays[25] including *Lysistrata* without the erotic erection scene.

Despite his mellifluous voice, some of Norman's friends thought he was the most unmusical man they knew but he thought they were being harsh – although he couldn't sing in tune, he protested that he 'was not unmusical'. He didn't hypocritically pretend to like 'Wagner's music or Rubens' pictures' because cultured people were expected to like them and he found opera and most piano concerts 'sleep-inducing'. He had an exceptionally keen appreciation of the beauty of the speaking voice (a novelist coyly refused to repeat the words Norman had used to

---

24   Mr Shiel, the MP for Tipperary, made this reply after Lord Lyndhurst called the people of Ireland 'aliens': *The American Monthly Magazine*, 3, 1837, 522.
25   University of Sydney Archives, 1919, listed Dr Norman Zions as one of 39 members of SUDS. Membership was open to all members of the university, whether graduates or undergraduates.

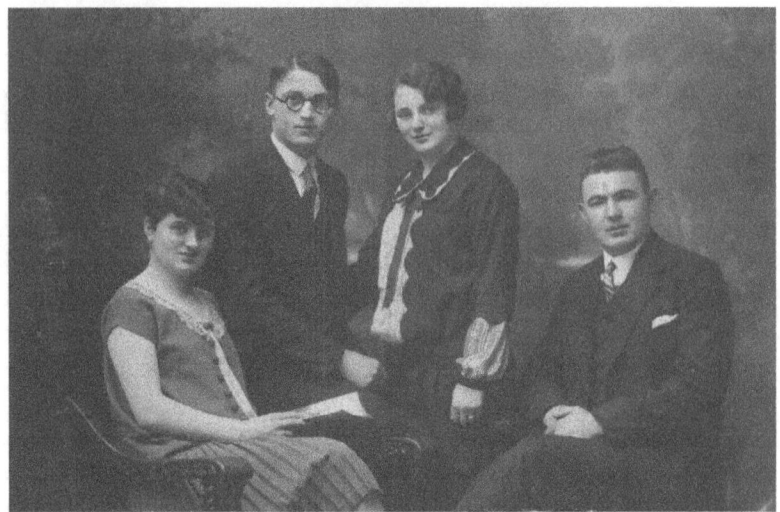

Figure 2.7. Four Zions siblings in 1916. Norman (second from the left) with Bert and two of their sisters.

describe Paul Robeson's glowering, smoulderingly sensual voice[26]) and he was stirred by the 'curious cadences' of the Mohammedan priest, the Jewish Cantor and Indian songs being sung to the accompaniment of a cheap little harmonium. He was also powerfully affected by 'many of the songs of Rimsky-Korsakov, Grieg's *Solveig's song*, a good deal of Debussy, and some Hungarian folk songs'. Once he had had to rush out of a Dresden cafe with tears streaming down his face because a customer had taken out his violin and played some wistful melody. A musical friend explained that most compositions he disliked were in a major key and most which pleasantly stirred him were in a minor key. He was also passionate about books and became the honorary librarian of the university's Medical Society in his final year.

Norman's graduation may have been a 'war pass'; all the university's courses were accelerated at the request of the Department of Defence

---

26 Landy and Fischer (2004, 202) quote Ethel Mannin as saying, 'The best description I ever heard of Robeson's voice was from Norman Haire – but unfortunately it is unprintable, since sexual imagery in this country is *verboten*, in spite of the fact that sex is life, and all art sexual'.

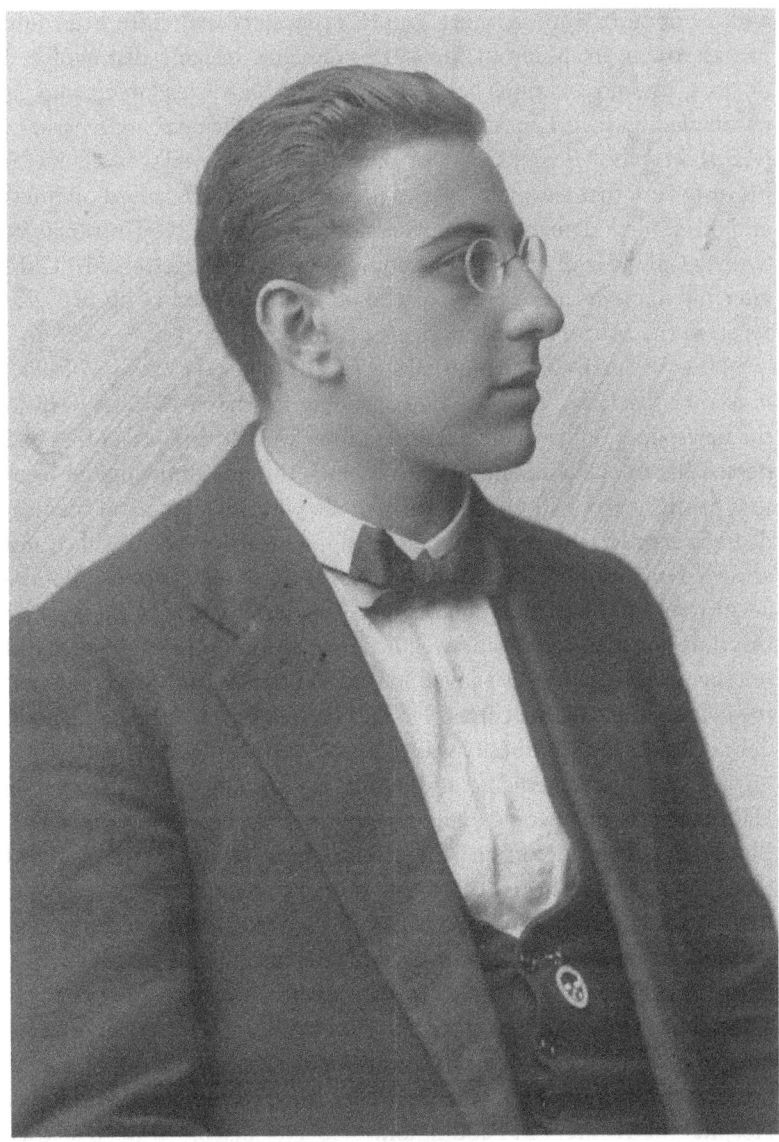

Figure 2.8. Norman Zions as a medical graduate, 1915. Note the Sydney University crest on his watch chain.

and, as doctors were in short supply, examiners may have been told to pass them all. Many of the 1915 graduates became distinguished doctors, the most famous being Sir Norman McAlister Gregg who, as chronicled by Paul Lancaster in the *Australian dictionary of biography (ADB)*, won the Military Cross for gallantry and received world fame for his discovery that German measles in early pregnancy caused cataracts and other birth defects. Norman's results appeared in the University of Sydney Calendar of 1915 and he could now write the letters MB ChM after his name because every candidate who qualified as an MB also received the Master of Surgery degree (ChM).[27]

He gave details of the unusual start to his medical career in *Through a doctor's spectacles*. On a Monday evening in March 1915 he went to the newspaper office where a friend's father worked and learnt that he'd passed his final examinations. At 9 o'clock the next morning he went to a printery and had visiting cards made with his name and medical degrees. Armed with these, he rushed to the theatrical agent's office and scrawled on one of the cards 'I have come to claim your promise' but the agent reminded him that doctors were needed because of the war. By this time Norman was 23 and weighed over 16 stone (102 kg) which did not favour his chances as a juvenile lead so he reluctantly accepted that medicine would be his career. He had ballooned from being a small, delicate child and his obesity was to become a lifelong problem.

He combined medicine and acting (as Dr Zions and then as Dr Haire) and many people remembered him as blustering Sir Ralph Bloomfield Bonnington in *The doctor's dilemma*, George Bernard Shaw's play in which the solution to corrupt medical self-interest was to eliminate private practice. In this role he perfected the technique of method acting *before* it became fashionable, insisting he *was* Sir Ralph. Norman held various medical positions during the war: in 1915 he was a Resident Medical Officer at the Hospital for Sick Children in Brisbane; in 1916 he worked as a Medical Officer in three New South Wales mental hospitals and in 1917 he was the Chief Medical Officer at the Royal Hospital for Women, in Paddington.[28] He later discussed the disparity

---

27   This degree was replaced by the MB BS in 1927.
28   A secret memorandum dated 2 August 1940 from HE Jones, Director of

between the clean orderliness of the hospital and the squalor in the slums. There were the normal problems with home birth of having to supply sterile supplies and being without backup doctors or nurses who could help if necessary. He recalled going out to his first confinement in a miserable, poverty-stricken home in Newtown. He and his colleagues entered a poorly lit room where the labouring woman was on a double bed jammed against the wall which made assistance difficult and the bed's sagging mattress meant that most of her muscular energy was wasted while she was giving birth.

In Paddington's obstetric hospital he saw deformed babies born to 'defective' parents; some to mothers worn out by incessant childbearing and others who were damaged by backyard abortions. He was particularly depressed by one woman who, after giving birth, suffered from puerperal insanity and was admitted to a mental hospital more than a dozen times only to be released as cured and become pregnant once again. Norman's suggestions to senior medical staff that such patients should receive contraceptive advice were 'very coldly received'.

When he joined the Australian Army Medical Corps (AAMC) in 1915 he was commissioned as a captain, as shown in figure 2.9. For the next four years Captain Zions had a part-time position near his home at the No. 4 Military Hospital, Randwick; it was initially equipped for 420 beds and was based in a former benevolent asylum for destitute children which the army had requisitioned. He called this period 'the unhappiest years of my life' and there are several possible reasons for this. First, he might have been a victim of the hospital's maladministration which was exposed by a special board of inquiry in January 1918. The ten-man committee compiled two contradictory reports, both of which gave details of the hospital's dirty, inadequate facilities and the feuds between its most senior administrators. Senator GF Pearce, the Minister for Defence, was so concerned that he took the very unusual steps of making the report public,[29] dismissing the

---

the Commonwealth Investigation Branch, Canberra, to the Secretary, Attorney-General's Department, Canberra, gave his educational qualifications and his hospital appointments (NAA A 367/1, C 69409).

29 Reports of the Advisory Committee for Military Hospitals and Convalescent

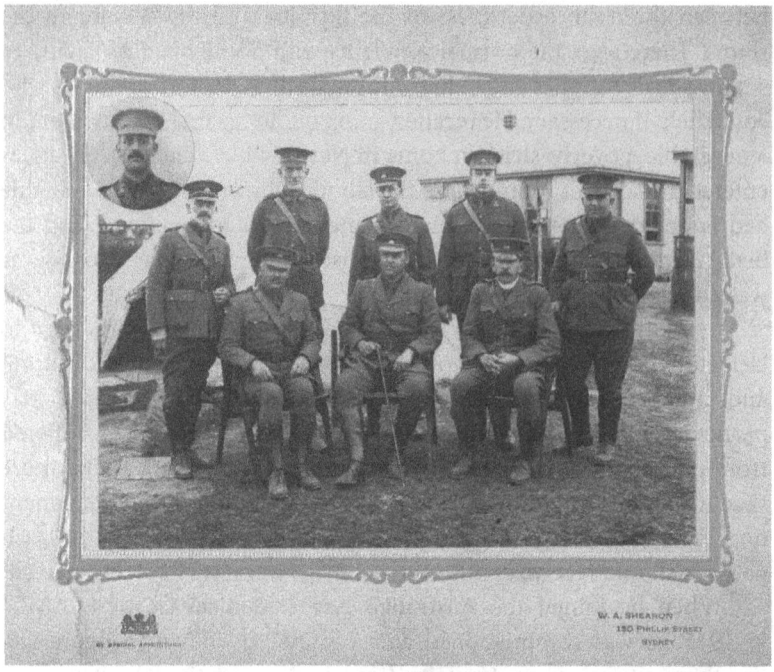

Figure 2.9. Captain Norman Zions at Australian Army Medical Corps Headquarters, Liverpool Camp, NSW, August 1915 (standing, second from right).

hospital's three senior staff[30] and introducing changes to improve medical administration in the Randwick hospital and in every hospital in the state. Second, Haire may have been grieving over the war deaths or he could have been discouraged because military doctors were treated as second-rate citizens within the medical profession who preferred not to treat wounded warriors and 170,000 sick or maimed soldiers had returned to a country that was unused to disabilities and

---

Homes, New South Wales, was reported in *The Advertiser* on 7 January 1918.

30 On 15 January 1918 *The Argus* provided details: 'The termination of the appointments of the following officers at No. 4 Australian General Hospital Randwick, NSW is announced as from January 7: Colonel Edward Sutherland Stokes, as Principal Medical Officer; Lieutenant-Colonel George Lane Mullins as Officer Commanding and Captain FE Ware as Registrar'.

embarrassed by them.[31] Adjacent to the hospital's main building in the old asylum were rows and rows of hastily built huts beside a road which the patients sarcastically called Easy Street, the name it still has. It was hard for everyone: soldiers' injuries turned them into mere home-duty men and medical staff worked long hours in makeshift hospitals, but, in addition to these wartime woes, Zions had others.

A third reason for his unhappiness (and probably the major one) is a workplace catastrophe that is discussed in the next chapter.

---

31 Discussed by Ford (1980, 73–74).

3

Zions the Scapegoat

Norman Zions spent his first years as a new medical graduate working in various hospitals in two states and as a part-time army captain at the Randwick Military Hospital. The sketchy details about his early career were discussed in the previous chapter but they do little to create a picture of him. This changed when he took a job as house doctor at Newcastle Hospital and his previously obscure medical career soon became headline news. This book is about sex so it is appropriate to repeat Oscar Levant's quip that he knew Doris Day *before* she was a virgin[1] and to say that this chapter is about Newcastle Hospital *before* it became Royal Newcastle and Norman Zions *before* he became Norman Haire.[2]

Port cities are very vulnerable to infectious diseases and, although Newcastle's first hospital was built in 1817, it still lacked an isolation hospital a hundred years later. In 1878, after the city's unhealthiest year on record (with 101 diarrhoea deaths, 54 from typhoid and 47 from scarlet fever), Newcastle's politicians appealed to the NSW Parliament for help. In 1882 the state government offered Newcastle hospital £3000 to build a contagious diseases hospital but the hospital board rejected this because the proposed site was 'unhappily situated' near the cemetery. In 1891 the hospital's secretary asked the Minister for Lands for £6000 for renovations because there was only one small isolation ward and they were forced to nurse patients with typhoid fever next to patients who had undergone major operations. This plea was ignored and, despite having had to treat bubonic plague patients in 1902 and

---

1 Oscar Levant (1906–1972), actor, composer, musician, wit and writer had appeared with Doris Day in her first film, *Romance on the high seas* (1948).

2 Most information in this chapter comes from the *Newcastle Morning Herald & Miners' Advocate* (*Newcastle Herald*), the *Newcastle Sun* and the Newcastle Hospital Archives in the Auchmuty Library, Newcastle University.

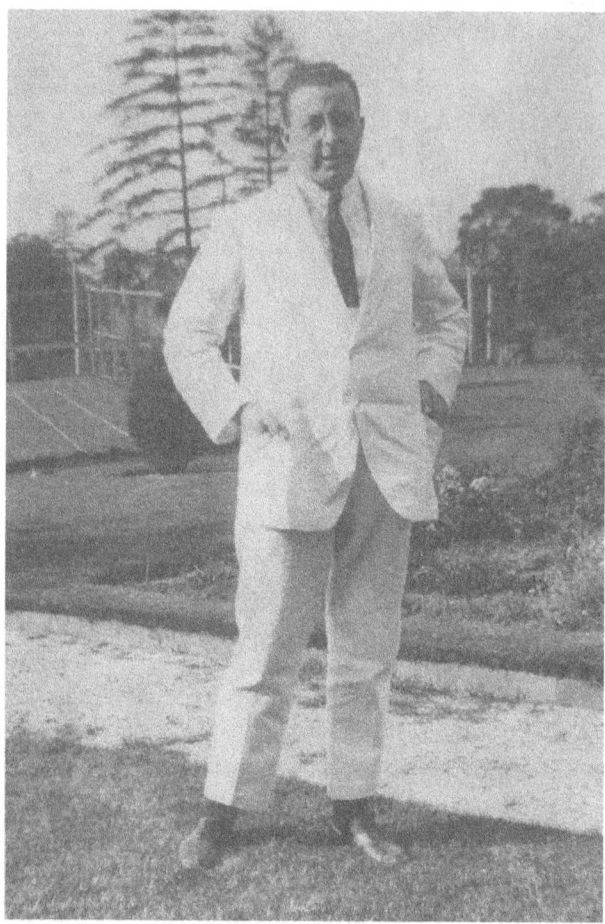

Figure 3.1. Dr Norman Zions at Newcastle Hospital.

1905, the hospital still had rats in the kitchen, pigeons under the roof and only two small isolation wards.³

Local doctors probably boycotted this troubled workplace but Zions was from Sydney and he would have been unaware of the hospital's

---

3 Champion (1978, 345) said these two small isolation wards were only 2160 cubic feet – half that provided in a modern hospital room. Nor were they provided in the new wings built in 1884 and 1913.

accommodation and financial difficulties, its inability to retain nurses[4] and the board's fearsome reputation. It was a medical minefield and superintendents were lucky to last a year – in 1913 there was a turnover of five doctors who 'lived in fear of the board' which was apt to give them a month's notice or dismiss them on the spot as they did to Zions' predecessor (Marsden 2005, 62, 90).

The 26-year-old Zions was soon promoted to the hospital's top job as their medical superintendent and the welcoming comments by hospital chair AA Rankin were published by the *Newcastle Herald* on 15 February 1918. He said 'how lucky they were' to have such a well-qualified administrator who, in a few short months, had 'shown them organising such as they had never seen before' and was eradicating the hospital's chaos and creating 'a state of order and discipline'.

This euphoria evaporated during the superintendent's very first week: a nurse complained to the matron that Zions had 'falsely accused' her when he reprimanded her for breaching the cardinal rule of infection control by mixing contaminated and clean items. Zions reported this to the board on 21 February, saying he had gone into the pan room which contained a sink, a slop sink, and a hand basin and discovered that the sink and slop sink were empty but the hand basin contained some '*very* soiled' dressings and a leaking bed pan. When he asked the nurse if it 'was customary' and she said it was, he replied, 'Well it is a custom that must stop at once.' He reported her to the matron and stressed the seriousness of such practices, particularly in a ward where there was 'at least one' typhoid patient; if nurses put dirty bed pans in the basin, the contamination could be transferred to a person's hands and cause a typhoid epidemic.

He was also critical of the hospital's 'great lack of care' and the 'large number of wounds' which became infected; if this happened in a 'city' hospital they would hold an inquiry to find out its cause. While a lower standard of medical care was more likely to be tolerated in a provincial

---

[4] Champion (1978, 347) noted that the hospital did not appear to be in favour with the Premier or Minister of Health in 1905; it was £700 in debt, the first time since its birth as a modern hospital in 1891.

hospital, his criticism showed that he did not understand what impact these remarks would have on his working relationships. Tensions increased when he said 'carelessness and deceit' by the nurses 'would cause a scandal' if these failings were made public. He thought these matters should be suppressed 'in the interests of the hospital' and would 'not . . . say anything further about this unless pressed.' His accusations and the implicit threat may have made the board start considering ways to avert a scandal, including silencing the bearer of such unwelcome news, and they were unsupportive on 5 March when they considered the bed pan incident. They conceded that some nurses had 'erred' but stressed that 'they had unknowingly breached hospital instructions' and, while they commended Zions 'for stopping the bad practice', they felt he could have handled this 'misunderstanding' with 'a little more tact.'

Outwardly, relationships seemed cordial at the hospital's annual meeting on 28 March when Rankin first commended Zions for his 'very satisfactory' work and skilful patient care and then directed his anger at the government's 'scandalous' and 'illegal' failure to provide them with an isolation block despite the 'strong letters' they had sent 'over many years'. Some of the hospital's other problems were discussed at their 16 May meeting and they were reported in the *Newcastle Herald*, including such sensitive details as criticism of the 'dreadful state' of the hospital's finances, with 'a deficit of £9349', and the charge that 'no other hospital in the country' was 'so expensively managed'.

In August 1918 Zions applied for a position as medical superintendent at Sydney Hospital and the board supplied him with glowing references, including the secretary's praise for his 'excellent service in re-organising various departments, establishing new ones, and . . . making our hospital everything that a modern up-to-date hospital should be.'[5] If Zions had won the Sydney job he would have been saved from a great deal of unhappiness, but his escape bid failed

---

[5] Zions received references from several Newcastle doctors. Dr Joseph Foreman, who had taught Zions and worked with him at Sydney's Royal Hospital for Women, found him 'zealous in his work' and said his 'record has been uniformly good.' Referees said Zions was of good character, praised his achievements and excellence as an administrator.

and soon Newcastle Hospital's troubles multiplied when a pneumonic influenza pandemic reached Australia where thousands died[6] in what was to become 'our greatest peacetime disaster' (Horsley 2007).

Australian health officials had received warnings about the dangers in October 1918 but Newcastle Hospital was totally unprepared. On 28 October the hospital's board warned the New South Wales Minister for Health about these very real dangers. On 19 November Zions reiterated his warnings about the hospital's inadequate facilities and, on the same day, the board doubled his salary (from £300 to £600 per year), noting at the board meeting that Zions had expressed thanks but, when asked if anyone had interfered in his duties, he replied that 'no board member had done so'. This question would not have been put if the board had had a good working relationship with Zions.

World War I had killed around ten million people in four years and, almost immediately after, influenza caused millions more deaths in a single year,[7] with some groups being more likely to catch and die from the disease.[8] It struck Britain in May 1918; then America and South Africa where it killed 139,471 and in October New Zealand had 6601 deaths.

When influenza struck New Zealand, the Commonwealth Quarantine Department began to quarantine ships with influenza outbreaks for seven days' observation and *all* ships which had come from New Zealand and South Africa. When a ship from New Zealand

---

6 In the six months from February to July 1919 there were 11,552 pneumonic influenza deaths in Australia, almost half of them in NSW, according to the *Official year book of the Commonwealth of Australia* (1920, 192).

7 Kolata (2000) cited estimates of the global mortality rate from influenza as from 20 million to more than 40 million.

8 The Influenza Report (1920, 144, 147) noted influenza was more lethal for non-Europeans, the overweight, alcoholics and those with TB. Burnet and Clark (1942, 73) noted that 26.6 per 1000 Maoris died compared with five per 1000 Europeans in the October 1918 epidemic. Graham (1921, 28) described a 1919 outbreak at an Aboriginal camp on NSW's north coast which affected 65 out of 110 with 12 deaths, while in nearby Alstonville only 31 out of 400 caught it. Cumpston (1919, 48) noted that on ships with European and 'coloured' crew, the latter were particularly vulnerable.

arrived in Sydney on 25 October carrying influenza sufferers, the passengers were detained in the hospital at Sydney's North Head Quarantine Station, which from that date until 30 January 1919, recorded 326 influenza cases and 49 deaths. The hero was the Commonwealth's Director of Quarantine, JHL Cumpston, who 'saved more Australian lives than any other person ever.'[9] He was responsible for this massive quarantine operation which involved 149 uninfected vessels (7075 passengers and 7941 crew) and 79 infected vessels (2795 patients, 48,072 passengers and 10,456 crew). Afterwards Dr Cumpston called it probably the country's most extensive and the most successful maritime quarantine exercise but believed it was 'improbable' that the enforcement of such large scale measures would ever be needed again (Cumpston 1928, 319).

Health authorities prepared huge amounts of vaccine during the three months the disease was contained offshore. The maritime barrier eventually failed, in Victoria;[10] on 23 January 1919 a soldier jumped ship and caught a train from Melbourne to Sydney where he was admitted to hospital with influenza. A week later, Sydney had four definite cases and about 18 suspicious cases who were all admitted to the Military Hospital in Randwick. However, this did not contain the disease and it 'invaded' Deniliquin (near the Victorian border) on 8 February and then spread, with Newcastle to be struck on 2 March, in an epidemic which lasted in Australia until 12 July 1919.[11]

Newcastle newspapers began their warnings in November 1918; a month later they were printing official health warnings and

---

9 Horsley (2007) gave the mortality rate in Australia as 228 per 100,000 – half that of other countries.

10 This caused great resentment in New South Wales. *The Triad* (1919) claimed that, as a result of ineptitude on the part of the federal and Victorian governments, 'pneumonic influenza has got loose in Australia.'

11 Influenza Report (1919, 166–67, Table 6): 'Towns of NSW in the order in which they were invaded by influenza in 1919. The first date indicates the date of first invasion. The second is that on which the epidemic came to an end.' Statistics are listed on p. 152: NSW had 21,731 influenza cases which had been notified under the *Public Health Act* – 11,922 in the metropolitan area, 2558 in the Hunter River District and 7251 in the rest of the state.

advertisements for quack remedies.[12] On 3 December the hospital board warned the minister again and then gave the story to the *Newcastle Herald*, including the chair's claim that the 'wholly inadequate' isolation facilities were 'a serious indictment' on the state's health department. The matter was raised in the New South Wales Legislative Assembly on 11 December by Labor politician Albert Gardiner who, in an uncharacteristically short question,[13] asked the Chief Secretary (George Fuller) whether the Minister for Health was aware of the newspaper reports, 'the very serious statement' made by the hospital superintendent and the 'voluminous' letters from the hospital to the health department requesting these facilities. Fuller promised to draw the minister's attention to this 'if notice was given' and Gardiner retorted that Fuller had been promising this 'for the last twelve months'. 'Grave public scandal' news was reported in the *Newcastle Herald* on 19 December and the *Sydney Morning Herald* noted that when Newcastle Hospital's northern wing was built, the old isolation wards were demolished and temporary buildings were built so close to the hospital that they were in breach of the *Public Health Act*.

This continued inaction infuriated Dr Martin Doyle who resigned from the hospital board and told the *Newcastle Herald* on 16 January 1919, that the board of directors were tired of suffering from the 'stigma of the scandal, for which they were not responsible'. He blamed the Minister for Health and the state government for their 'almost criminal negligence' of patients with infectious diseases despite being a Labor appointee to the New South Wales Legislative Council and the government's representative on the hospital board. The minister expressed his regret about Doyle's resignation and then offered that age-old excuse which politicians still find convenient: a 'half a century old' mistake was 'not the fault of this generation'.

On 29 January the *Newcastle Herald* published Zions' dramatic news that the epidemic had 'definitely broken out in Sydney' and was 'to

---

12 *Newcastle Herald*, 1918, 5 and 6 December, 30 January and 4 February 1919.

13 Mark Lyons (1981) noted that Gardiner's overnight speech of 12 hours 40 minutes in 1918, the longest ever in federal parliament, forced the introduction of a time limit on parliamentary speeches.

be expected in Newcastle at any moment'. Zions advised people to wear masks, avoid public gatherings and be inoculated; the hospital's patients and staff were vaccinated and he and other staff would 'do everything possible' if it arrived. Two days later Zions received a midnight telephone call about a suspected case of influenza and because the motorised ambulance was 'out of commission' he had to use the horse-ambulance. When another flu suspect was isolated in the hospital on 3 February, the chair made a proposal that lacked benevolence but was probably necessary: they should evict the old people from the Benevolent Home at Waratah and house influenza patients there.

There were more shock headlines on 10 February after the *Newcastle Herald* revealed that men from the troopship *Argyllshire* had escaped from Sydney's Quarantine Station. One soldier had returned to his Newcastle home and his friends arranged a welcoming party but it was broken up by police who quarantined all 11 of the revellers in the house. They were acting on evidence supplied by Zions, who must have had very good sources of information to have known about this. The bad news continued and on 3 March the *Newcastle Herald* confirmed citizens' fears – influenza had broken out in Newcastle and Frederick McAlister, a 28-year-old seaman from the island-trading steamer *Ooma*, had died from it in the hospital and others were infected. The board's chair hurriedly convened a meeting to consider the serious situation they faced after the man's death, which was first thought to be from 'enteric fever' (typhoid) and then thought to be from pneumonic influenza. After much discussion the board agreed on the diagnosis and that the five sick nurses who had been in contact with the seaman were also suffering from the disease. They decided to close the outpatient department, to refuse non-urgent admissions and 'as far as possible' to quarantine D Ward where he had been. They did not carry out tests for typhoid[14] and decided it was 'not necessary to bring up a Board of Health doctor to confirm the diagnosis' although his services would be 'required for public health purposes'.

---

14 The Widal test, devised in 1896, was a quick and accurate diagnostic test for typhoid. Typhoid has characteristic inflammation of bowel, known as Peyer's patches, which would have been picked up in the autopsy.

In his report to the board, Zions said that the ship had had two doctors onboard, a husband and wife named McNaughton, who had observed the seaman for a fortnight and diagnosed his illness as typhoid. Dr Hubert Harris had attended the ship as the government's representative and he had agreed with their diagnosis and recommended the man's admission. The seaman was placed in D Ward and 'showed no strong chest symptoms until shortly before his death'. Two nurses with similar symptoms, and three other nurses with abnormal temperatures, were sent to the old linen room which was now the hospital's makeshift isolation ward. A wardsman and an honorary doctor were also isolated there. The details Zions provided were later collaborated by Cumpston in the official 1919 quarantine report:

> *Ooma* – Steamer, tonnage 3991. Passengers, nil; crew, 56. Vessel left Melbourne 6.45 pm on 21 February; was medically examined in accordance with the routine at outward inspection at commencement of voyage in Melbourne for Newcastle district. On 22 February one of the seamen became ill and was [immediately treated by the ships' two medical doctors and on arrival in Newcastle on the 25th he was] examined by a quarantine officer and a state health officer. The vessel was held under quarantine detention until the expiration of four days from Melbourne. The case was diagnosed as typhoid, and dealt with on that basis. [The patient was then admitted to] Newcastle hospital without any special isolation, and died on 3 March. The diagnosis on post-mortem examination was made to be pneumonic influenza, though no suspicion of the diagnosis had occurred before death. Sixteen cases were alleged to have been infected from this case, all being either members of the hospital staff or patients in the same ward.

The Director of Quarantine's final sentence, about the 16 cases 'alleged to have been infected' suggests he doubted this claim. Questions can be asked about the inadequate isolation; if the seaman caught influenza in the hospital from those who had been admitted with it in February; if the postmortem findings were wrong or deliberately lost.[15] The board may have decided it was too risky to ask for a Board of Health official's

---
15 McAlister's autopsy report is not held by NSW Archives.

opinion because he might have ordered a typhoid test or said that the man *had* died from typhoid. Reports of such medical disagreement in the newspapers would have sparked a political inquiry and damaged the hospital's reputation and its source of funds. Zions had discovered serious hospital irregularities and it is likely that his threat to make them public 'if pressed' made the board decide to act first to prevent this.

The day *after* the death, the hospital was notified that the Benevolent Home, now called the Waratah Influenza Hospital, would 'receive all influenza patients and contacts'. And, in the first of a series of inflammatory editorials, the *Newcastle Sun* stressed the citizens' 'unease' about the 'serious outbreak of pneumonic influenza at the local hospital'. It blamed the doctors for admitting the seaman and had 'no doubt' that the government's advisory committee would 'closely investigate' his death so that in future, 'if travellers from an infected port developed high temperatures, they would be placed in special isolation'. The editorial did not consider the hospital's obligations to treat the sick or the uncertainty about the diagnosis and ignored the lack of adequate isolation facilities in the hospital or anywhere else in Newcastle.

In surprising contrast, on 5 March the *Newcastle Sun* published the first of two sympathetic, well-informed articles about the problems doctors faced in attempting to treat this disease which was notorious for its confusingly varied symptoms, including a condition called a 'typhoid state' which could show symptoms of meningitis, pneumonic influenza, or any one of a series of diseases. Little was known about pneumonic influenza which was comparatively new and the 'germ' had 'not yet been satisfactorily isolated' despite the ravages it caused. In clear, carefully chosen words, the author argued that in such a case the doctor taking over from other doctors who had had it under observation for 'a fair period' would be wrong to disregard their conclusions. The two ship's doctors said McAlister had typhoid fever and the port quarantine doctors saw no sound medical reason to disbelieve their diagnosis. The man was accordingly sent to the hospital where he was treated for typhoid fever. In four days the patient 'sank towards death'. But when suddenly the patient developed 'symptoms that were somewhat suggestive of pneumonic flu', the doctors treated him for that. 'It was the eleventh hour for McAlister, but no effort was spared to save him, the doctors failed: the man died'. He had not 'died in vain' because the medical staff had gained experience from the tragedy which could save the lives of others.

The *Newcastle Sun* resumed its attack on 6 March with a front page report about two Cessnock coal miners who went to the hospital for treatment of their eye injuries and caught influenza there. A spokesman for the miners' union deeply resented this and could not understand why the men had been allowed to develop 'the worst scourge of all.' There was also an item tucked away on the back page of the paper about 'a well-known Newcastle doctor' who, after developing a raised temperature had followed the correct procedure of reporting the matter and isolating himself in his room and was then admitted to Waratah Infectious Diseases Hospital with suspected flu. The *Newcastle Herald* identified the 'well-known' doctor as Zions, saying that he and Dr LA Kortum from D Ward had been placed in isolation.

On 11 March the *Sun* published a second atypical article which questioned the received wisdom by asking if the first victim really did have influenza. This, and the previous sympathetic article, have Zions' stamp on them and it is amazing that he had managed to persuade the editor to publish them and that, despite his serious illness, he could have written two such logical, well-argued pieces – one during the feverish early stages and the other from his hospital bed. He stressed that the *Ooma,* after leaving Newcastle was declared 'a clean ship' when it arrived in New Zealand. If McAlister had had influenza on its Newcastle run, other crew members would almost certainly have caught it.[16] The author said that because there had been no 'instance' of influenza on the ship, it was 'being asked locally' if McAlister 'might have caught it in the hospital'. It was also questioned if any definite evidence of pneumonic influenza was found postmortem since 'all that was apparent' was 'a slight congestion of one lung and the bowels' which was 'not absolute

---

16 On the *Ooma*'s previous voyage, from 25 January to 10 February 1919, 89 percent of the crew caught influenza. A new crew, hired in Melbourne, was used for the 21–25 February voyage (Cumpston 1919, 164–65).

proof' that he had died of influenza.[17] The *Newcastle Sun* then resumed their hunt for someone to blame, their hostile editorials reaped trade union support and on 14 March Newcastle's Labour Council resolved:

> That the Minister for Health be asked to have a searching inquiry into the cause of the spread of influenza in the Newcastle Hospital and district; and, further, that should there be shown negligence or want of ability on the part of any person or persons, the Government take such action as it deems necessary in the public interest.

On 20 March the board's inquiry was deferred 'owing to illness of some of those intimate with the circumstances.' Like a hanging committee, they waited for Zions to recover before they delivered their verdict. Martin Doyle said it was the 'most important' meeting of the board's whole existence because it concerned its principal administrator and 'if the board had not held the inquiry the Government would have done so'. He was tacitly instructing his fellow directors to make a decision that the government would like or otherwise the government would make a decision the board would not like. Doyle, a former medical superintendent with strong Labor Party links, had once castigated the government for the hospital's woes but after his whistle-blowing resignation from the board in January 1919 he had been renominated for the position by the Minister of Health and his reinstatement was reported in the *Newcastle Herald* on 8 February. Doyle's action on 11 April suggests there had been a secret deal with the minister: as a reward for his speedy return to the hospital board, he would shield the government from criticism and Doyle kept the bargain by alleging that:

> Zions had made a very great error which caused a great deal of pain, trouble and death. Thirty-five cases had arisen from the one in question

---

17 No postmortem record remains and, as the doctor who attended the death was 'unregistered' – probably a recent medical graduate on the hospital staff – less reliance can be placed on the diagnosis. Frederic McAlister was born in Hamilton, Victoria, and is buried in the Roman Catholic Cemetery at Sandgate. His death certificate lists: '(1) Cause of Death: Pneumonic Influenza; (2) Duration of last illness: About 10 days; (3) Medical attendant: JM Ford, not registered; (4) When he last saw deceased: 2 March 1919.'

and 25 others are indirectly traceable. The medical superintendent is paid £600 per annum, and is absolutely in charge, and he placed the patient in a ward with nearly forty beds and kept him there nearly a week.

The cynical motive for increasing Zions' salary three months earlier may have been to use it in this denunciation. Doyle had proposed an even more drastic motion that: 'Zions had displayed an utter want of administrative capacity in admitting to a large general ward, full of patients, a seriously ill patient, just arrived from the heavily infected port of Melbourne, thereby causing the spread of pneumonic influenza'. This motion was defeated although the matter *was* clearly contentious: one board member sent an apology, a second did not vote, a third wanted to defer the matter and a fourth would not pass such severe judgement on Zions because although he 'had made a mistake, others were not altogether free' of such mistakes, none of the honorary visiting doctors knew anything about the case, the honorary in charge did not say that the seaman should be removed, nor did he inform Zions of any concerns.

After Doyle's pre-meeting directive, the board was under pressure to deliver a government-pleasing verdict by firing Zions but they also had to convince the Medical Board and Health Department that their decision was fair and open. The government and hospital representatives considered the voluminous evidence and finally agreed that 'the conduct of Dr Zions in admitting this case and treating him in the general ward was, looking at all the circumstances, indiscreet'. There were seven votes in favour and three against this motion which the board needed as their justification for getting rid of Zions.

An entry in Zions' chequebook stub relates to the day when his life unraveled: 9 April 1919 payment of '£22.10.0, LA Kortum bet'. He had made a huge bet with his colleague in the confident belief he would keep his job and was totally unprepared for the blow. The board must have believed that the hospital's crisis (and theirs) ended on 11 April at their special meeting when 'the resignation of Dr LA Kortum, senior resident medical officer, was received and accepted. A request from Dr Norman Zions, medical superintendent, for a month's holiday was granted'. These words disguised the reality that the board had sacked their chief administrative officer, although it is unclear if Kortum left in disgrace or disgust or at the end of his contract.[18]

On 15 April the *Newcastle Sun* continued to clamour about citizens' uneasy feelings but conceded these would be 'partially allayed' by the board's report about Zions' indiscretion in admitting McAlister and treating him in a general ward. Their submerged message had been to incite citizens to find out who brought influenza to Newcastle and punish them. When Zions resigned because he had become 'completely run down under the strain of work', the newspaper seemed disappointed that as a result the board 'got off lightly'. The editor warned them to ensure that the next administrator would 'have the confidence of the public in this hour of trial'.

Zions left the hospital immediately and was so traumatised by his experience that he never spoke about it. George Williams, the hospital secretary, sent him a friendly letter on 21 May hoping he was 'OK' and wondering if he had had a relapse or if he had got away as medical officer on a steamer. Williams had tried but could not induce them to grant any further severance pay. His letter concluded: 'Hoping to hear that you have fully recovered and with kindest regards, I am yours fraternally, Geo N Williams, Sec.'[19] 'Yours fraternally' was the greeting used between Masons[20] and, as the chair AA Rankin, board member Martin Doyle and the four resident doctors were Roman Catholic, the deep-seated rivalry between Catholics and Masons may have added an extra layer of tension to this dysfunctional hospital.

After Zions' March and April illness, he became sick again after he left Newcastle but it wasn't influenza. Once again his chequebook provided the evidence, with a 6 May cheque for £6.6.00 'paid to Sydney

---

18   Ludwig August Kortum, MB ChM (Sydney University, 1917) was listed in the *Medical directory for Australia* (1935) as an RMO at Royal Prince Alfred Hospital, Sydney. In his final, 1938 entry he was listed as an Honorary Medical Officer at St Joseph's Hospital, Auburn, NSW.

19   'Yours fraternally' is also a Labor Party and union movement salutation.

20   Haire listed the Masonic Club in Sydney as his club in the 1944, 1947 and 1950 issues of *Who's Who in Australia*.

Hospital for two weeks illness there'.[21] He planned to leave Australia and requested and was given the customary letter from Sydney's Lord Mayor on 30 May introducing 'Doctor Norman Zions a well-known medical practitioner in this city', who was visiting China, 'in connection with his profession'. It added that any courtesies shown to him would 'be appreciated and regarded as complimentary to the City of Sydney'. It sounded impressive but a City of Sydney archivist said that until 1991 these letters were given to anyone who made a written request and enclosed a reference from a suitable third party.[22] Zions' chequebook had entries on 20 May for £1.13.3 for socks and handkerchiefs for his father; on 30 May he gave his mother £5. He settled his tax bill on 24 June.

There is a strange link between Zions' plight and that of another harshly treated man. The story was told by an old Newcastle man who had been a junior doctor when Zions was superintendent. He said Zions was a good administrator and looked after the patients well but was 'inclined to antagonise people'. This was inevitable in a hospital of over 100 staff, including 62 nurses, who would have resented the reforms Zions tried to implement, particularly his move to stop their bad work practices. The man said that Zions 'used to entertain sailors at Newcastle's Mission to Seamen in his time off'.[23] While this may sound salacious, it was completely chaste and charitable. Robert Close wrote in his autobiography that in the 1920s his lonely life as a teenage apprentice had been brightened by the 'mild entertainments' such as recitations by Zions, Sunday night teas, picnics up the river, knitted gifts and being able to flirt with the well-chaperoned girls in activities arranged by the Mission Chaplain, 'Reverend Mr Vicory' [sic]'.[24] Close holds a tragic

---

21 Sydney Hospital keeps medical records for 20 years so there is no record of his illness. Zions must have been treated for some other illness because he would have been sent to an isolation hospital if it had been influenza.

22 The same applies to his Justice of the Peace (NSW) qualification which Haire listed in the 1939 and 1940 editions of Britain's *The medical directory*.

23 Ian Cope (1998) did not give the name of his source.

24 Canon Hadden Vickery was chaplain to Newcastle's Seamen's Mission and Port Chaplain to the Royal Australian Naval Reserve from 1922 to 1928.

record in Australian literary history as the only author to be jailed for his writing when the true-to-life novel *Love me sailor* was judged to be 'obscene libel'.[25] After ten days in jail, he began a 'self-imposed exile' from Australia which lasted 25 years. Zions' exile lasted for 20 years.

By 12 July 1919 the epidemic was over and Zions had left the country. Doctors in other towns were not blamed by their peers, publicly humiliated and forced to resign when influenza hit their locality in an epidemic which killed thousands of people throughout the state. Newcastle decision-makers were unique in their venal response to the crisis. Zions' punishment would be inexplicable without a consideration of the complicated politics surrounding the crisis. It would have been embarrassing to be seen as the source of an epidemic and it was a sensitive topic; shortly before the outbreak, the *Newcastle Herald*'s 16 August 1918 editorial had boasted about the city's improving health statistics and had indignantly denied a town planning lecturer's claim that slums and overcrowding had caused an increase of disease in Newcastle.

The normal stages of an epidemic are denial, fear, panic and finally rational response, but in this case the decision-makers did not accept that the outbreak of influenza was inevitable. When it struck, Newcastle's newspapers, employers and unions looked for someone to blame and their hostility focused on the hospital and the government but both escaped censure by blaming Zions. The hospital board and health officials got away with it because there was no public support for him, and his dismissal allowed all involved to deny the facts by blaming outsiders for the scourge: troops returning from overseas, a seaman from Melbourne and a doctor from Sydney.

Memories of the 1919 crisis were fading by the time the New South Wales Department of Public Health published its 160-page 1919 Influenza Report in April 1920. It did not mention Zions (or the shameful

---

25 The book is reviewed in *The Journal of Sex Education (JSE)* (April 1949) and Moore (2002, 316–29). It became a bestseller when it was published in France but, when there was an attempt to import an English edition of the book into Australia in 1951, Customs referred it to the Literature Censorship Board, which recommended it but their decision was overruled by the minister.

way he was treated) nor was it mentioned in the first two histories of the hospital.[26]

---

26 Champion (1978); Lewis (1997). Marsden (2005, 90) mentioned this episode in her history, quoting Wyndham (2000). The hospital has been relocated and in 2006 the New South Wales government sold this prime Newcastle waterfront site to developers.

4

Haire the Phoenix

Zions joined the flood of doctors, scientists and other intellectuals leaving Australia; he made his exit as a surgeon on the SS *Changsha*, a Chinese cargo ship which sailed via Borneo, the Philippines and Indo-China arriving in Hong Kong on 5 July 1919. On his first overseas trip he developed a lifelong love for Oriental art, crafts and music and, while other crew members blocked their ears, he listened attentively to the plaintive songs accompanied by Chinese instruments. He returned to Australia briefly and on 18 August *The Argus* reported that he was 'on his way to London'. His last cheque on 25 September was £1.6.0 for packing made out to his married sister Estelle Jacobson. An official letter from Sydney's Victoria Barracks arrived at his family house in Paddington, dated the day *after* his departure, indicated he was 'permitted' to leave.

He sailed from the Victorian port of Geelong as surgeon on the SS *Lucie Woermann*, owned by a German-East African shipping company. He was fascinated by the different cultures on his voyage via Borneo, the Philippines, China, French Indo-China, South- and South-West Africa, Sierra Leone and Holland to Britain. In every port he asked, 'What was being done about human breeding?' and the reply was always the same: 'Nothing at all – everywhere children of chance, not choice'. He arrived in London on 28 October and, while butterflies emerge in spring, he made a wintery metamorphosis by changing his name to Norman Haire,[1] explaining in his 1941 entry to *Who's Who in Australia* that he'd done so because 'during the war many people thought that it was a German name.' There were also strong anti-Jewish feelings in Britain[2] and one of

---

[1] Norman Zions' change of name by deed poll on 2 December 1919 to Norman Haire was published in *The London Gazette* (1919). His father Henry had changed his name to 'Zions', which is the anglicised and phonetically spelt version of 'Zajac'. It means 'hare' in Polish.

[2] McLaren (2007), quoting Holmes (1979, 104–74); Lowenstein (1993) and

his relatives, Gillian Shenfield, believed that could have been the reason. Norman's brother Bert, followed his example but his daughter, Gloria Saville, said he forgot to check the spelling and became Bert *Hare*. In his 1996 entry for Haire in the *ADB*, Frank Forster commented:

> He took what he regarded as a more acceptable surname. One would like to think that the insertion of an 'i' was a display of Norman's ego, for he always had plenty of that.

Ivan Crozier believed he sought a name 'that did not betray his Jewish heritage. The "I" was added for its Irish flavour. This could perhaps be seen as part of Haire's lifelong effort to have a stage name.' Ironically, a few decades earlier, a celebrated British actor had changed his name to Hare.[3] Discrimination against Germans made Britain's royal family exchange their German titles and surnames for English ones in 1917 but, if it worried Zions, it would have made more sense to change when the war began. Haire might have added the 'i' to differentiate himself from an animal but this did not prevent one cartoonist drawing him as a hare. His ego was not a sign of vanity but an indication of his strong character which sustained his quest for sexual reform.

When Haire registered as a doctor on 10 December 1919[4] he was living at 19 Lavender Vale, Wallington in Surrey; he moved to London and began working as a junior doctor at Hampstead General Hospital. He wrote to ask Havelock Ellis' advice about his plan to work in his field and, because he was an Australian, he was immediately welcomed by the philosopher who invited him to his tenement flat in Brixton. They met in January 1920 which was a death and life month for Haire: his

---

Rubinstein (1996, 192–223).

3   Sir John Hare (1844–1921), the famous comic actor and manager of the Garrick Theatre in London, was born John Fairs.

4   Haire registered in a supplement to the *Colonial List* on 10 December 1919. Sands (2008) said practitioners with recognised diplomas from British possessions could register without examination in the UK as their names were already on the *Colonial Register* (which became the *Commonwealth List* in 1948) and Haire's name remained on these lists until his death.

father died, and a friendship began between Havelock Ellis (the master) and Haire (the disciple) which lasted until Havelock Ellis' death in 1939. Haire was meeting the man whose writing he had admired for years, so it is not surprising that his emotion poured out.

In May the 28-year-old thanked the 61-year-old Ellis for supporting his application to join the British Society for the Study of Sex Psychology (BSSSP) but foolishly said he was 'a little disappointed' in this group which had just agreed to have him. He hoped to 'find many at whose feet' he could 'sit and drink in wisdom' because he always looked 'for a guide to lean on' and distrusted his 'own unaided efforts' but felt that his knowledge equalled theirs. He poured out his distress, saying that for a long time he had been intensely unhappy with 'great disharmony' in his 'psychic life'. He was sure Ellis would understand this because of their conversation in January but fortunately 'that time of *acute unhappiness*' was over.[5] Even so, his mental life still lacked balance if physical or psychological strain lowered his resistance. He had recently experienced both: physical strain from influenza and mental strain from the Newcastle incident. He asked Ellis about psychoanalysis since he distrusted his 'urgent impulse' to try it because he was often given to 'impulsiveness and enthusiasm' which he sometimes regretted later. The 'absolute denuding' of his conscious and unconscious mind to another person was not to be undertaken lightly and he needed to be sure of the 'absolute secrecy of the analyst' – his medical experience had taught him that 'professional secrecy' was often ignored.

---

5 This is why the acute stage was over: Henry Zions' death certificate records his death from carcinoma of rectum on 4 January 1920. Years later, Haire discussed his terrible dilemma in *Woman* (1947). Haire left home on learning his father had inoperable cancer, because as a medical graduate, if he had stayed he would not have been able to abstain from providing his father with a painless death. Haire repeatedly wrote to his medical attendant (Dr Michael O'Gorman Hughes), asking him to relieve his pain and hasten the end with large doses of morphia. But the doctor had religious scruples and Haire received harrowing letters from his family: the man's agony in the nine months it took him to die was so great that he used to scream for a merciful death, and threaten to throw himself out of the window or off the balcony, because the pain was too great for him to bear.

Haire later told a novelist that he had been 'a mass of diffidence and shyness' until he discovered his organising talent and began to succeed in his medical work and gradually gained confidence.[6] He must have impressed Havelock Ellis who was often 'at home' to his acolyte while refusing to see others, and the philosopher sent him patients and gave him professional and publishing contacts and, in return, Haire provided him with patient case notes, some of which Ellis used in his books.[7] This mentoring seems odd given the older man's anti-Semitic views,[8] and their age and personality differences, but it was based on usefulness, not friendship and, as Haire noted in an obituary tribute, he had been 'a revering disciple' and 'did not know him intimately'.

Havelock Ellis was also mentor to America's pioneering birth control crusader Margaret Sanger who was later denounced by American televangelist George Grant in *Grand illusions*, 'the best-selling pro-life book of all time.' Grant portrayed her as an unbalanced, sexually promiscuous woman who supported crank 'Malthusian offshoots' such as 'Freudians' [sic]. He continued:

> Margaret's English exile gave her the opportunity to make some critical interpersonal connections as well. Her bed became a veritable meeting place for the Fabian upper crust: HG Wells, George Bernard Shaw, Arnold Bennett, Arbuthnot Lane, and Norman Haire. And of course, it was then that she began her unusual and tempestuous affair with Havelock Ellis.[9]

Grant included Norman in this list of 'bed' relationships Sanger enjoyed as 'a fugitive from justice' in Britain in 1914–1915, despite the fact that he did not arrive in London until 1919. Such errors litter this attack on birth controllers, but, during George W Bush's presidency, Grant's work

---

6 Ruck (1935, 165).

7 Havelock Ellis (1937, 232–35) included a woman's description of her menstrual cycle 'kindly furnished to me by Dr Norman Haire which is interesting as it seems to show careful and precise self-observation'.

8 Ellis' oblique anti-Semitism distressed Margaret Sanger in 1926 when he wrote 'Wonderful how Jews are sometimes capable of intelligence, receptivity & enthusiastic appreciation!', quoted in Grosskurth (1985, 348).

9 Grant (2000, 76).

influenced the American government's decision to stop funding birth control projects.

Sanger, like Haire, was one of 11 children and, after her 48-year-old mother died of tuberculosis, became an almost fanatical birth control crusader. According to her grandson, when her son and daughter-in-law were expecting their fourth child she said, 'You've disgraced me. I'm going to Europe.'[10] As a young woman, Sanger was an extroverted charmer who could show good sense or be 'impossibly difficult'. Havelock Ellis often sent Margaret Sanger snide comments about their mutual friends and mentioned the problems he was having with 'Jane Burr', daughter of the millionaire Guggenheim family who used this pen name when writing about women's rights. They had met in 1921 after she published a best-seller; during her September 1922 tour she had scandalised Londoners by wearing 'knickerbockers' and she now wanted Havelock Ellis to 'help her to find herself'. He told Sanger that he didn't think he could because she worried him; although he had faith in her possibilities and admired her 'large and fine' qualities, they didn't come across properly in her actions and she seemed to have 'made an awful impression in America. She is just a little too Jewish – like Norman Haire, whom she knows and criticises justly but is a little like him in a feminist way only nicer' (10 December 1922, MSP – LC). Havelock Ellis disliked their 'strident' crusading which he attributed to their Jewishness – he had rigid ideas on race and always attributed certain characteristics to the Jews (Grosskurth, 1985: 295). A few months later his antipathy towards activists had become non-sectarian: he told Sanger he was afraid birth control advocates 'are rather objectionable people, what with Marie Stopes and Norman Haire' (9 February 1923, MSP – LC). He was not alone in these views: birth control stalwart Bessie Drysdale said Stopes was powerful and disagreeable with a catty way of making tremendous publicity.[11] Others felt Marie was quite contrary,

---

10 Alexander Sanger (1995).
11 Benn (1992).

'unbalanced'[12] and 'perhaps, not quite sane'.[13] The movement was filled with such tensions and, after Dr Alice Vickery Drysdale's death in 1929, Edith How-Martyn (a birth control and women's suffrage pioneer) regretted she had not 'had the recognition she deserved from feminists but petty jealousies spoil much in life.'

In 1920 Haire signed a rent agreement with Dr Halliday Sutherland for a consulting room at 26 New Cavendish Street. It was an advance for Haire who made it clear on his stationery that the address was only '2 doors from Harley St', but while the landlord was strongly opposed to birth control his tenant was a stout supporter. Haire's income tax return for 1921–22 shows that he went into debt to start his own practice:

Fees to anaesthetists	£ 19.19.0
Chemical dressings, gloves, vaccines, sera, suture, materials for operations & replacing instruments etc	£ 75.17.0
Travelling expenses in connection with professional work	£ 50.00.0
Rent of consulting room	£145.0.0
Telephone	£ 10.0.0
Stamps & stationery	£ 10.0.0
Insurance	£ 1.10.0

His work in the Hampstead hospital had ceased and these were enormous expenses considering that his sole income that year had been 34 guineas he earned for three months' night shift work, once a week at the London Lock Hospital, treating women and children who had venereal disease. The clue to his readiness to spend this money is a receipt for a £200 loan from the Countess of Hungary (the wife of Count Albert Apponyi), a feminist who held several League of Nations

---

12 Hall in Bland and Cross (2003, 218) quoting Stella Browne's letter to Havelock Ellis (BL, 6 March 1922).

13 Ferris (1993, 109).

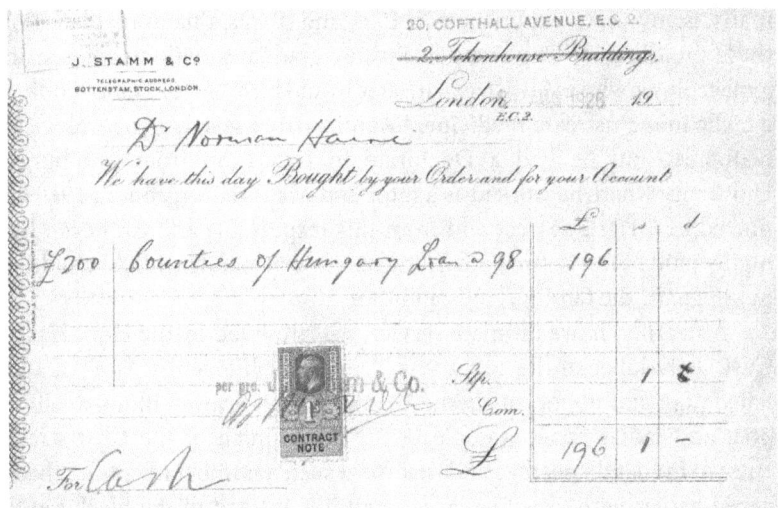

Figure 4.1. Countess of Hungary's £200 loan cheque to Haire.

positions and supported many welfare and women's interest groups (Zimmermann 2006).

Although Haire had trained and worked in obstetric hospitals, he had no specialist qualifications because obstetrics and gynaecology were not taught when he was a student, even though the University of Sydney's veterinary school did provide training in animal obstetrics. On hearing this, Millicent Preston-Stanley, New South Wales' first female politician, is said to have demanded 'Horses' rights for women', a slogan coined by Judge Ben Lindsey (1920). Haire asked his university if he could be examined in England for their Doctorate in Medicine but they refused in March 1922 because candidates 'had to be examined locally'.

In middle age Haire reminisced that when he started practice as a specialist he never knew where his 'next quarter's rent was coming from' and barely managed to keep his head above water. He had been glad to earn a guinea working in a friend's practice in the evening – perhaps with Dr Solomon Jervois Aarons who performed artificial inseminations (AI). Haire waited two decades to discuss his work which produced a 'number of heirs for titled people' and 'humbler people at the other end of the social scale'. Haire began to benefit from the older man's 'many years' experience' in 1921 and it was a natural alliance of these multilingual University of Sydney graduates with an interest in gynaecology, who as Jewish expatriates would have had difficulty finding a niche in mainstream medicine.[14] Aarons wrote several gynaecological textbooks and he had a Doctorate in Education from Edinburgh University where he worked as a tutor and obstetric surgeon. In 1916 he moved to 6 Harley Street and from this respectable address began his highly paid secret service providing barren aristocrats with AI children to safeguard the family's lands and title.

An earlier, more intimate service was provided by the Hon. Harry Cust, 'lady-killer of the century,' a 'delightful philogenist [sic]'[15] and a failed poet and politician (Leslie 1972). Wilfred Scawen Blunt, a fellow poet and ladies' man, was pleased that 'so much of the Cust strain entered England's peerage and that from such a number of cradles there gazed babies with eyes like large sapphires instead of the black boot-buttons of their legal fathers.'[16]

Years later Haire's surgery was equipped for gynaecological procedures, including AI (Lehfeldt 1981), a procedure in which a husband's sperm (AIH) or donor sperm (AID) was syringed into the woman's vagina. Society often blamed women for infertility problems and some hid their partner's problem with donor-assisted pregnancies. The British surgeon John Hunter achieved the first successful human artificial insemination in 1785 by using sperm from the woman's husband but it was considered a fluke. Carl Hartman removed the guesswork in 1938 when he calculated that the most fertile period for women with a 28-day menstrual cycle was 11 to 14 days after the first day of menstruation.[17] Even so, there were still medical, ethical and

---

14 Dalby (2007) found Aarons' 1916 entry in *The London medical directory* but not in *Munk's roll*, indicating he was not a Fellow of the Royal College of Physicians, possibly because he operated outside the accepted boundaries.

15 It should be philogynist, a lover of women.

16 Leslie (1972, 279) said that Lady Diana Cooper, the beautiful socialite daughter of the Duke of Rutland, acknowledged that Harry Cust was her 'real father'.

17 Haire (HC – 21, 57) stressed that while AI was useful in the treatment of sterility, it was not always suitable. 'Sometimes it was only successful after many

legal problems and, when reports of assisted pregnancies appeared in medical journals in the 1940s, the Archbishop of Canterbury called for the procedure to be made a crime – a suggestion which Haire, who found it preferable to adoption, considered 'a monstrous impertinence'. The British government was not prepared to ban AI but agreed it was 'undesirable and not to be encouraged' and in 1945 *Time* magazine emphasised the problems:

> Adultery? Blackmail? Johns Hopkins' Dr Alan Guttmacher has reported success in no less than 20 out of 36 attempts. But the problem of possible charges of adultery against the mother, illegitimacy against the child, and blackmail by donors of semen remains unsolved. For their own as well as their patients' protection, US doctors usually seek refuge in a rigmarole of anonymity and secrecy.

In 1970 Dr Arthur 'Bung' Hill, a well-regarded Melbourne gynaecologist, described his experience from 1946 to 1967 in treating 21 women for infertility (16 by AID and five by AIH), as a result of which 18 healthy children were born. Some doctors provided AI but would not write about it because of 'timidity, inexperience, distaste, fear of legal implications, religious or other reasons' – he broke this silence.

Another 80-year-old secret was revealed in 1981: Dr Ralph Worrall, a noted Sydney gynaecologist, provided successful AIH treatments in 1901 and 1904 for a woman 'whose husband was impotent (sexually infantile). She had a boy who died in infancy, but the second, also a boy, passed away only a few years ago' [in the 1970s]. This was revealed by 'J Westone, Canberra' who apologised for her shaky writing in a letter which was hand-delivered to Sydney's King George V Hospital, marked for the attention of the Clinical Superintendent. Worrall had secretly supported Marion Piddington's crusade for 'Celibate Motherhood' (AI) in his 1918 pamphlet, *Facultative motherhood without offence to moral law*,[18] allegedly by 'Dr Henry Waterman Swan' – a *pen* name which is a double pun referring to the Waterman and Swan brands of fountain

---

attempts, lasting over many months, have been made'.

18 The title was a synonym for artificial insemination; others included scientific motherhood, eugenic, celibate or facultative (optional) motherhood and, later,

pen and to the female swan which is called a pen. Piddington, the wife of Judge AB Piddington, ran a Sydney clinic offering counselling and contraception.[19] As 'Lois', in her *Via nuova or science & maternity* pamphlet, she proposed that women left childless by the war should be artificially impregnated by eugenically suitable donors. Critics called it 'conscription of the virgins' and one feminist claimed that 'bastardry under the hedge' was preferable.[20] Haire later distanced himself from her campaign: 'Before the end of the last war a well-known Sydney woman published a little book, called *Vita nuova* [sic],[21] in which she advocated artificial fertilisation as a means of enabling unmarried women anxious to have children to do so artificially. Many people were inexpressibly shocked at her suggestion'.

Haire credited Havelock Ellis, HG Wells and George Bernard Shaw for helping to shape his interests and was gratified to discover that his views on birth control and eugenics were shared by the four-decades-old Malthusian League which he joined after hearing Margaret Sanger address them in May 1920. He claimed disingenuously that he had 'no experience of public speaking' and had been 'pressed into service' by the Malthusians who urgently needed speakers but he must have relished the opportunity. Ellis introduced him to 'the best medical authorities on the subject' and to the groups concerned with the social aspects of sexual problems, and sensibly warned him to 'beware of the opposition and persecution which were still the inevitable lot of any writer in the

---

eutelegenesis and now euphemistically called a method of assisted reproductive technology.

19 It was called the 'Institute of Family Relations' which Edith How-Martyn dismissed in 1933 as 'a money making concern' and called Piddington a 'rather unbalanced' woman who had earlier 'made the movement look rather foolish by her strong advocacy of artificial insemination'. Information supplied by Lesley A Hall.

20 Mary Elizabeth Fullerton, Vice President of the Women's Political Association in Victoria, said this at the WPA's August 1919 meeting and it sparked lively correspondence in their magazine *Figaro*.

21 The title was *Via nuova* (Latin for 'new way') but Haire was probably thinking of Dante's *La vita nuova* (Latin for 'new life') and the book title may also allude to this.

new sphere of sexology'. One group he joined was the Society for the Study of Orthopsychics which offered a three-year course on normal and abnormal psychology and psychogenesis and it also included psychoanalysis and supervised work with patients (Raitt 2004).

The British Society for the Study of Sex Psychology (BSSSP) was briefly interested in psychoanalysis and some Freud advocates joined and then resigned when the BSSSP began to advocate the views proposed by their own members: Magnus Hirschfeld, Havelock Ellis and Edward Carpenter (Waters 1998). The minutes of the BSSSP 21 March 1921 meeting include Haire's statement that the psychoanalytical group was 'moribund' and they agreed to bury it because work pressures had forced him to resign as secretary. In the same month he joined the Eugenics Society which keenly interested him. When he joined the Malthusian League, he agreed to work two or three afternoons a week as the honorary medical officer in their birth control clinic.

The League began their plans for a clinic in 1917 but these stalled until they received funds from the philanthropic Sir John Sumner, who made his fortune from Ty-Phoo tea, and finally the clinic opened on 9 November 1921 at 153a East Street, Walworth. Haire commented that Marie Stopes 'and her equally courageous and public-spirited husband' had opened their clinic nine months earlier and the Malthusians were reassured because 'nothing alarming happened', the police did not close it down and the consulting medical officer was not struck off the medical register. Stopes' clinic was the first in the British Empire (but not the first in the world) so the League always emphasised that theirs was the first English clinic where birth control instruction was given under medical supervision. Two American researchers, Norman Himes and his wife Vera, said these two clinics 'opened up a new period in the history of the movement aimed at the emancipation of women from their slavery to the reproductive function'.[22] They helped relatively few patients in 1921 but this was a victory and, as two British historians made clear, 'the year was one of the most important in the whole history of birth control simply because of their very existence.'[23] They were meant to

---

22 Himes and Himes (1929).
23 Wood and Suitters (1970, 161).

be the models for local authorities to emulate but government-funded clinics were not introduced in Britain until July 1930.

Despite their powerful external enemies,[24] birth controllers quarrelled among themselves: Stopes and Sanger were rivals, Stopes battled with the Malthusian League and Haire fought with Dr CV (Charles Vickery) Drysdale and his wife Bessie, the League's primary sponsors. The Drysdales had strong links with Margaret Sanger who, when charged with four criminal counts carrying a maximum jail sentence of 45 years in the United States, fled for London in 1914. Her obscenity trial was aborted after 'prominent men and women' from both sides of the Atlantic appealed to the American President.[25] The Drysdales advised her to write to Havelock Ellis and soon she was his 'Darling Woman' and he was her 'Dear Twin'[26] in a relationship which 'was both intellectual and erotic' (Nottingham 1999, 153). Sanger, who had visited Holland in 1915, said she suggested the clinic idea to Bessie Drysdale and Norman Haire in 1920 by talking 'clinic, clinic, clinic' to convince them it was more effective than written advice.

Three months before the Malthusians' clinic was due to open, Haire wrote to Sanger on 15 September 1921 to beg for her support. He said that he and Mrs Drysdale had 'nearly quarrelled' because she wanted to advertise the clinic in all the papers, and have a 'grand opening ceremony' and he wanted nothing to do with it in those circumstances. He was sure her 'unwise' actions would antagonise the medical profession and asked Sanger 'to find some opportunity of saying so tactfully'. He sent his letter from Berlin on the first day of the First International Congress for Sex

---

24 Opposition was fiercest in America; on 15 November 1921 *The Times* reported a serious riot in New York when the police stopped a meeting of the American Birth Control Conference which Sanger was to have addressed. *The Times* later reported the police ban and that Sanger's arrest had been ordered by Patrick Hayes, New York's Roman Catholic Archbishop.

25 Mrs Anne Kennedy, 'Greetings and reports. United States of America', in *Fifth Neo-Malthusian conference* (1922, 19). Rose (1992, 91–92) noted that Stopes had organised a petition, signed by influential people including Arnold Bennett, HG Wells and Professor Gilbert Murray, begging President Wilson to drop the charges against Sanger.

26 Grosskurth (1980, 242–45).

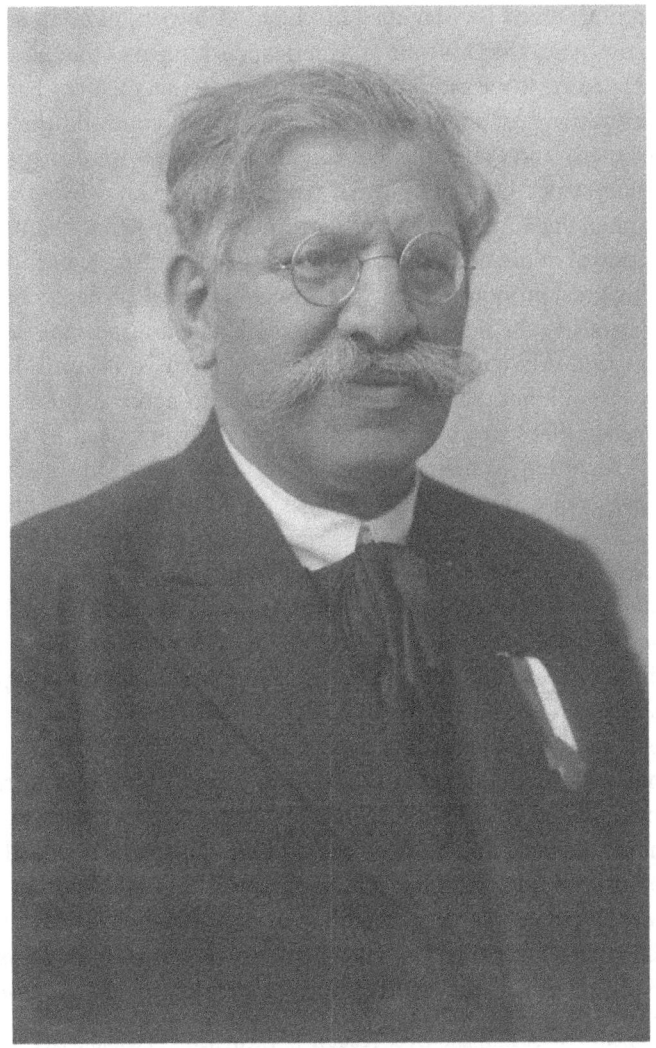

Figure 4.2. Magnus Hirschfeld, the 'Einstein of Sex'.

Research arranged by Magnus Hirschfeld, 'a Jewish, gay and socialist sexologist', who, after his tour of America was known as the 'Einstein of Sex'.[27] Haire made the astute comment to Sanger that the British medical profession was 'just about ready' to take up birth control if they could do so 'quietly and gracefully' but might resist if they were antagonised by the Drysdales' publicity. He may have had inside knowledge because in October the King's physician, Lord Dawson of Penn, championed birth control in his 'Sexual relationships' speech to Anglican Bishops.[28] After his 'great pronouncement' the press and publishers began 'opening their portals to the new message' and it became a respectable topic of conversation. Although the Bishops conceded that 'birth control is here to stay', it took another nine years for them to agree at the Lambeth Conference that birth control was acceptable if practised by married couples according to their consciences and under medical supervision.

Haire sent a second plea to Sanger on 1 October with a dramatic opening: 'September was a disastrous month for Birth Control in London.' He then gave *his* version of events because he knew Mrs Drysdale would send her a 'dreadful account' of him. He had been 'staggered' by Mrs Drysdale's news that the centre was to have 'a grand opening day' with reporters interviewing *him* which was 'quite opposite' to his plans and he had maintained firmly that it would antagonise the doctors 'instead of persuading them gently and tactfully.' Mrs Drysdale became very rude and sent an 'insulting letter' asking him to resign, which he did in 'a polite but very frank letter such as I am sure she had never received in her life before' and the centre was now without a doctor and would be run like a Marie Stopes clinic. Although he knew that Mrs Drysdale was 'very difficult to work with', he was amazed by her sudden change after the pleasant time he had spent with the Drysdales and Sanger in Holland in 1921 and very disappointed because 'she

---

27 Kennedy (2003, 123) and Dose (2005). Einstein had just completed a tour of America. However, as Hirschfeld was a complete unknown, his tour manager cashed in on Einstein's popularity by billing Hirschfeld as the 'Einstein of Sex' to generate interest in his lectures. Information provided by Ralf Dose, copies of the 1930 press clippings can be found online at: www2.hu-berlin.de/sexology/GESUND/ARCHIV/TRIP01.HTM.

28 Dawson's speech (1922), quoted by Hauck (2003, 228).

seems now to be anxious to outdo Marie Stopes in the matter of self-advertisement. Alas, alas, alas! She now believes that I was connected with the clinic merely for the object of making my fortune and fame out of it. She really suffers from delusions'.

The Drysdales had a 'three-week's special campaign' in south London, 'both indoors and out', and a mass distribution of leaflets. Haire had been right to worry and their publicity generated a near-riot in the clinic's first days: 'rotten eggs, apples and stones were thrown, windows smashed, the clinic doors battered and graffiti (Whores) scrawled on the walls.'[29] Dr Drysdale later told Sanger that the clinic had to be made independent of the Malthusian League because otherwise 'Dr Haire would dominate everything' and Mrs Drysdale claimed they had 'chucked' him from the clinic.[30] Haire put it differently, saying that after he 'withdrew', the Drysdales installed a doctor who wanted the money but knew little about birth control and had 'no great enthusiasm for it'. She had few patients and after a few months the Drysdales asked him to take over and reorganise the clinic which he did. He ran lectures on birth control, anatomy, physiology and hygiene 'for poor women', and similar ones for men, several nights a month. These 'aroused great interest and brought a large number of new patients' so he soon ran the clinic three afternoons a week, often seeing 40 patients in an afternoon.

Despite Haire's careful observance of medical ethics, he had to justify himself to the Britain's medical regulatory body for revising the League's leaflet, *Hygienic methods of family limitation*.[31] Haire wrote an appeasing letter, saying he had 'always respected the authority of the General Medical Council and endeavoured to conform to the spirit of its regulations' even when this prevented him participating in propaganda which he felt was vitally important for society's welfare. He had frequently refused to write signed articles for the lay press

---

29 Rose (1992, 156).
30 Benn (1992, 213-14) and Ledbetter (1976, 159, 220-22).
31 *The Lancet* noted on 24 December 1921 that after 45 years as *The Malthusian*, it would be renamed *The New Generation*. In January 1922 the Malthusian League became the New Generation League and its journal continued until October 1949 although the League itself ceased in 1927.

where there was any chance that people might think he was 'seeking advertisement'. In particular, he had refused when invited by 'at least two very distinguished members of the medical profession' to contribute a signed article to a series in *John Bull*. He was 'surprised and disturbed to find that an article written by me for the poor in all good faith nearly four years ago and now long out of print, has been deemed to require explanation by your Council'. Copies of the League's 1911 *Practical leaflet* (and Haire's 1922 revision) were restricted[32] and, to receive a copy, the individual had to write their name on the leaflet and agree:

> I, the undersigned, hereby declare that I am over twenty-one years of age, that I am (a) already married, (b) about to be married; that I consider the artificial limitation of the family justifiable on both individual and national grounds; and that I have applied to the New Generation League for a copy of [its] Hygienic methods of family limitation. And I hereby declare that I will hold myself entirely responsible for the proper use of the information therein contained, and for keeping it out of the hands of unmarried persons under twenty-one years of age.

In Britain publications about birth control were strictly regulated but in America they were banned as an anonymous reviewer made clear in the June 1922 issue of Sanger's *Critic and guide*. She described Haire's paper as '*practically* the most valuable of all the papers' at the BSSSP Symposium because it described the 'actual means of prevenception, with illustrations', condemning some and stating which methods and appliances were best. The reviewer wanted to publish the paper 'but, alas!' this would breach the anti-contraception statute, render the issue 'unmailable' and subject the editor and publisher to the same penalties as those 'meted out to people convicted of arson, burglary and homicide'. They already had their 'share of trouble' and would not print Haire's paper 'for the present' in their 'free country'. Printing

---

32 The British government opposed birth control advice and services and would not promote either until the 1960s (Kiernan 1998). Contraception and the dissemination of birth control information was banned in America after Comstock's law in 1873 made it an offence to post any 'obscene, lewd, or lascivious' book. Remnants of these restrictions remained until 1972.

was allowed in 'benighted monarchical countries, such as England, Holland, Italy, Norway, Sweden and Denmark' and such papers could be printed 'with perfect impunity' in Germany or Austria. Sanger, who was almost certainly the reviewer, mused that in 30 years the restrictive American statute would be 'dead and buried' and she would publish the paper and her own supplements. It is strange that the title of Haire's paper was changed to *Practical methods of prevenception* which is an ugly euphemism, but choosing an apt alternative is difficult: 'family limitation', 'family planning' and 'Malthusianism' are too vague and while Lord Dawson believed 'conception control' might please those seeking 'strict accuracy', others were shocked by its explicitness. When Sanger's young friend Otto Bobstein suggested 'birth control' in 1914, this memorable juxtaposition became the punchy slogan for Sanger's campaign because she liked it despite the opposition from some of her friends who did not care for 'such strong meat'.[33] The editor of America's *The Birth Control Review* said the decision to become the American Birth Control League was very valuable to their progress: a name such as the League for Responsible Parenthood 'could be spoken and written without any of the shock produced by Birth Control' but it would not have got the idea across to most people, who would have allowed it to slip by without attention and without interest' (Porritt 1922).[34]

Marie Stopes' well-publicised address on birth control at a public meeting in London attracted an audience of over 2000 on 31 May 1921. Stopes was a non-medical newcomer and, despite joining the Malthusian League, she criticised other members for their choice of contraceptives and was annoyed by their reverence for Charles Bradlaugh and other secular birth control pioneers such as Annie Besant, Charles Knowlton, Charles Robert Drysdale and his partner Alice Vickery Drysdale, and

---

33 Chesler (1992, 97).

34 In 1942 the Birth Control Federation of America felt their title contained 'fighting' words and became the Planned Parenthood Federation of America (Chesler 1992, 292–93). They masked their timid name-change by running a competition and declaring the new name as the winner; other entries included POP (Parents On Purpose), Don't, Chosen Children and Heir Care (Suitters 1973, 25). In 1939 Britain's National Birth Control Council changed its explicit title to the Family Planning Association.

their son Charles Vickery who was the husband of Bessie Drysdale. When the League opened its clinic, a newspaper scoffed that Stopes was 'a talented lady who has been advocating birth control so effectively that she is inclined to suppose that she is the inventor of it'.[35] Stopes angrily resigned her membership and in 1921 formed her own Society for Constructive Birth Control and Racial Progress which was 'less economic and more sentimental in its appeal' and stressed the health and eugenic benefits of birth control (Himes 1936, 258–59).

The Roman Catholic Church was particularly opposed, especially Dr Halliday Sutherland,[36] a Scottish professor (once Haire's landlord) who attacked Stopes as 'a doctor of German philosophy (Munich) who had opened a Birth Control Clinic and was exposing the poor to experiment'. Stopes retaliated with a defamatory review of his book in the May 1922 issue of *Birth Control News*, saying 'Dr Sutherland's book will impose only on those who are more ignorant than he is. It is nicely calculated to encourage the biases in their prejudices, for now, when speaking against birth control, they can say, "A doctor says so!" They will probably forget he is a Roman Catholic doctor. The omissions from the book are quite as remarkable as its lies'. When he declined Stopes' invitation to a debate, she foolishly sued him and the *Stopes v Sutherland* libel suit generated huge interest and lasted two-and-a-half years; Stopes lost the first round, appealed and won and then she lost again in the House of Lords.

Haire played a crucial but reluctant part; initially, he had admired her work and asked to visit her clinic. She promoted the 'Gold-pin' wishbone-shaped pessary (one of the earliest intrauterine devices – IUDs) and the eugenically named 'Pro-Race' cap, a French cervical cap which she modified by adding a higher dome. The Malthusian clinic favoured a modified Mensinga pessary (an occlusive pessary) because

---

35 Ruth Hall (1977, 199).

36 When Sutherland toured Australia, *The Rationalist* commented in May 1940 that 'any persons who speak against Birth Control are in the same position as advocates of flat earth; nobody takes them seriously'. In June they objected to Sutherland's boast that he 'had gone from one end of Australia to the other but not one opponent of any note or any kind had come forward to challenge him.' Haire did not return to Sydney until September.

it was effective and easy to insert and Haire repeatedly warned Stopes about the dangers of the Gold-pin pessary. Haire's experience came from removing those which had been inserted by other doctors (Australian doctors joked about IUDs being 'inserted in Melbourne and removed in Sydney'). As the name suggests, they were made of gold although Haire repeated an unlikely tale about a 'Harley Street surgeon' removing a platinum one 'studded with diamonds.'

When Stopes asked him to accept two of her patients who wanted to use the Gold-pin pessary, he declined and warned her that it could act as an abortifacient (also a possibility with modern IUDs).[37] He warned her on 26 May 1921 and again on 6 June saying he was sorry to see her 'give any grounds for a possibly successful attack by the many bitter enemies'. He earnestly begged her to be very careful about the device and was sorry that he could not try it but thought she would find that, any other reputable practitioner would take the same attitude, especially those who 'had any knowledge of gynaecology'. When prosecution lawyers asked Stopes if Haire had refused to use the Gold-pin pessary because of the risk of abortion, she claimed, 'On the contrary, Dr Haire came to my clinic personally and asked me to send him subjects for the Gold-pin.' The defence subpoenaed Haire who was angered by her lie and by the suggestion that he had been canvassing for patients. While her 5 June letter to Haire did not prove that she had 'experimented on the poor', it damaged her credibility when he was forced to read it to the court:

> As regards the 'Gold-pin' . . . I hear from American women it is entirely satisfactory. I should therefore like very much for you, if you don't mind, to take on two or three cases which you could watch carefully, and if these yielded unsatisfactory results, we will then drop it. On the other hand, if it does have, as reported, so many advantages, I should be sorry to discard it without proper investigation. [She asked] May I send these to you definitely? [She had written to the two women, stating]: 'I would warn you that the method being a new one, we are not yet quite sure whether

---

37 Haire wrote: 'When I first heard of this method in 1921, the description given to me ... inclined me to try it, but ... before I had actually used it in a single case I heard of two cases in which it had caused septic miscarriages. As a result, I have always advised against it' (HC – 21, 62).

the result would be entirely satisfactory, but Dr Haire will watch the case carefully and remove the spring if it seems advisable and recommend some other method'. I particularly hope that you will investigate this method impartially, and should be very glad to hear from you details of it.

The two women did visit him and Haire wrote to Stopes on 8 June saying that he had refused their requests and had told them to return to her clinic for a check pessary. Haire was more explicit in his 19 June letter which warned Stopes 'that if in one single case' it could be proved that contraception caused abortion, 'an enormously damaging blow will have been struck at the whole birth control movement, and *your work and that of others will be largely nullified*'.[38]

Despite his embarrassing court evidence, on 6 August Stopes invited Haire to serve on her society's Committee of Research into Contraceptives. He agreed but stipulated that his name should not be used in any publicity; he had to comply with medical ethics because he was a 'young man, not far over the threshold' of his career and had to be very careful 'not to give the slightest opening for criticism'. Later on he might be able to 'act more independently'; but at present his usefulness and livelihood depended on ensuring that his conduct was beyond reproach. Haire was not going to be upstaged by Stopes and invited doctors at the 1922 Neo-Malthusian Conference to join a Medical Society for the Study of Contraception which *he* hoped to form.

When Stopes asked Haire about 'the clinic' and whether he had been misreported in *The Lancet*, he confirmed in his cordial 5 January 1922 reply that the report was accurate. He added that he had 'not yet met a case where the Gold-pin pessary has not caused trouble'. He assumed she meant the Malthusian League's clinic and said he had withdrawn from his position as honorary medical officer before it opened because of a 'lack of sympathy & incompatibility with Mrs Drysdale and her methods'. He told her 'in confidence' that although Mrs Drysdale was very enthusiastic and her motives were 'impeccable', he did not agree with her tactics. He was being either naïve or cunning to confide in

---

38 In a typed postscript to a letter to Stopes he warned that in 1898 a doctor was charged with using the Gold-pin pessary and sentenced to four months' imprisonment (5 January 1922, BL, ff 42–43).

Stopes but he may have felt that these small confidences would win her support. He said how sad it was that (at least in public) most gynaecologists opposed birth control because 'we would all benefit so much by a conference on *method*, with an exchange of our experiences'. He explained that he had not joined the Society for Constructive Birth Control and Racial Progress earlier because he disagreed with her on some details; but then added chattily: 'after all, we are both working for the same end and details are insignificant when one remembers how much you have done to bring the birth control question out into the open'. She had asked to have a chat with him and, after this flattery, he said he would be pleased to see her at any time.

Haire was also busy in another venture: rejuvenation, and the fountain of youth fantasy[39] became the wellspring for his wealth in the 1920s. It might appear that rogue rejuvenators were making money from gullible patients but initially the 'rejuvenation' surgeons believed in the technique developed by Eugen Steinach a physiologist, hormone researcher and biology professor who became the Director of Vienna's Biological Institute of the Academy of Sciences in 1912. The lure of juvenescence began in the 1920s[40] and, by the 1930s, newspapers were filled with 'defeat of old age' stories about rejuvenated hedge-hopping octogenarians and San Quentin convicts escaping over prison walls. Rejuvenators said 'sex was life itself' and it was controlled by the 'sex glands'[41] and, in his analysis, medical historian Chandak Sengoopta (2006, 8) noted that, despite the controversies surrounding these early studies, no one had ever charged the authors with deliberate deception.

The first in a trio of renowned rejuvenators was Charles-Édouard Brown-Séquard, an eminent 19th-century researcher who trained in France[42] and is known for his scientific triumphs and fiascos. He became Harvard's first professor of physiology and neuropathology

---

39 Sengoopta (1993, 55), quoting Grmek (1958) and Trimmer (1967).

40 Discussed by Gilman (1999) and Groopman (2002).

41 Sengoopta (2006, 186), quoting historical studies.

42 Charles-Édouard Brown-Séquard was born in Mauritius (then part of the British Empire) to a French mother and an American father and so he could claim nationality for all three countries.

and is honoured as the 'father of endocrinology' but he was scorned as a rejuvenator and risked disrepute at the age of 72 when he injected himself with extracts from the testicles of guinea pigs and dogs, claiming they made him stronger, brighter and more sexually potent.

The second was a charlatan: Serge Voronoff, known as 'the monkey-gland doctor', was a 'dapper, effervescent' man who claimed that gland-grafting operations would produce more 'sex hormones' and give men 'vim, vigour and vitality'. In 1920 he performed an ape-to-man testicular transplant and in 1925 he boasted of being able to 'add thirty or forty years to human life.' Within five years, 300 men had received these expensive, dangerous and useless grafts. Scientists were sceptical but his fame was assured by his skilled media-handling and his 'lucid, persuasive [self-published[43]] books' (Sengoopta 1993, 62).

Haire adopted the techniques of the third one, Eugen Steinach, who began his animal experiments in 1894 and discovered that by injecting hormones, or transplanting rats' ovaries and testicles, he could rejuvenate them or change their sex. Since the rats responded to hormones from glands ('puberty glands'), he thought it might work in humans and that vasectomy (cutting the vas deferens) or vasoligation (tying it) would reduce or stop the reproductive functions and the hormones would reduce or reverse senility so that instead of giving life to children, old men would give life to themselves. Steinach claimed 'a man is as old as his endocrine glands' and that men with 'sexual insufficiency' from hormonal or 'psychic influences' would be improved by being injected with synthetic male hormones. His announcement in 1920 was greeted by the eugenic proposal that rich old men should produce children to try and redress the wartime loss of fit young men. Steinach also proposed to 'reactivate' post-menopausal women and in 1917 he even claimed to have cured an 'effeminate, passive homosexual man' (LeVay 1996).

---

43 Haire told his publisher that he had approached Octave Doin (Voronoff's publisher) about a French translation of *Rejuvenation*. Doin published the books at Voronoff's expense and suggested doing the same for Haire who was horrified and 'did not accept of course' (AUC, 9 January 1925).

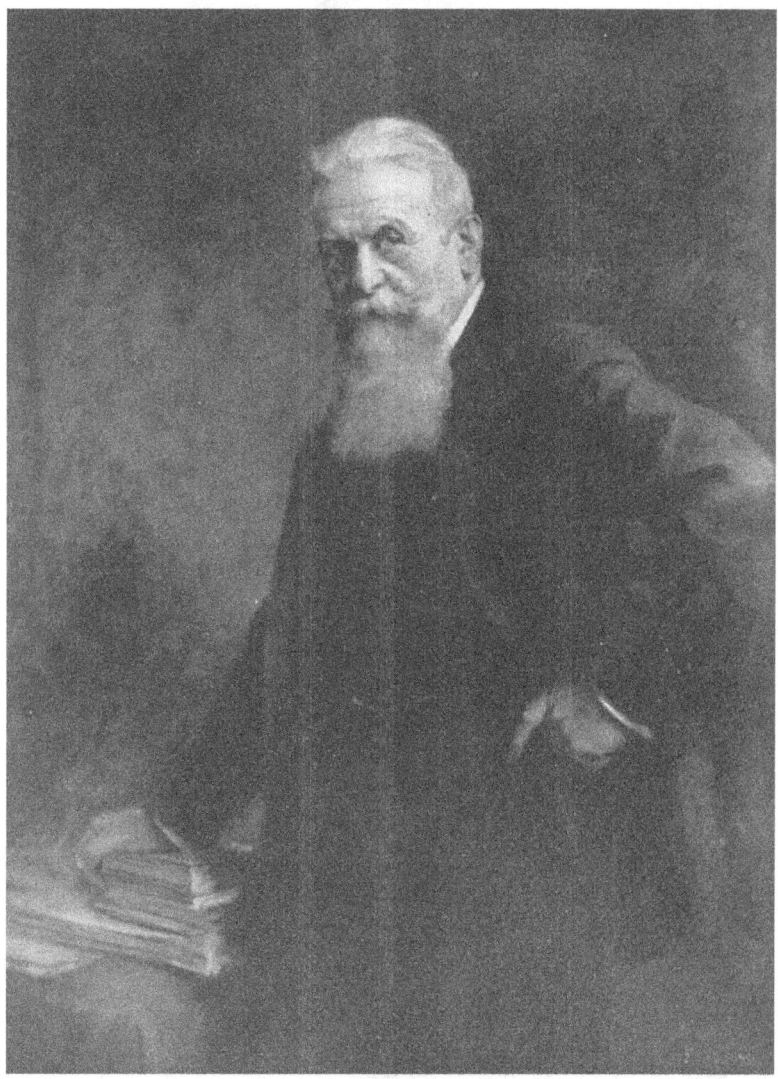

Figure 4.3. Eugene Steinach. Published with permission of Wellcome Images. Photograph by J Scherb.

A limerick stressed this quickly discredited aspect of Steinach experimentation:

> Ah, Vienna, the fortress of Freud!
> Whose surgeons are always employed;
> Where boys with soft hands
> Are provided with glands,
> And two-fisted girls are de-boyed. (Baring-Gould, 1970, 129)

Steinach's fame was assured by his slim 1920 book on rejuvenation and his 1922 film.[44] The 9 February 1922 headline of the *New York Times* announced 'Dr Steinach Coming to Make Old Young' but the trip was cancelled. He received six nominations for the Nobel Prize in Physiology[45] but he never won and this might explain his moodiness, despite the wealth he earned from 'Steinached' men. Henry Benjamin, in a June 1944 obituary for his colleague, attributed this gloom to his enforced exile in Zurich and the 'unjust criticism' of his rejuvenations and emphasised the 'enormous impetus' his work had for biochemists to concern themselves with all the endocrine glands.

Vasectomy had been used to treat men with prostate problems, or to cure masturbation, punish criminals or sterilise the 'unfit', but now it had a new purpose. *The Lancet* (24 December 1921) reviewed Hirschfeld's First International Congress for Sex Research in Berlin and found it 'valuable' for containing recent verdicts on Steinach's 'well-known work'. However, this remained controversial until Professor Carl Benda (a famous pathologist and a former Steinach opponent) endorsed rejuvenation in 1926 at Albert Moll's Conference in Berlin which he, in defiance of Hirschfeld, called the First International Congress for Sexual Research. The first Steinach surgeons made the snip during an unrelated operation without telling the patients, saying they did not want their expectations to influence the outcome, but Dr Eden Paul complained in a speech to the British Society for the Study of Sex Psychology in 1923,

---

44 *The New York Medical Week*, 13 October 1923, reported the only American showing of the Steinach film and in 1927 *The Triad* reviewed a December 1926 showing of the film in Sydney.

45 Sengoopta (2000, 456, fn 197) listed the six nominations from 1921 to 1938.

that such 'liberties' were 'quite impossible' in their 'stolidly conservative land'! Haire's 1922 report about rejuvenation was published in *Medical Life*, the journal of New York's American Society of Medical History. However, research and evaluation was unsophisticated then as this puffery in a 1920 issue of the *Scientific American* shows:

> It seems that the magic hand of science has found that Elixir of Life ... for which Faust bartered his soul. But now the new method of rejuvenating senile men and animals lies in the knife of the surgeon rather than in the vial of the apothecary ... Old men thus operated on not only looked fresher and younger, but felt an increase in strength and vigor, while aged trembling hands grew steady, feeble tottering steps became firm and failing masculine instincts and impulses acquired new vitality.

In Vienna alone, 'well over a hundred university professors and teachers, including Freud', had undergone this 'reactivation', the term that Harry Benjamin urged Steinach to use instead of 'rejuvenation'. Haire felt the term was 'unfortunate' and 'too sensational' but it was difficult to find a satisfactory substitute and 'youthing' sounded childish and ugly.

March 1922 marked a change in fortunes for the 30-year-old Haire – it was the date of his first Steinach rejuvenation operation and from this time he was freed from having to abide by other people's rules for running a birth control clinic or the need to provide clandestine artificial inseminations. His father had forced him to abandon his theatrical dreams and study medicine but now he could control his future – if he prospered he could also achieve his humanitarian goals. He shrewdly chose a new field and, thanks to the vogue for rejuvenations, fame and fortune soon followed. He was a pioneering surgeon in this field and did much to promote rejuvenations in Britain where he soon became the acknowledged expert. Within nine years he had Steinached 'rather less than 200' artistic and intellectual men (WLSR 1930, 563).

Erle Cox explored the theme in his futuristic book *Out of the silence* about a perennially young, extraterrestrial woman who planned to rule the world, and rejuvenation added a fashionable frill to many books in 1923: the criminal in Arthur Conan Doyle's 'The adventure of the creeping man' had overdosed on monkey-gland hormones; there was a rejuvenated monkey in Aldous Huxley's *Antic hay* and Gertrude Atherton's biographical novel *Black oxen* was the tale of a young suitor who was desperate to marry and have a child with the rejuvenated heroine, not knowing she was 60. *Black oxen* topped the *Publisher's Weekly*'s best-selling fiction list and her idea was sparked by Harry Benjamin's fanciful claims that 'women were running to the Steinach clinic from all over Europe, among them Russian princesses who sold their jewels to pay for treatments [to] restore their exhausted energies and enable them to make a living after the jewels had given out' (Sengoopta 2006, 90–91, quoting Atherton 1932: 538). There were not many princesses after the Russian revolution but that did not worry Atherton who became Dr Benjamin's first female patient, and despite his 1932 warning in *The New York Times* that it would not change 'oldsters into youngsters', she claimed his treatments – irradiating her ovaries eight times – proved that old age could be deferred; at 64 her creativity had slowed but was restored after a month of treatment and she produced some of her best work in the following decade (Atherton 1933). The *Los Angeles Times* (1924) had misgivings but her anti-age message prompted more than 70 New York women, 'some of them well known in society, on the stage and in the arts', to have rejuvenations. Famous Steinach surgeons included Victor Blum, Robert Lichtenstern and Peter Schmidt in Germany, Harry Benjamin in America and Norman Haire in Britain.

There were also medical sceptics such as Morris Fishbein, who edited the *Journal of the American Medical Association* and in 1927 likened rejuvenation cures to finding gold: once the 'cry of "gold, gold" was taken up by Steinach enthusiasts' and famous actors, physicians, and financiers had the operations, the newspapers reported their good news stories and there was an additional rush of applicants. Fishbein reminded readers the pre-Steinach vasectomies on old men with enlarged prostates had not produced rejuvenations, emphasised the part the mind plays in sexuality[46] and criticised the lack of scientific controls

---

46 Such improvements, which arise from patients' expectations rather than from effective medical treatment, were to become known as the placebo effect; this is

in Steinach surgeons' records. In 1930 Peter Schmidt complained that Fishbein had 'stifled' rejuvenation by 'malicious scorn' even though 'the excellent objective clinical works of H Benjamin were regularly sent to him'.

Chicago urologist Edwin W Hirsch wrote a scathing report on the procedure in 1936 and, despite his own involvement, Haire included the study in the series he edited, 'The international library of sexology and psychology'. Hirsch said the operation was 'ridiculously simple' to perform and this enabled rejuvenation surgeons to treat so many patients. In addition, media promises that old men could become young within a few minutes promoted a 'mad rush of decrepit recruits' who had been assured that 20 to 40 years could be added to their life by this 'wonderful operation'. Hirsch said the patients were either 'sexual neurotics' or had 'inveigled' the rejuvenating surgeon because they wanted to become sterile. Tellingly, 'not one of these cord-ligators has given a reliable account of having succeeded in rejuvenating himself'.

Haire's interest was sparked by Eden Paul, a communist doctor and translator who, in his rejuvenation presentation to the British Society for the Study of Sex Psychology in January 1921, said Ponce de Leon 'searched for the Fountain of Youth not the Fountain of Passionless Senility'. Haire read Steinach's book, learnt the technique and wrote about it. He also employed Voronoff's techniques and told Havelock Ellis he had a man waiting for a testicle transplant 'as soon as he could get a testicle'.[47] There is no record of this but in February he treated a man with 'injections of extract of bull's testicles and at first there seemed to be a slight improvement sexually'. He performed his first rejuvenation operation on 20 March and told Ellis that he usually used a local anaesthetic for the procedure which took around 15 minutes.

---

discussed in Chapter 9.

47 G Frank Lydston, an American urologist, performed transplants on four men in 1916 by using testicles from criminals and people accidentally killed, hoping to 'cure eunuchs, eunuchoidism and homosexuals'. On 28 January 2002 the BBC reported 'Testicular Transplant First' on a man who had had tissue taken from his testicles and frozen before being made sterile by cancer. It was later re-implanted and his wife became pregnant. The results were 'encouraging but not conclusive'. Retrieved 1 May 2008 from: news.bbc.co.uk/2/hi/health/1787030.stm.

In April Haire enclosed a card of introduction from Eden Paul with his request to meet Stanley Unwin and the meeting led to a productive relationship between Haire and the publishers Allen & Unwin. Soon after, Haire offered the BSSSP £10 towards the costs of publishing Dr Paul's paper (plus one of his own) and the two papers were published in 1923.[48] Haire also advocated sterilisation for people who were 'unfit' or wished to limit their families and said at the Malthusian's 1922 conference that men and women could be confident that their 'health, sexual desire, and sexual potency' would not be damaged.

Haire became President of the Contraceptive Section of the Neo-Malthusian and Birth Control Conference, he was elected to the British Society for the Study of Sex Psychology's Executive Committee on 11 May 1922,[49] he invited the editors of mainstream medical journals and newspapers to attend their February symposium and convinced *The New Generation* to publish the papers.[50] He had successfully promoted three of his passions: eugenics, teaching birth control in medical schools and having birth control clinics run by doctors. Haire, in an 8 July letter to *The Lancet*, signed 'President, Contraceptive Section, International Conference on Birth Control', invited medical practitioners and students to attend the Malthusian League's 11–14 July 1922 conference. Sanger's 'handsome personal gift' had helped fund this jointly run historic event.

Haire later said that many doctors had begged for their names to be kept secret when they wrote for tickets but, on learning that Lord Dawson of Penn and Sir Arbuthnot Lane would attend, they became braver. The conference did not discuss the ethics of birth control because, as Havelock Ellis had observed at the 1921 American conference, it was

---

48 BSSSP archives recorded Haire's £10 offer on 8 June 1922. On 10 May 1923 the 111th Management Committee noted payments by Haire and Porter towards publishing pamphlet no. 11.

49 BSSSP archives, 98th Management Meeting, 6 April 1922 listed Haire's nomination which was proposed by S Halford, and the 99th Management Committee minutes 11 May 1922 note Haire's agreement to serve on the Executive Committee.

50 BSSSP archives, 95th Management Meeting, 12 January 1922, listed those who were approached: *The Lancet, British Medical Journal, The Times, The Telegraph* and *The Manchester Guardian*.

'idle to discuss whether or not it produces minor evils. No doubt it does' but 'the reckless disregard of Birth Control produces evils that are vastly greater than those produced by its observance'. The breakthrough came in Haire's address to a large gathering which included many of the profession's more eminent members.

Haire's address was midway between an apology and a boast: he believed it was the first British medical conference on contraception. Although he had only had seven years' experience in the field, he had accepted the presidency of the session because the organisers were unable to find any doctors specialising in this subject 'who would publicly avow their interest in birth control'. After criticising harmful and ineffective methods, Haire discussed the 'best contraceptive method available', including two types of rubber pessary the Dutch had been successfully using for 40 years and which he had used the previous year in nearly 200 cases without a single failure 'either among my private patients, or among the less intelligent patients at the welfare centres.'

Haire prefaced his remark by saying the audience might think him 'dogmatic' in his claim 'that all methods but one are faulty' except the one which had a success rate of 100 percent. Methods which sometimes succeeded were 'not of much practical use' and, as well, they had to be 'sure, safe and simple'. He announced: 'I know such a method'. He meant the eponymous Haire pessary, which he introduced to England at the conference; it was a modified version of the vaginal diaphragm Dr Wilhelm Mensinga had invented in Germany in the 1870s.[51] It was an overstated boast, which he later had to retract.[52] However, in his overview of the conference, the President, Dr CV Drysdale, was right to praise the medical sessions, because medical opinion was previously supposed to be against contraception. The Contraceptive Section, which was attended by 164 members of the medical profession (few of whom

---

51 Dr H Arthur Allbutt (1887) referred to the Mensinga diaphragm in his sixpenny pamphlet and Himes (1936, 252-53) believes this is the first such reference in a birth control tract published in English.

52 Haire (1936, 17) conceded that 'no contraceptive method ... can be guaranteed as 100 percent sure, though at least one of the "combination" methods [of a Gräfenberg ring or a diaphragm plus contraceptive jelly] approached very nearly to complete security.'

had any previous connection with the movement), proposed and passed a resolution[53] with only three dissentients. This was 'of vast importance' as it showed the change in medical opinion and would do much to allay many groundless fears. Drysdale said that those people who studied the proceedings carefully would 'realise that the case for carefully exercised Birth Control is irresistible', and would help spread the 'only scientific doctrine which has been devised for the uplift of humanity'.

Haire spread the uplifting message from the conference podium and continued it over lunch when he asked the British Minister for Health, Sir Alfred Mond (later Lord Melchett) why he did not authorise the giving of birth control at government-funded maternal welfare centres. He replied that politicians did not form public opinion, they followed it. 'My boy', he said 'it is your job to educate the public to demand that this information should be given at state-aided welfare centres, and, when the demand for the information is more insistent than the demand that it shall not be given, then you will find that the Government will authorise it'.

Midwifery professor Abraham Wallace congratulated Drs Haire and Drysdale and said he was glad to see so many young doctors in the audience. He mused about Drysdale's father, Dr Charles Robert Drysdale, 'who many years ago earned the scorn of a host of people' by advocating birth control: 'If he could see today such a distinguished company of men [had come] to listen to this excellent paper, he would be very pleased indeed.' Haire answered questions which continued until 'the lateness of the hour' forced him to close the session. The published proceedings include congratulations for Haire's paper by such luminaries as W Arbuthnot Lane, Lord Dawson and Dr Frances M Huxley, a gynaecological surgeon and a founder member of the Medical Women's Federation. Dr C Killick Millard, the Medical Officer of Health for Leicester, who chaired the conference's general medical issues session, considered Haire's address on technique to be 'of the

---

53 'That this meeting of the medical members of [this conference] wishes to point out that Birth Control by hygienic contraceptive devices is absolutely distinct from abortion in its physiological, legal and moral aspects. It further records its opinion that there is no evidence that the best contraceptive methods are injurious to health or conducive to sterility.'

utmost value' and 'the first serious attempt to approach the question in a scientific spirit'.

Haire's paper on sterilisation was accidently replaced in the conference proceedings by a 'very elementary and sketchy' one which had already appeared in *The New Generation*, in the first American birth control conference's proceedings and in the February 1922 issue of *The Birth Control Review* where Sanger omitted his final sentence: 'I hope the time is not far distant when any individual who considers himself unfit for parenthood may apply at a public hospital for surgical sterilisation, with a reasonable prospect of having his request granted'. In an apology for printing the wrong version of Haire's paper, the British editor said the complete one would appear in his forthcoming book by the Oxford University Press. By March 1923 Haire's *Manual of contraceptive technique for medical practitioners and students* was ready for the press and he asked Havelock Ellis for permission to quote 'rather abundantly' from his work (Haire to Havelock Ellis, 20 March 1923 – HC 3.16).

The book was not published, however, and in 1936 Haire gave details of its stillbirth: 'A well-known firm of medical publishers' invited him to write a manual on birth control for medical practitioners and students but when in 1922 it was about half written, without reading a word of it, they decided to refrain from publishing a book on 'such a questionable subject' and paid him 'a considerable sum' to cancel their contract. He was disappointed that Marie Stopes' medical text in 1923 had deprived him of 'the distinction of being the author of the first English text-book on the subject'. Havelock Ellis said reassuringly that it would not matter and it would have been a libel issue *not* to cull it. Although the book contained useful information, numerous small errors had occurred as he and others had experienced in their writing (Havelock Ellis to Haire, 14 July 1923 – HC 3.16). Haire changed publishers and in 1924 Allen & Unwin accepted his revised manuscript and, when it finally appeared in 1936, it was based on his much broader experience.

The book's cancellation by Oxford University Press shows the sensitivity of the topic. Haire asked for Stopes' help on 28 July 1922 after hearing that a politician had given notice of two questions he planned to ask in the House of Commons suggesting that birth control literature should be restricted. Haire urged 'all those working for birth control' to forget their minor differences and unite 'against the common foe', who in this case was Augustine Hailwood, a politician from Manchester, 'an RC by religion, a baker by trade and the father of three children'. Haire had been 'working at very high pressure' lobbying politicians and for several days he had been 'almost without sleep'. He had sent out calls for help in 'various quarters' and his strategy seemed to have succeeded, judging from the politicians' questions and answers in the 1 August issue of Hansard[54] which Haire posted to Stopes the next day.

Hailwood first asked Edward Shortt, the Home Secretary, 'what steps, in the way of criminal proceedings' he proposed to take to check the 'seriously increasing output of obscene literature' about the prevention of conception and whether the government intended to introduce legislation, 'on the lines of the French law of 1920', making it an offence to 'publish or distribute' material which advocated or taught contraception or to advertise or offer such articles for sale. Shortt said it was the duty of police to act when obscene books were circulated, but it could not 'be assumed that a court would hold a book to be obscene' merely because it dealt with contraception and he added that there was no intention of introducing legislation. When Hailwood asked if he was 'aware that many of these books contain positively obscene drawings', Shortt replied, 'this it would be a question of fact in each case whether a book was obscene or not'. Another politician adroitly changed the subject by asking if it was possible 'to prevent the publication in the newspapers of very undesirable matter which is given in evidence in the law courts'. This was greeted by shouts of '*News of the World*' and one member asked rhetorically 'is there anything published in any book worse than the proceedings of the Russell divorce case?' He meant Bertrand Russell's May 1921 divorce from his first wife Alys which was also reported in *The Times*. Haire told Stopes that he was delighted with the 'very satisfactory' response and thought it would make a 'good central square for the front page' in the next issue of her newsletter.

---

54 Great Britain. Parliamentary Debates, House of Commons. 'Birth Control 20 and 46', 1 August 1922, 1244–45.

Haire's reference at the conference to 200 successful birth control cases prompted Stopes to boast in *The Lancet* on 12 August that her clinic had dealt with a *thousand* cases with about 0.5 percent of failures in women who had been fitted with the small occlusive cervical cap she used. Haire responded in *The Lancet* on 19 August: 'Mrs Marie Stopes, DSc, PhD', was a 'non-medical woman' and patients at her clinic were examined and treated only by a nurse, although she referred some to a consultant doctor who did not attend the clinic regularly and saw only a small fraction of cases. As the conclusions were mostly made by a nurse and were uncorroborated by medical evidence, 'neither data nor conclusions have much scientific value.' In addition, 'her ignorance of medical matters had led her to advocate, in her books, at her clinic, and elsewhere, the use of the Gold-pin pessary, which had been condemned by British medical men and women as indisputably dangerous, giving rise to sepsis and abortions'.

Haire was supported by Ettie Rout who had started work as a pioneer stenographer, became deeply involved with the union movement and recognised the need to fight venereal disease in World War I when she saw the huge impact it had had on troops stationed in Egypt. Havelock Ellis said she was 'rather similar to Haire' and he was right: they were newsmakers, witty, hated cant and campaigned for tolerance, while their dislike of humbug did not earn them full marks for tact. Jane Tolerton's excellent 1992 biography *Ettie* describes this brave New Zealander who met troop-trains in Paris, issued condoms to soldiers and guided them to safe medically inspected brothels. While she was their 'guardian angel', a bishop called her 'the wickedest woman in Britain', her own country scorned her and the French gave her a medal.

Marie Stopes found 'certain physiological objections' to the occlusive pessary Rout recommended in her book so there was a personal element in Rout's letter objecting to Stopes' methods which appeared in *The Lancet* on 19 August 1922 below Haire's letter. Rout described herself as 'an experienced official reporter' who had collected all the available evidence about contraception and made it available to Sir William Arbuthnot Lane and other medical authorities. Her rebuttal had a Haire-like sting: 'May I suggest, without offence, that Dr

Stopes' 1000 local adherents and 10,000 corresponding ones, recorded by fill-up-a-form methods, do not furnish "clinical experience." It is not "evidence" at all – except as to the popularity of birth control. Contraception is a branch of medicine and it must be studied and applied in the same way as any other branch of medicine – otherwise it deteriorates into quackery. "Science" – not "Christian Science" – must be applied to this problem if the general public is to obtain any real and lasting benefit'. In her 1922 book, *Safe marriage*, Rout called the Gold-pin pessary 'an instrument, the arms of which spread out within the womb, and the gold spring keeps the mouth of the womb open, thus facilitating infection and conception. It is claimed as a "preventive"; it is really an abortifacient, and cannot be too strongly condemned, as causing septic miscarriage.'

Once more Stopes responded in *The Lancet* on 2 September and denied using the Gold-pin pessary, claiming to have advocated it only once, in her book *Wise parenthood*, 'for abnormal cases only'. She childishly attacked Haire in the 9 September issue of the journal and claimed that her clinic's contraceptives were better than his. Haire's sarcastic response was printed in the same issue: he was sorry that she should think he had any intention of 'jibing' at her as 'nobody realises more than me the immense service of Dr Stopes in popularising the knowledge of birth control in this country'. After this preliminary sweetener, he observed acidly that she had 'abandoned her scientific attitude and discredited herself in scientific circles with her volume entitled *A new gospel to all peoples* (1922), in which she makes the explicit announcement that she is a prophet, and claims to have received a direct revelation from God on the subject of birth control. A person who is capable of deluding herself, or seeking to delude others, with such a belief, is no longer to be treated as a scientific investigator'. *The Lancet*'s editor closed the correspondence because 'it has got into regions of personal and more or less unassociated controversy where few can want to follow it'.

After working in two London hospitals and at the Saffron Hill Welfare Maternity Centre, Haire had established his own practice and combined

HAIRE THE PHOENIX

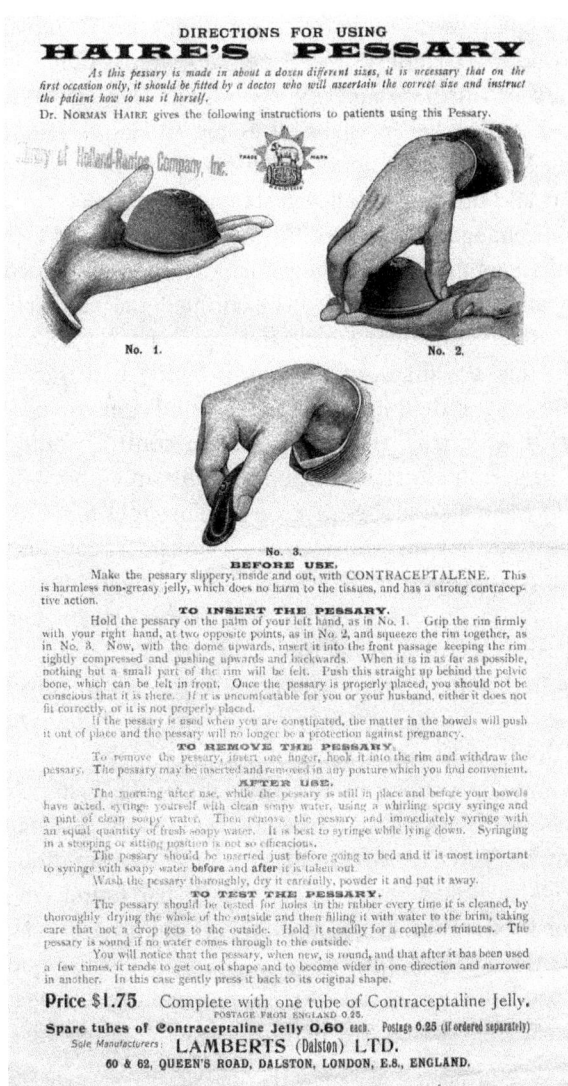

Figure 4.4. Haire pessary. Published with permission of Sophia Smith Collection, Smith College, Northampton, MA 01063. Description: Advertisement for Dr Norman Haire's pessary from Lamberts Ltd, London, circa 1920s [Illustrations and instructions for using pessary] (Margaret Sanger Research Bureau Records).

this with unpaid work in birth control clinics. By 16 September 1922 Haire moved to 71 Harley Street,[55] perhaps after reading *Birth control: a statement of Christian doctrine against the Neo-Malthusians* by Dr Sutherland. A reviewer (perhaps his ex-tenant Haire), said his 'method of refuting Malthus was to quote Malthus as having said something he did not say and proving the alleged statement untrue.'

In an exchange of letters in *The Lancet* on 7 and 14 October 1922, Haire challenged the findings of Dr Richard H Vercoe, a medical officer of health and school doctor, who examined the medical records of an unspecified number of Colchester's primary school children and concluded that the firstborn child in a family had the worst health 'whilst the best is definitely the *eighth* child and upwards' (Vercoe, 759). If this were true, the case for birth control would have been seriously undermined. Haire responded with an authoritative rebuttal in *The Lancet* on 14 October: Vercoe had 'brought forward some very interesting data but his omission from consideration on one vitally important factor absolutely invalidates his conclusions'. Vercoe had referred 'only to *children who have not died before the age of 18*'. To highlight this error, Haire referred to figures Professor Alfred Ploetz quoted in 1912 at the First International Eugenics Congress taken from Arthur Geissler's studies of miners' children; the mortality of children was least in the first four children, and then increased steeply – the first child having a 23 percent chance of death in the first year while the risk to the twelfth-born child was 60 percent. Haire also mentioned the 1910 study of 1600 Chicago families by Dr Alice Hamilton, an icon of occupational health and women's rights, who had found a mortality rate of 118 per thousand in families with four children or less, increased to 303 per thousand for nine or more children. He also quoted Emma Duke's study[56] and concluded, 'if Dr Vercoe would investigate the child mortality statistics among the families whose children are included in

---

55 Haire moved to number 90 Harley Street in 1923, staying until December 1927 when he bought the lease of 127 Harley Street.

56 Duke's study of 5617 births in Johnstown, Pennsylvania, conducted for the US Children's Bureau in 1913, found a mortality rate of 133.3 per thousand for the first and second-born children, increasing to 201 per thousand for the ninth and subsequent children. Sanger cited this study (1920, 13).

his recent investigation, his conclusions would have to be very greatly modified, if not absolutely reversed'. No one convincingly challenged his scholarly rebuttal.[57]

Haire received high praise from an American expert who said the Dutch Mensinga pessary was 'the device which had found most universal acceptance clinically' when used in combination with a spermicidal paste or jelly. The compliment came from Norman Himes who later wrote the seminal *Medical history of contraception*.

The scholarly Himes noted that from about 1922 Haire had popularised the use of the eponymous Haire pessary (a modification of the Dutch one) and he had 'done much to push this improved technique in England, and was among the first to use it there'. In addition, Haire was one of 'the most important physicians' to have written both for academic and popular audiences at a time when medical opinion on this subject was 'confused.'[58] Another reviewer, who happened to be Haire's doctor, criticised another such history that did not mention Haire's important contribution or the Cromer Welfare and Sunlight Centre which, as the Malthusian League made clear, was 'the first one opened in England by, and under the supervision of, a medical man' (Avery 1965, 10).

Provocatively, Haire begged the medical profession to study contraception to rescue it from the hands of 'quacks and charlatans and non-medical "doctors" who write erotic treatises on birth control conveying misleading information in a highly stimulating form'. Angrily Stopes paid a friend to publish a biography and demanded the right to veto anything she disliked. It was a rash decision and Aylmer Maude's hagiographic book, *The authorised life of Marie C Stopes*, was ridiculed and sold poorly (Hall 1977, 261). In contrast, Haire's success was increasing, with reports of it even appearing in *The Sun*, a Sydney

---

57   John Brownlee MD DSc, UK Medical Research Council's Director of Statistics, made this unconvincing claim in *The Lancet*, 1 November 1924, 925–27: 'There was no evidence that large families were more unhealthy than small ones, and the statement that it is better to have three healthy children than six unhealthy ones has no apparent foundation'.

58   Himes (1936, 210–11, fn 3) about the pessary. Himes (1936, 322–23) about Haire's academic and popular audience.

newspaper which on 16 July 1922 wrote about the Malthusians' London conference and quoted this resolution which delegates passed: 'It is of the greatest importance that provision for hygienic birth control instruction should become part of the recognised practice of the medical profession'. *The Sun* also reported Haire's statement that there was a growing realisation of the need for 'sterilisation of the unfit in the interests of the race' and that soon 'all but the very lowest would practise birth control' and, when this happened, citizens would turn on the reckless breeders and insist on their compulsory sterilisation. This seems horrifying now, but before genetics was understood this view was widely held, and Haire, Stopes and Sanger used eugenic arguments to justify the use of contraception.

In 1922 Haire suggested to Havelock Ellis that Britain's birth control movement needed a 'beautiful personality' like Sanger, to which he replied: 'I am sure Marie Stopes would say, "What more can you want than ME."'[59] Haire never thrust himself forward for this role but he must have been gratified when medical journals discovered 'the gap in medical knowledge' and started to discuss contraception; the first was *The Lancet* which, on 26 March 1921, timidly suggested that any qualified doctor should 'inform himself about the arguments for and against contraceptives' and learn to anticipate 'the relative degree of nervous wreckage' they might expect in patients who used the methods.[60] *The Lancet* had grown bolder by the time it reviewed Sanger and Drysdales' joint British–American conference in 22 July 1922: it was the first time the Drysdales agreed to such explicit words in the title of a conference and the first *international* conference to deal with birth control. The *British Medical Journal* followed with an article on the subject and, in July 1923, *The Practitioner* published its special contraception issue. In their 1970 history of contraception, Clive Wood and Beryl Suitters noted that these early years marked the 'real breakthrough in contraceptive acceptance in Great Britain', led by Lord Dawson of Penn whose brave address was reported in *The Lancet* on 14

---

59 Havelock Ellis to Sanger, 6 October 1922, in Grosskurth (1985, 374).

60 *The Lancet*, 29 November 1924, incorrectly claimed in an editorial that the 26 March 1921 issue urged for medical students to be taught contraception.

January 1922 and by two pioneering birth control clinics in 1921 run by Marie Stopes and the Malthusian League. Haire was the major catalyst for this acceptance.

In 1921 Haire was unknown, in debt and working sporadically in fields which were shunned by those in mainstream medicine. Within a year the fees from rejuvenation operations ended his poverty and his triumphs at two medical conferences brought him recognition within the medical profession. He had become a leading figure in Britian's birth control movement and, in the next three years, he was to gain a worldwide reputation in the new field of sexology.

5

MAKING HIS MARK

Satisfying people who yearned for longevity made Haire rich. The craze appealed mostly to men and it was really only a vasectomy (women had their ovaries irradiated) but, until the medical claims were refuted, hopeful patients paid high fees to revitalise their sex lives or defer senility. On 20 March 1923, exactly a year after his first rejuvenation operation, Haire was 'astonished and delighted' to find his patient, a former novelist, was 'transformed.' He elaborated in his 1924 book, *Rejuvenation: the work of Steinach, Voronoff, and others*, before the operation the patient could not write but postoperatively he was eating and sleeping well and 'had written a new book, several short stories, and some one-act plays.' The man and his wife said their sexual intercourse was 'entirely satisfactory' and 'the mental condition of the whole family' had improved. Despite the destruction of Haire's patient records, we know that two of his rejuvenation patients were WB Yeats and Field-Marshal Plumer.[1] In *Sex talks* (1946) Haire alluded to a 'famous poet' having written 'his best poetry' after the operation, 'though he had for many years before that, written nothing at all'. He had also 'seen a world-famous statesman, one of the leading figures in the war, restored from senescence to renewed activity'. They were his patients but he masked this by saying he had 'seen' them.

Haire sent a draft paper about the technique to Dr WJH Sprott (a Cambridge psychologist and intellectual known as Sebastian to his friends) and asked if he should discuss animals in a revised version

---

1 Frank Forster (24 August 1993) confirmed the identity of Sir Herbert Plumer (later Baron Plumer). Despite looking like David Low's Colonel Blimp and being called 'Daddy' by his men and 'Drip' by officers because of his sinus problems, he is revered as the British army's best general in World War I. He later became Governor and Commander-in-Chief of Malta, then High Commissioner in Palestine and was active in the House of Lords.

so he could 'say more without evoking the condemnation of those unemancipated from ancient taboos'. Perhaps he should include humans, even sex-change operations. Sprott published Haire's paper in *The National & The Athenæum* on 4 August 1923 and in it Haire dismissed the myths about 'monkey-glands' and confessed that at first he was 'very sceptical' of Steinach and his co-workers' claims but he had seen 'some amazing results' and no longer doubted that in some cases the operation caused a 'real rejuvenation'. In his thank you letter to Sprott, Haire offered to send another paper on birth control or sterilisation, asked about research funds, invited him to see Steinach's film and promised that he would be amused by a lecture to husbands at the Walworth Centre. Haire, who was teaching the men 'a little about marital relations', had learnt a lot from their questions and difficulties and was sure that his 'really quite unique' work would interest Sprott. He added the enticement, 'I think Hugh Dalton is coming.'[2] Haire also asked Sprott to let him know when he could dine with him and invited him to stay the night 'at any time' because he had 'a wonderful concealed bed here!'[3]

In June, a few days after Haire sent his invitation to Sprott, Havelock Ellis gave him a letter of introduction to Magnus Hirschfeld with the reassurance that the famous German sexologist would 'be kind and anxious to be helpful'. Haire immediately began to prepare for his visit to Hirschfeld's Institute for Sexual Research (*Institut für Sexualwissenschaft*) in Berlin and planned to arrive ten days early so he could refresh his German. However, he had to wait because the publishers of the magazine *The Practitioner* had sponsored a special symposium on contraception and he was to present the key paper, 'Contraceptive technique: a review of 1400 cases'. The magazine editor declared that birth control would never be taught to male medical students although medical schools for women would teach it because

---

2   Hugh Dalton (Edward Hugh Dalton, Baron Dalton) was a British Labour Party politician. His biographer, Ben Pimlott, said that he was mentor to various (mostly heterosexual) young men and may have been a repressed homosexual. Sprott and Dalton were friends of John Maynard Keynes.

3   Moggridge (1992, 354) described Sprott as being part of the Bloomsbury Group and John Maynard Keynes' lover so he may not have been interested.

'women are more practical and less hypocritical'. His strange statement was more pro-women than those of his colleagues 40 years earlier who tried to exclude women from medical courses altogether.[4]

These symposium papers had marked an important medical advance as two experts assessed many years later: Norman Himes said in 1936 that Haire's paper was the only one 'to surpass a mediocre level'.[5] The Queen's surgeon-gynaecologist, Sir John Peel, elaborated in 1964 and allocated praise and criticism. He quoted Haire's paper approvingly but disapproved of the others by 'distinguished gynaecologists and consulting obstetricians': three claimed that contraception caused sterility, a fourth alleged that it caused 'mental derangement in subsequent offspring' and a fifth 'equated birth control with masturbation' and said both practices 'were distinctly dangerous to health'. These distinguished men 'backed up their obviously limited medical knowledge with aphoristic moralizing, eugenic and demographic prognostications and totally unsupported generalizations regarding parental motivation'. Peel described Haire as the only contributor with practical experience and said the others were either opposed to contraception or confused by it.

Haire advised in 1923 'there is no method which is at once harmless and certain' and they were all unreliable, except the Dutch Mensinga pessary, which if used with contraceptive jelly, was nearly 100 percent safe. Haire warned that prolonged breast feeding would not prevent pregnancy and stressed that withdrawal (*coitus interruptus*) caused great mental and physiological harm: although it was widely used, because it 'costs nothing, requires no apparatus and no previous preparation', it had resulted in more babies 'than the failures in all other birth control methods put together'. Condoms were not nearly as safe as people thought and 'interfered with sexual satisfaction'. He risked religious wrath by warning that the 'the so-called safe period', the only method the Catholic Church sanctioned, offered 'little security'. It offered none

---

4 Wood and Suitters (1970, 175–76). There was another shift in the 1970s when female doctors had fewer work options as a result of childcare responsibilities and some male colleagues were condescending about the work they did in family planning clinics, because it was part-time work.

5 Himes (1936, 304).

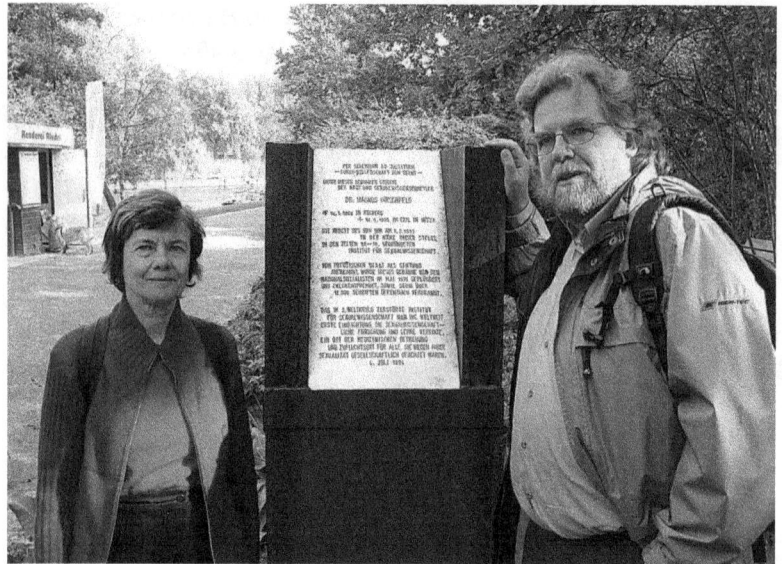

Figure 5.1. Diana Wyndham and Ralf Dose at the Magnus Hirschfeld Memorial in Berlin.

at all to those women who followed Dr Halliday Sutherland's advice in 1922 that the safe period was 'mid-menstrual period'. Sutherland subsequently conceded that women are most fertile at this time but he offered 'no apology to anyone who owes his or her existence to that error'.[6] Haire called this a 'typical example of the Roman Catholic attitude' and said additional words were superfluous.

Later Haire gave sensible and humane advice in his book *Birth-control methods (contraception, abortion, sterilisation)*, saying that douching 'often fails to prevent conception' and was 'extremely unromantic' and 'physiologically harmful' because 'a woman should not be expected to get out of a warm bed on a cold night to prepare hot water for a douche'. New Zealand historian Hera Cook selected

---

6   Haire meant Sutherland's book *Birth control* (1922, 4) and his 1936 essay on the 'safe period' in *Laws of life*. Ironically, in 1942 the Irish Censorship Board banned the essay for being 'indecent and obscene' because it dealt with the 'safe period' (O'Faolain 1953).

quotes from the book but she either misunderstood his writing or was intentionally dismissive when she claimed 'it was obvious that Haire was not talking about working-class women. This was the experience of the privileged middle-class women who came to his Harley Street practice'. When Haire discussed the disadvantages of this method at the 1922 birth control conference he made it clear douching was out of the question 'in the case of the lower middle classes and the poor', because they lacked privacy and had inadequate bathroom and heating facilities. In the 1920s Haire and Australian-born speech therapist Lionel Logue had been charging wealthy patients high fees in Harley Street so they could treat poorer ones without charge.[7] Haire's generosity prompted Bernard Hesling (1960, 12) to call him the 'Ned Kelly of Harley Street' although the bushranger was not noted for his charitable works.[8] In contrast, Stopes' advice was *only* for the rich and she gave them tips on how to instruct the servants to fill a douche bag with warm water and hang it on a hook outside the couple's bedroom door for use after intercourse.

After giving his keynote paper at the London symposium, Haire travelled to Berlin to meet Hirschfeld and see his Institute for Sexual Research. Hirschfeld (1935, xvi) had bought the former residence of Prince Hatzfeld, Germany's Ambassador to France, in 1918 and described it as one of Berlin's finest 'architecturally speaking'. Visitors to the Institute were greeted by the inscription *'Dolori et Amori Sacrum'* above the door which translates as 'dedicated to love and pain' (Tamagne 2004, 63). The Nazis demolished it and Ralph Dose and I posed at the building's site beside the memorial which is dedicated to Hirschfeld and the Institute.

---

7   Suzanne Edgar noted in her *ADB* entry for Lionel George Logue (1880–1953) that he taught elocution, public speaking and acting; practising as a speech therapist at 146 Harley Street from 1924. He became famous for treating the Duke of York's stammer. There is no record of any relationship between these two mavericks who established themselves in Harley Street.

8   Bill Gammage (1998, 362–63) noted the difference between the images of him as murderer and a public icon: although Kelly identified with the poor and did not rob them, the poor did not benefit from his year of bushranging.

On 20 August 1923 Haire wrote to Havelock Ellis and sent 'warm thanks' for his letter of introduction, confirmed that Hirschfeld had been kind and helpful and described the visit: he saw 'two interesting cases of transvestism' and in the evening a young man acted as his guide and conducted him to 'several interesting Lokals' (bars) where he was amazed by the 'openness of homosexuality'. On Sunday, Hirschfeld collected him from his hotel and they made a small excursion to Charlottenburg. After dining together, they visited another male Lokal and Hirschfeld booked a lesbian guide for an outing the following night to 'an enthrallingly interesting female one'. Next morning Haire saw more cases and saw and spoke to many lesbians that night. Haire planned to return to London on 4 September and invited Ellis to have lunch or dinner with him at his flat because there was much to discuss and he particularly wanted to talk about the 'possibility of founding such an institute – or a satisfactory substitute – in London'.

This idea was too radical for Britain and, despite Berlin's daring cabarets which made WH Auden say its reputation as the 'sin capital of sexual freedom was well deserved' Hirschfeld was in danger because he was Jewish, openly homosexual, left wing and had links to a film promoting gay rights. He was attacked and badly wounded in 1920, the next year he was almost killed by anti-Semitic thugs and in November 1923 he had to flee to Holland and turned to Haire for help. Haire was shocked by Germany's escalating anti-Semitism but he was unable to offer him a bed because it was already being used by a bankrupt relative from Frankfurt. Haire asked Hirschfeld to deliver a message to his 'Dutch friend' (Willem van de Hagt) and offered to help him contact his old friends in England – Havelock Ellis, Lowes Dickinson and Maynard Keynes. Havelock Ellis replied that he was about to go to Cornwell for some months but was not surprised by the news that Hirschfeld was getting away as Germany seemed to be getting worse not better (Havelock Ellis to Haire 14 November 1923 – HC, 3.16).[9]

Haire also discussed the British Society for the Study of Sex Psychology in his letter to Havelock Ellis. Although he had been a

---

9 Maynard Keynes was the noted economist and Goldsworthy Lowes Dickinson was a British historian and pacifist. Both were homosexual.

member since 1920, Haire was dissatisfied with the BSSSP. This is not surprising and years later Australian-born intellectual Gilbert Murray described its *metier* as a 'disinterested enthusiasm for sexual misconduct in all its forms, from obscene language to unnatural vice' (Hall 1995, 673).[10] American educationalist Homer Lane called its members (or psychoanalysts in general) 'hairless perverts with twitching lips' (Wills 1964, 201) and in her diary entry for 21 January 1918 Virginia Woolf noted Lytton Strachey's 'amazing account' of the Society which met in Hampstead where '50 people of both sexes and various ages' discussed questions 'without shame' and had the appearance of 'a third variety of human being'. She considered joining but refrained because 'it's unfortunate that civilisation always lights up the dwarfs, cripples, & sexless people first. And Hampstead alone provides them' (Hall 1995, 670).

French historian Florence Tamagne (2004, 1: 117) described the performance of the BSSSP, 'Britain's only homosexual movement', as 'lackluster' because 'English homosexual militancy was characterized in the 1920s by its great discretion' and, although in July 1920 its 234 members began a program of 'timid reformism', their influence remained 'within the progressive intellectual milieux'. Bold reform was more Haire's style and some BSSSP members feared it might become a 'Haire publicity society' (Hall 1995, 673). Lesley A Hall, a British archivist, historian and Stella Browne's biographer, described how these tensions boiled over in a fight about the choice of BSSSP premises when Browne complained on 20 June 1923 about Haire's attempt to 'jockey' the Executive to choose premises he liked.

She conceded that the rooms 'are excellent' but, at '£15 a year, rather expensive'. Haire had told her over the telephone that Halford approved of taking the rooms, but since he had already inspected them rather surreptitiously with Miss Bailey she was disinclined to take his word.

---

10 Lesley Hall (26 May 2007) sent me details to 'clarify the rather confusing collation of cites by several different authors' caused by 'editorial limitations on the number of endnotes. The quote is from an anonymous article in the Society's archives which appears to be [Reginald Wellbye's] "A constructive view of sex psychology as a humanistic study" [given 27 March 1930], cited by Gilbert Murray, without further attribution (from the BSSSS archives)'.

Haire was furious to hear that Stella had said that 'we would *not* take them'. (Hall 2011, 118)

Hall does not say who made the inspection, why it was done in secret, who Browne complained to and whose word she doubted. Although an office in central London would cost more than their rooms in Hampstead, it was likely to attract more members. Haire's complaint was justified if Browne had made the decision alone and bypassed the Executive. Browne often had money troubles and lived frugally, which would have influenced her to favour an inexpensive office, but Haire wanted a more stylish, easily accessible one in the hope that additional members would offset the extra expense. Hall took Browne's part when she said that Haire's plans for the Society 'verged on the grandiose' while 'Stella had her feet more firmly on the ground'. Haire's plans for the BSSSP could be better described as 'verging on the brilliant' and Browne herself later praised the similar marketing tactic which Haire and Dora Russell used for the World League for Sexual Reform (WLSR) 1929 congress: their expensive publicity campaign was successful and, as a result, they had enough money to hire the Wigmore Hall for five days.

Haire deplored the Society's low membership and stressed the need to boost the numbers in an appeal he sent on 20 June 1923 to fellow member Dr SH Halford: 'A certain element in the society is far too pronounced. Let us more normal people take the wheel and steer the society to success.'[11] Halford was a misogynist who had warned in his book *Population and birth-control* that the realisation of 'the full feminist ideal' would wipe out British and American intelligence within 'two or three generations' and understandably Stella Browne refuted this (1917, 243–57). Unfortunately, Haire was prepared to work with a dubious ally in his bid to unseat her.

Havelock Ellis was ambivalent about Haire and his behaviour switched from friendly encouragement to outright hostility. For instance, he made snide comments in response to Haire's 20 August letter, telling Sanger: 'As regards Stella Browne, a letter just received from Norman Haire (though we don't greatly admire him) very truly said

---

11 Letter provided by Stephanie Brody, 2010.

of her: "S.B. is clever and brave but unbalanced and indiscreet". Stella Browne was one of the founders of the BSSSP and had been a major force within it for many years, unlike Ellis who 'preferred to emanate approval from a distance' and did not join because he could rely on her to regularly provide him with BSSSP briefings. She had angrily broken off their friendship in June 1923 and this might explain the unkind comments Ellis made about this intrepid woman who embraced free love, Malthusianism, communism and feminism but rejected marriage and motherhood. Dora Russell, who campaigned with her, called her 'a holy terror' and felt she harmed feminists' fight for contraception and abortion rights although she admired her 'intransigence'. British feminist Sheila Rowbotham, in her 1977 Stella Browne biography, described her as a 'doughty Canadian campaigner for women's sexual freedom'.

Haire confided to Havelock Ellis in August that the BSSSP was not very useful because it was controlled by Stella Browne, E Bertram Lloyd who 'carries discretion to extremes', and George Ives who 'was as timid as a hare'. In fact Lloyd was a capable organiser and Ives became 'cautious and highly secretive' after being 'shaken to the core' by Wilde's trial.[12] After the rooms altercation, Haire fumed that as long as he was a member of the Society's committee, Stella Browne would '*not* rule as an absolute monarch' and she retaliated by saying that Haire's 'peculiar methods' had alienated him from the Malthusian League.

Two months later Haire tried a different tactic, telling Ellis the BSSSP was 'not very useful' because there were too few medical members. He argued it was essential to ally themselves with this 'powerful priesthood' because the BSSSP could achieve its ends more easily by working with the medical profession than against them.

Haire also gave Havelock Ellis a report on his hormonal contraception experiments which he had begun in May. He discussed them in *The Practitioner* and, while they sound unethical and misguided now, many years of hormonal research led to the revolutionary oral contraceptive pill. Haire was 'trying to sterilise about a dozen women by a course of hypodermic injections of human semen', a technique which had worked

---

12 Rowbotham (2008, 332–83).

on rats. It would be 'at least a year' before he could draw conclusions about this treatment and much longer before he would know whether it was permanent. In 2007 medical historian Yolanda Eraso referred to a 1940 study[13] which said (citing van de Velde) that in 1928 Haire was 'reputed to have been the first to apply biological sterilizations to women.' However, van de Velde did not make this claim[14] and Haire acknowledged in 1936 that his hormonal experiments had failed.

Surprisingly, Ellis was full of praise for Haire in his 15 September 1923 letter to Sanger: 'Did I tell you I had lunch with Haire the other day? He seems very flourishing and thinks of starting a clinic of his own, free from hampering supervision by committee. I think he is doing good work.' However, after Haire's bids to add new members and new life to the BSSSP failed, he wanted to resign, but on 4 October all but one of the Society's executive agreed to ask him to reconsider.

A contingent of BSSSP members wanted to change the laws and attitudes relating to homosexuality (Rowbotham 2008, 382) but Haire went too far in his 10 January 1924 lecture to the BSSSP, and Havelock Ellis warned him that, 'The usefulness of the society will be largely destroyed if it comes to be regarded as simply a homo-club.' After this Haire was carefully circumspect and five years later insisted that homosexuality should not be discussed be at the WLSR congress in London.

Unlike the humourless Marie Stopes who came across as arrogant,[15] argumentative and litigious, Haire would debate with anybody and never sued anyone. He even called the anti-Semitic, anti-feminist and

---

13 Yolanda Eraso told me in 2009 that she was quoting Perez (1940) translated from Spanish: 'Talking of Van de Velde, Norman Haire was the first to apply the method of biological sterilisation to the human species'. She was 'almost sure' Perez was referring to van de Velde's *Ideal marriage*.

14 van de Velde did not cite this in *Ideal marriage* (1926) or in his *Fertility and sterility in marriage* (1929) and he was sceptical about Ludwig Haberlandt's 'hormonic' sterilisation of women. Simmer (1970, 3-27) said Haberlandt was a physiologist who failed to interest doctors in the technique.

15 Rowbotham (2008, 384) described Bertram Lloyd's 1915 meeting with Stopes in which he had been exasperated by her arrogant high opinion of her own scientific credentials and her utter disdain of the BSSSP as amateurs.

arch-conservative Anthony M Ludovici his 'great friend', admired his work and invited him to dinner parties. He included Ludovici's *The choice of a mate* in his 'The international library of sexology and psychology' series with this disclaimer: 'Our ultimate conclusions about life are poles apart. He is essentially a believer in aristocracy and conservatism, I in democracy and liberalism'. Ludovici thanked Haire, because although they disagreed entirely about birth control, he really appreciated Haire's many kind hints and criticism. Ludovici boasted that he had taken his objections 'right into the heart of the enemy's camp' in his debate with Marie Stopes on 12 February 1923 and when he addressed the BSSSP on *The psychological objections to the use of contraceptives, and an alternative* and 'crossed swords with the eminent gynaecologist and advocate of birth control, Dr Norman Haire', but his lecture caused such an uproar that the BSSSP members decided never to invite Ludovici again.[16]

After his failure to hormonally sterilise women, Haire continued with the conventional methods of male sterilisation. In 1924, after mastering the technique and performing 25 rejuvenation operations, he wrote *Rejuvenation: the work of Steinach, Voronoff, and others*. An inscribed copy of the book was donated to the BSSSP's library by the Society's treasurer, Captain Evelyn Broadwood, the director of his family's piano manufacturing company. On the flyleaf Haire acknowledged that he would not have written the book if he had not heard the paper on Steinach's work which Dr Eden Paul read to the Society. Haire hoped his book would stimulate interest in a subject which had been 'too long neglected'.[17] It impressed HG Wells, a rejuvenation enthusiast and a Haire patient (perhaps a rejuvenated one) who prophesised a more mature, graver society in future with 'active and hopeful children' and adults 'full of years' where none will be 'aged'.

---

16 Hall (1995, 673, fn 26) cited the BSSSP minutes of 8 April 1926 in which Haire had suggested another Ludovici lecture but 'the committee felt it was not advisable to agree to this at present'.

17 Beat Frischknecht (2008) bought the book in Zurich and sent me a scanned copy of these details from his signed copy which is inscribed 'Norman Haire, Harley St, 13 March 1925'. It is stamped 'British Society for the Study of Sex Psychology' and has a library classification 'III.9'.

The catalyst for Haire's book was a sensational American book *Rejuvenation: how Steinach makes people young*. The author was 'George F[our] Corners',[18] the punning pseudonym chosen by George Sylvester Viereck, a German-American whose surname in English means a square or four-sided figure. He was a charlatan who suggested that men should have their first rejuvenation between 40 and 60 and then repeat it until death came 'pleasantly, as in a dream'. He even claimed the operation would have saved the lives of Presidents Harding, Roosevelt and Wilson. In contrast, Haire used quaintly Biblical language to play down sex and emphasise health in his book, saying many ageing men were 'glad to be rid of what has been at times a disturbing element in their life, glad to have reached an age at which they are no longer troubled by the lusts of the flesh, and yet are loth to lose their physical and mental efficiency'.

In his 2 March 1924 letter to Haire, Havelock Ellis said that Viereck had sent him a copy and asked if Haire would like to see it. It had a galvanic impact on Haire who thought the American's book was attracting the wrong sort of attention; Haire may have wanted to restore *gravitas* to rejuvenation to protect his livelihood and he may have been irked because his name was not among Corner's list of 'eminent rejuvenators'. Haire wrote his 'little' book (twice the size of Corners') to inform the educated layman because he could only find one British publication on the topic (the BSSSP papers he and Eden Paul wrote). He also wanted to rectify the 'unfavourable impression' made when the rejuvenated Alfred Wilson was found dead in his bed on 11 May 1921, the day of his lecture at the Royal Albert Hall: *How I was made twenty years younger*. According to Haire, disaster struck because Wilson ignored warnings and tried to live like a 20-year-old. Wilson, a wealthy ship-breaking septuagenarian, 'formerly of Australia and well known

---

18   Wolff (1986: 396) identified George F Corners as the pseudonym used by George Sylvester Viereck who was later unmasked as Hitler's highest-paid American propagandist and spent four years in jail in the 1940s (*The Chicago Daily Tribune*, 1940 and *The New York Times*, 1942). Ironically, in the 1940s a renowned medical historian, biographer, humanist, anatomy professor and philosopher called George W Corner supported the US National Research Council's funding of Alfred Kinsey's research.

in Sydney',[19] complained about chest pain. It was a heart attack but his doctor thought it was caused by Wilson's chest-thumping displays of virility.

The inquest learnt that Dr Steinach had charged Wilson £700 for his rejuvenation in Vienna. Steinach may not have been the surgeon because Harry Benjamin said although he was 'present during all operations' he only operated on animals.[20] Dr Sengoopta, who has made an extensive study of this field, told me in 2006 he felt that Benjamin 'put the matter rather too mildly' as Steinach's letters to Benjamin suggest that he was not just present at the operations but supervised them. Steinach wanted to ensure the procedure could not be dismissed as a vasectomy and emphasised his particular methods of tying off the vas. Sengoopta added that a cynic might consider two other reasons for his presence: to impress the patients and to justify his high fees, £1000 in one instance.[21] There have been similar deaths: healthfood publisher JI Rodale[22] died of a heart attack in 1971 on the Dick Cavett Show after proclaiming he would live till 2000; Dr Stuart Berger, who wrote *Forever young*, died at 40 and Jim Fixx, the jogging pioneer, died while jogging at the age of 52.

Haire had begun to translate Dr Johannes (Jan) Rutgers' book *The sexual life in its biological significance as a dominant factor of vitality in man and woman, and in plants and animals*. He blamed the publishers and his over-busy schedule for taking ten years to complete it, but the urgency may have vanished when Rutgers died in 1924. Aletta Jacobs and Jan Rutgers were pioneers of the Dutch Neo-Malthusian League which promoted birth control but Jacobs and most other doctors wanted contraceptive advice to be given by doctors or midwives; however, he had trained lay women to do the work. As a medical student Rutgers had attended a lecture by a professor who opposed birth control on economic, moral and medical grounds but mostly because he feared it 'would lead to the replacement of love by lust'. While Rutgers had

---

19   Wilson's death was mistakenly described by the *Sydney Morning Herald* on 14 and 16 May 1921 as 'Rejuvenation. Thyroid gland treatment'.
20   Hamilton (1986, 46–47).
21   Sengoopta (June 2006, 9) quoting Hamilton.
22   JI Rodale, the son of Polish immigrants, was born Jerome Irving Cohen.

enthusiastically reviewed this lecture, later his medical work convinced him of contraception's benefits.

The League was opposed by Holland's Roman Catholic Federation for Large Families whose motto was: 'Better war, disease, death, poverty, or famine than Neo-Malthusianism' (Brandhorst 2003, 42). Britain's counterpart was the League of National Life which championed the 'honour and blessing of parenthood', said contraception degraded women, lied that clinics used corrosive products such as Lysol and denounced contraception as 'a deadly evil'. While claiming to be non-sectarian and non-political, the League was both; 'it was largely Roman Catholic in inspiration and membership' with 'a handful of High Anglican members' to give it 'a rather spurious inter-denomination air' (Simms 1975, 712). The Catholic convert Dr Halliday Sutherland was a founder and extremely active member who continued to hold Nazi views in 1944 and advocated the death penalty for contraceptive manufacturers.[23]

If their opponents told lies, birth control advocates invented some myths of their own and Haire searched in vain for the alleged plethora of Dutch birth control clinics, writing on 21 June 1927 to the Hon. Marjorie Farrer at the North Kensington Women's Welfare Centre because he could not find *any*. He confirmed this four years later in *The Eugenics Review*, saying he had visited Holland 'about fifty times in the last ten years', and had been in touch with the leaders of the birth control movement there and had never discovered that 'any birth control clinic exists, or has ever existed, there'. When he attended a small birth control conference in Amsterdam on 29–30 August 1921 with Dr CV Drysdale, Bessie Drysdale and Margaret Sanger,[24] they visited a labourer's wife who gave contraceptive advice. Dr Rutgers had shown her how to fit rubber pessaries and she had a notice on her house with her name, the words Neo-Malthusian League and the consultation hours. Haire was

---

23   Simms (1975, 713) quoted Sutherland (1944) who commended the 1936 Nazi Penal Code for making 'public ridicule of marriage or of maternity, and all propaganda in favour of birth control and abortion' criminal offences.

24   Margaret Sanger (November 1921, 11) listed the other delegates: 'Mme de Beer-Meijers, Mynheer and Mme Kiersch de June, Mr de Vries, Mr S Ten Cate and Dr Risselade (Holland) and Dr E Goldstein (Germany)'.

assured by Rutgers, Jacobs and others that 'this was a typical example of what propagandists in other countries describe as the Dutch clinics'.

In her autobiography, Margaret Sanger placed their visit in context. Convinced that birth control clinics were more effective than printed information, she and the Drysdales had made the visit with:

> Dr Norman Haire, Australian born, a gynaecologist who had settled in London, sensed the public interest in birth control, informed himself thoroughly on the subject, written a great deal about it, and become prominent in the movement advocating contraception from his Harley Street office.

She found that birth control services had deteriorated since her previous visit in 1915. In those six years, 'during the reorganisation period of Europe' there had been a Russian influenced tendency for 'young laborites to be in charge' who had ousted Dr Rutgers and the Dutch Neo-Malthusians and replaced them with workers' clinics. However, the new lay boards did not realise the need for technical knowledge and experience such as Rutgers possessed and he became sad and 'profoundly discouraged' by the odds against him;[25] he had no successors when he resigned from the Neo-Malthusian League in 1919.

Haire's comments about the 'fairy tale of the fifty Dutch counselling clinics' were repeated in 1932 by Dutch psychiatrist Coen van Emde Boas at the WLSR congress in Brno. He said there was only one clinic, the Aletta Jacobshuis (Aletta Jacobs House), which did not open until 1931 and he was one of the medical officers in charge (Brandhorst 2003, 50). A similar myth was fed to Americans by Dr S Adolphus Knopf, a prolific author and birth control advocate. He claimed in 1921 that birth control was widely available and almost universally used in Australia and New Zealand, which produced brave and fearless fighters in World War I whose physical endurance was probably superior to their 'English brethren' where 'birth control was frowned on by the legal and nearly all the ecclesiastical authorities'.[26] These mythical good deeds in

---

25 Sanger (1970, 290–91). See also Van Poppel and Röling (2003).
26 Knopf's and Johannes Rutgers' views reflect those of the NSW Royal Commission on the Decline of the Birth-Rate (1904). After extensive analysis,

remote countries were meant to motivate, the Dutch legend did inspire Margaret Sanger to open her birth control clinic in New York and they made the Malthusian League think about opening theirs.

Haire's 1924 diary survived his executors' destructive zeal and it contains an interesting list of his friends and colleagues including Dr Eden Paul and Michael Davidson, a newspaper editor, homosexual and mentor to WH Auden.[27] The first diary entry was for an afternoon appointment at the Overseas Club on 6 January, followed by a rehearsal on the 8th and on the 10th he gave the BSSSP lecture which created such a stir. There is a mysterious diary entry for the 15th: '6.00 pm, dinner with Mr Bruce, Hotel Cecil'; this hotel on the Embankment was London's largest and grandest and the formal wording, 'Mr Bruce', suggests it was for business not pleasure. Was it a ritzy dinner-for-two with the Australian-born Stanley Bruce, who spoke with a Cambridge drawl, wore spats and hated being called by his first name?

On 3 February 1923, a week before he became Australia's Prime Minister, *The Times* published a profile of this 39-year-old, noting that he looked years younger and 'for some mysterious reason' had been known as 'Janey' as a student at Melbourne Grammar. Haire really knew people in high places if it *was* Stanley Bruce, who was representing Australia at the British Empire Exhibition.

'The intellectual snob society of the day was the Heritics', according to Ivor Montagu, a son of the wealthy banker, Baron Swaythling. After Haire lectured there on 21 January this Australian outsider continued his duckling-to-swan transformation by becoming a fêted speaker at this prestigious Cambridge University society. Montagu wrote:

Rutgers (1923, 129) concluded that 'In recent years birth control has made such strides in the different provinces of Australia, that it is amongst the white population, that the decrease in the birth rate has become more marked than in any other country in the world.' Haire translated Rutgers' book in1924 but seemed unaware of the earlier one.

27 Auden sent his poems to Davidson who then gave helpful criticism. Davidson also helped with gifts of poetry books and literary criticism and he gave Auden's poems good reviews in his newspaper.

The Heretics managed to induce on to its lecture list an astonishing series of the intellectual lions of the day, who, after performance, would proceed to someone's rooms in college where we could interrogate them far into the night. If young people got on with the lecturers it might be the start of long-standing fertile friendships. [There he met] Norman Haire, the gynaecologist and populariser of studies in sexual behaviour.[28]

Haire was now famous but fame did not go to his head and, after his 10 February 1924 speech to the Golders Green Ethical Society, having told Beatrice McCabe he liked the coconut cakes served at supper she sent him the recipe and a note: 'Dear Dr Haire, Mr McCabe thanks you for your offer to send an article' and he 'would have been glad to receive any you would send. But alack! *The Tribune* was not paying and would have to cease to exist.'

> Coconut Cakes: 1 lb desiccated coconut; ¾.lb castor sugar; Whites of four eggs; 12 or more drops of vanilla flavour. Separate eggs, & put whites into bowl & beat moderately, add sugar, beat again, and put in coconut. Stir well, add flavouring, & stir in thoroughly. Have ready two baking sheets – can be bought for as low as four pence ha'penny each – dip the hands into castor sugar, and take up about a table-spoonful of the mixture & press it firmly with the fingers into a cone shape. The sugar prevents it sticking to the hands. Bake in a moderate oven – not hot – for about a quarter of an hour. The yolks could be used in puddings. (HC, 2.18)

In 1925 Haire had his portrait painted by Chris Watt. He also wrote the foreword for Ludovici's book, *Lysistrata: or woman's future and future women,* and said it was 'stimulating' and 'a great pleasure' to read. However, he felt Ludovici was being very hard on the medical profession because, with the 'idiotic system of paying the doctor better for illness than for health', it was a wonder that doctors didn't have more

---

28 Montagu (1970, 222) also mentioned Haire's request, on behalf of a Vienna practitioner, to visit the Black Museum, Scotland Yard's collection of criminal memorabilia. It was arranged but the Police Commissioner said, 'We did not have much to interest him. I am afraid we do not study so carefully here those matters they seem to be interested in on the continent'.

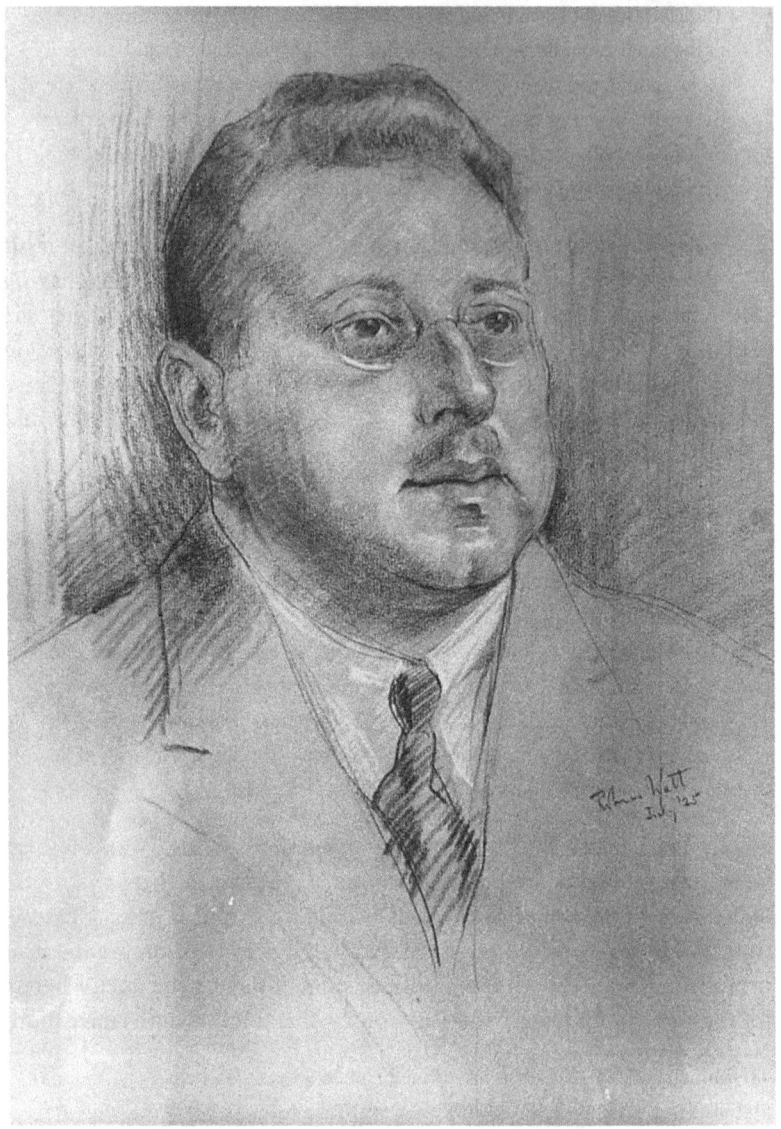

Figure 5.2. Sketch of Norman Haire by Chris Watt, July 1925.

faults. He prophesised that in 'a saner age' doctors would get a retaining fee to keep people well, and so they would aim to prevent disease rather than alleviating it.[29] Haire agreed with Ludovici's propositions that a good prenatal diet would help childbirth, babies should be breastfed and, although some women were happy and unmarried, 'sound and desirable women cannot be happy unmated.' He hoped Ludovici would 'trumpet forth' his view that 'moral depravity is no more voluntary than physiological depravity.' Haire felt his views about 'the unfit' and infanticide were 'splendid' and agreed that marriage needed some modification, probably 'concubinage', because although people claimed to be monogamous, eventually they would 'admit that men are polygamous' – best summed up by William James' epigram:

> Hogamous higamous
> Men are polygamous;
> Higamous, hogamous,
> Women monogamous.[30]

Haire's definition lacked this punch: 'Few men are monogamous, and few women polyandrous, but both are exceptions' and it would be better to allow all women 'half a husband' rather than give 'half the women a whole husband' while others had 'no husband at all.' Haire expected that Ludovici would 'be denounced as a daring and fantastic visionary' and that he would be 'blamed as an aider and abettor' but said that this did not matter if the book stimulated people to examine their values. Disappointingly, there was no shocked response because 'this style of book is quite in the fashion' according to *The New York Times'* 9 August 1925 review of 'two combative studies' written by Ludovici and Dora Russell.[31] A reviewer in *The Times Literary Supplement* thought

---

29   Haire was prescient about pre-paid health maintenance organisations which became popular in America in the 1930s and 40s and still operate, but after becoming more conservative he opposed Britain's new National Health Service in his articles in *Woman*, 24 January and 14 February 1949.
30   Rubinstein (1990, 195) attributed these lines to the psychologist William James. She did not give a source so the anecdote may be apocryphal.
31   These studies were Ludovici's *Lysistrata* and Dora Russell's *Hypatia*. Hypatia

her book was 'written in a temper' and it probably was, considering the conflict between her liberated views and the constraints on her life; in 1923 she had a difficult pregnancy, the marriage was strained after Bertrand became impotent with her in 1924 and she had to coordinate parenting, activism and writing with running the school.[32]

Haire was going on an American lecture tour in March and April of 1925 and wrote to Allen & Unwin on 9 January suggesting 'if available my book should sell well there at that time'. He meant *Rejuvenation* which was well reviewed in *The Lancet* the following day, although he complained on 13 January about the publisher's skimpy and haphazard advertising, and in his 16 January letter to Stanley Unwin enclosed a letter from 'a journalist friend in Australia' with the comment, 'I think you will see that I have every right to be disappointed.' The un-named letter-writer had had great trouble trying to find A & U's agent because he had moved and wasn't listed in the phone book. Finally, he discovered the address of the Australasian Publishing Co by a lucky chance. He went there and found that Stanley Bartlett was indeed Allen & Unwin's agent but he didn't stock Haire's book and didn't know anything about it or its author. Bartlett became interested when he was given the book and reviews from *The Sun*, *Bulletin*, and *Punch* and was told about Haire's visit to America. He promised to call on George Robertson from A & R (Angus & Robertson) to discuss stocking the book and he hoped it would soon get underway. Bartlett was a man of wide experience of books and book-selling who thought it was ridiculous'that his principals hadn't advised him about Haire's book.[33] After Unwin reassured him,

---

was a Greek scholar who headed Plato's Alexandrian school in Egypt around 400 AD and was the first notable woman in mathematics. She was killed by Christians who falsely blamed her for religious turmoil.

32 Brooke (2005, 149–50) quoting Monk (2001) and Griffin (2001).

33 For details, see Jason Ensor's 2009 paper. Ensor's paper discusses the tension between British and Australian publishers and the attempt in late 1930 to create a cooperative 'axis' between A & R in Sydney and George G Harrap and Co in London, with the Australasian Publishing Co (as part of the Harrap group) with Barrett representing both. In 1924 Barrett was an agent for Harrap and A & R and, consequently, he would have had little interest in promoting Haire's book for their publishing competitor, Allen & Unwin.

Haire posted 'a number of reviews' on 2 March and the publisher promised to supply him with others.[34]

On 12 March 1925, just as he was setting off on his American tour, Haire asked Unwin about possible German rights for his book and, rather cheekily, requested a letter of introduction to Macmillans in New York. Perhaps to make amends, Allen & Unwin advertised *Rejuvenation* in *The Saturday Review* in 1925 with a quote from the *New Statesman*: 'It is exactly what is required . . . The evidence is startling enough without being emphasised, and the book is not at all sensational'. A few months earlier Haire had committed an unwitting gaffe with the influential Dr RL Dickinson who made medical history in 1924 when his evaluation of contraception was published in the *American Journal of Obstetrics and Gynecology*.[35] Dickinson had said that he might ask Haire to lecture if some of his English friends gave him an endorsement; he meant Havelock Ellis but Haire did not know this and sent the American a 'fairly frigid letter pointing out that the more eminent gynaecologists were incapable, owing to ignorance, of either endorsing or controverting' his work. Haire ruefully confessed to Havelock Ellis on 24 February 1925: 'with [the maturity of] years perhaps I shall grow more tolerant.' Haire also hoped that winter had not tried the older man's lungs too severely because, despite his comparative youth, he woke each morning with 'organ pipes' in his chest.

On 14 March 1925 Haire sailed for New York as the British delegate at the Sixth International Birth Control Conference. He was one of the prominent speakers listed in the newspapers, along with Dr James F Cooper and Dr Hannah Stone (from the American Birth Control League) and Dr Aletta Jacobs (from The Hague). Delegates were entertained at

---

34   There was a note on the letter: 'Dr N Haire has not received reviews from the following papers; *New Generation*, December 1924; Church Times, 7 November 1924; *London Rotarian*, 1 November 1924; *Organotherapeutic Review*, November 1924; *Reynolds News*, 2 November 1924; *Medical Times*, November 1924, *Dental Record*, February 1924, *Times of India*, 11 February 1925'.

35   Himes (1936, 443) described Dickinson's article as a: 'Pioneer publication in the USA from any gynaecologist and obstetrical authority, giving details of methods and evaluation. It was a deliberate challenge to the Federal Postal Laws both as a journal article and a pamphlet, but was never questioned'.

a 'tea' given by Juliet Rublee, Sanger's friend and benefactor, and *The Washington Post* reported the Conference's highlight occurred when 1000 physicians, at a 'doctors only' session, had recommended that birth control should be included in all medical training programs. Margaret Sanger sent President Coolidge a telegram urging him to form a federal birthrate commission and on 6 April *Time* reviewed the congress and quoted Dr CV Drysdale who exuberantly hailed Sanger as 'the Joan of Arc and the Florence Nightingale of the birth-control movement': the topic was now respectable and had shifted from court rooms to drawing rooms. Haire told Havelock Ellis on 5 June: 'My visit was wonderfully interesting. The Conference was really a triumphant success. I addressed nearly a thousand doctors on contraceptive methods on the Sunday afternoon'.

Haire also spoke at the Brooklyn Gynecological Society where he mentioned his invention of a non-greasy contraceptive jelly of lactic acid and boracic acid for use with a vaginal pessary.[36] He lectured to the Toronto Academy of Medicine, the Hamilton Medical Research Association, a number of other medical meetings, and at Cornell, Syracuse,[37] and Buffalo universities. Havelock Ellis thanked him for his work on the conference and Haire responded by apologising for harassing him because, on taking on the job, he had been 'compelled to be very unpleasant at times'. There had been a great deal of work and although the 'gratifying' results 'far exceeded' his expectations, it was at the expense of his own work which he had neglected for more than nine months and he doubted if he would ever tackle a conference again. However, despite his intentions, Haire would take on an ever larger challenge four years later.

In her address to the Royal Institute of Public Health's August 1925 congress in Brighton, Margaret Sanger praised 'our friend' Dr Norman Haire, who 'in his quietly effective manner' stressed the need for birth

---

36 Haire (1936, 75–76) said that at the 1925 meeting, when he mentioned the contraceptive jellies he had devised about 1921, Dr William Carey, 'the well-known New York gynaecologist', said that he had devised a similar jelly even earlier.

37 In 1870 Cornell University was the first Ivy League college to become co-educational and in 1921 Syracuse University became non-sectarian.

control for the good of humanity and the nation. He also featured in an article about Australians living in London written by Thomas Burke, a now-forgotten author who was impressed by Haire's 'two or three valuable works on sex psychology' and his status as a 'specialist in Harley Street' which was even more remarkable because 'most men only arrive in Harley Street after many years in the wilderness, but Norman Haire has only just passed his thirtieth year'. Haire was six foot three (190.5 centimetres) and stocky so calling him 'tall and muscular' was euphemistic, but Burke was right about his 'Australian energy', direct speech and candid manner bringing a 'breath of strong air to the street'. However, while such behaviour is valued as the norm in Australia, it is often misunderstood and disliked in Britain where words and feelings are more controlled and complex. Burke's view of Australia stretched as far as emus, sheep, beachcombers, bush, Norman Lindsay and Nellie Melba but Haire's voice and opinions distorted this view and he wrote condescendingly: 'Unless you knew his country you could not name it. By habit he is cosmopolitan, and though I have studied him in one or two interesting talks, I have learned nothing about Australia. It seems that Australians lose their colour very quickly when away from home'.

Historians Roy Porter and Lesley Hall found Haire's rapid prosperity remarkable because, as well as being a foreigner, he was 'homosexual and Jewish which must have militated against him in medical circles'.[38] Although this success was remarkable, it was unlikely that the medical fraternity would have known about his sexuality, but even without this knowledge they would still have ostracised him. Haire's Sydney relative Professor Gillian Shenfield put it succinctly:

> The English medical hierarchy in London was a very closed shop and very snobbish, so to come to London in the early 1920s when you're Australian and Jewish and what you're trying to do is not respectable, to set up and be a successful practitioner is a testament to his personality because he must have been on the outer in the medical establishment. There is no way it could have been otherwise.

---

38 Porter and Hall (1995, 352 fn 47) wrote: 'For further details about Haire, see Weeks, *Coming out*, 128–43, 151–55'.

For most people these odds would have been insurmoutable but Haire relished the challenge and established links with British and overseas specialists and soon became world famous, helped by mass marketing of his books.[39] As well as being mentioned in *The Times* on 30 May 1925 when he discussed birth control at the Brighton congress, and lectures in the US and Canada, in October 1926 he had presented an important paper at the First International Congress for Sex Research in Berlin.

The difference between Haire's progressive views and the conservative norm is shown by the report *The Lancet* printed on 13 February 1926 about a parliamentary decision. The House of Commons had (by 167 votes to 81) refused to introduce a bill authorising local authorities to 'incur expenditure' and provide birth control information to married women.[40] On 18 November *The Times* claimed the words 'birth control' were offensive and, in the first of two pompous letters, Sir Arthur Newsholme, the Chief Medical Officer of England, agreed with birth control opponent Sir James Marchant that the advocacy of birth control was 'extremely undesirable before a general broadcasting audience.' On 19 November *The Times* published the BBC's claim that 'no talk has been given on this subject', a reference to it in a radio debate had been 'entirely inadvertent' and was 'at variance with' their policy, and action had been taken 'to prevent its recurrence.' *The Times* added: 'The statement of the BBC seems to render unnecessary the publication of any further letters, of which a number have reached us, on this matter.'

---

39   Haire informed Stanley Unwin (Haire, 17 April 1925, AUC) that his secretary had posted circulars to about 6000 medical men in London and needed 5000 more in order to be able to send them to doctors in the rest of Britain. Haire said he had spent over £50 in postage in the first year after *Rejuvenation*'s appearance 'to say nothing of envelopes and his secretary's time' and could not afford to spend any more on it.

40   When Ernest Thurtle, a British Labour politician, sought leave to present the bill to the House of Commons, he was given ten minutes to make his case for making this expenditure on birth control and argued for it on the grounds of gender and class equality. Thurtle was a member of the Workers' Birth Control Group, along with Dora Russell and Frida Laski, the wife of Harold Laski, a Marxist economist and professor at the London School of Economics.

There was also a difference between Haire's weight and the norm – Thomas Burke said diplomatically that he had a 'Dominion physique' but many people were openly rude about it and Haire mused: 'If I drank as much as I eat, people wouldn't notice it at all. Over drinking is fashionable – overeating isn't.'[41] He had got very drunk when he was 19 and it made him so sick that he resolved never to do it again; he had no moral objections and wasn't a teetotaller but he disliked the taste of beer and spirits (although he liked a few liqueurs) and he didn't like the effects of alcohol. This was healthy but his smoking and eating habits were not. People with distant or cruel fathers often seek solace in food and it may have been a response to his inner turmoil and his only permissible outlet in an era when homosexuality had to be hidden.

Although he shared Queen Victoria's food gobbling heartiness,[42] he was both a gourmet and gourmand who worked hard, entertained generously, read widely, and was interested in the arts generally, but, above all, he was passionate about the theatre. Cartoonist Bernard Hesling (1960) reminisced about their theatrical 1926 meeting at London's Gate Theatre; he was impressed when the bald, 'vast' 34-year old doctor introduced himself as Norman Haire and later, when they went to the Cafe Royal after the show, Hesling, then a 21-year-old actor, was horrified because Haire, 'famous in Europe as he never was in his native land', envied him for being an actor. The stage manager worried that 'a young innocent from the provinces' had gone off with Haire 'a professed homosexual' but joked: 'watch out for him, he's a good bloke but never ask his advice about sex or he'll send you a bill.' Haire was not bald but Hesling tended to embellish stories and this habit once led to his dismissal.[43]

---

41   Haire quoted by Hesling (1960, 14).

42   Wilson (2001, 48–49).

43   Robert Hughes (2006, 208–09) said Donald Horne, the editor of *The Observer*, fired Bernard Hesling in 1958 for writing a savage review of a William Blake art exhibition he had not attended. Horne gave the job to Hughes and it marked the start of his career as an art critic. Peter Coleman (2012) said he was there and that Hughes' account was not true: the newspaper proprietor was a friend of the Hughes family and was determined to give Robert a job. Hessling's review had nothing to do with his sacking.

Haire did not seek to make money from his writing but translations helped to introduce the work of German and French sexologists to English-speaking audiences. Haire and his Australian collaborator Ernest Jerdan were skilled linguists and rationalists so their translations were free from religious bias. It is easy to spot mistakes in English, such as Germaine Greer's (1984, 314) sloppy statement that Haire was born in 'Australia or New Zealand' but they are harder to see in other languages. Mistakes of bias are even harder to detect and Heike Bauer (2003, 381–405) showed the consequences of such 'multilations' in a splendid analysis of English translations of the works by three pioneering German sexologists: Karl Ulrichs, Richard Krafft-Ebing and Magnus Hirschfeld.

In 1924 Haire and Ernest Jerdan had translated *Woman: a treatise on the anatomy, physiology, psychology and sexual life of woman* by Viennese gynaecologist Dr Bernhard A Bauer. Havelock Ellis had not seen it but suspected it was 'of a useful rather than original character' (Havelock Ellis to Haire, 4 February 1924 – HC 3.16). In the introduction Haire elaborated on one of his key themes: 'the outlook on sexual matters is terribly muddle-headed and wrong' and caused enormous and unnecessary suffering with 'most marital unhappiness being linked to ignorance and bigotry. He said we persecute the unfortunate sufferers from all sorts of sexual aberrations, instead of treating them as *ill* people needing care and attention', which sounds like a veiled reference to his sexuality and Jerdan's deteriorating mental health. Haire assumed readers' knowledge of poetry when he said Bauer's work had 'a striking resemblance to that of Pope as expressed in his *Moral essays*, Epistle 2: *Of the characters of women*, and is diametrically opposed to the concept of the Victorian age, which invested women with a halo.' Haire meant Alexander Pope's 1735 poem that described an 'estemable woman' as being witty, refined, soft-natured, cunning and silly who incorporated 'the best kind of contrarieties'. An anonymous reviewer liked Bauer's appendix on prostitution but felt it would anger 'those queer fowl – the Feminists'. They had every reason to object to this diatribe about 'the insatiable woman who lives only for sex' and 'can wreck not only one man but many. Physically, mentally and morally, but especially morally', whole peoples would be sacrificed by lust-crazed men once they fell into the clutches of 'she-vampires who would suck the life out of them'.[44] A reviewer in the *British Medical Journal* on 4 June 1927 found it hard to understand why a barrister [Jerdan] and a medical man [Haire] had spent so much time in translating a verbose book such as *Woman*.

In April 1926 Norman Himes received a fellowship from America's Social Science Research Council to study 'The history of the birth control movement in England with special reference to the development and growth of the clinics' and asked Margaret Sanger for a list of the leaders in the field, saying 'you will immediately think of Dr Norman Haire, Dr Drysdale and others'. Haire must have relished his status as an expert and he responded warmly to Himes' request, invited him 'round for a chat' and offered to provide him with 'a good deal of information about the movement in the last six years, particularly about the commencement of the clinics' because he was 'one of the founders of the Walworth Clinic'; Himes would find details in *Who's Who*.

Havelock Ellis wrote to Haire on 11 September, saying he could not meet Magnus Hirschfeld because language barriers would make talking a little difficult and asked Haire to explain this to Hirschfeld, stress his very high regard for his work and send his best regards. Haire replied that he understood the difficulty and 'would put it nicely to Hirschfeld'. Havelock Ellis was relieved because, at their previous meeting in London, Hirschfeld had delivered a long address in German on his own special doctrines. Havelock Ellis could not easily follow spoken German and had found it very difficult to understand or make intelligible replies. Haire passed on the explanation and then 'motored them down' to Harold Pickett's[45] for the weekend but found the atmosphere 'very queer and distasteful' because Hirschfeld and his young secretary had 'only one topic of conversation, which soon palls'.

Haire contacted Norman Himes on 30 September 1926 on the eve of his departure to attend the First International Congress for Sex Research in Berlin where he would present his paper on the comparative value of

---

44 Bauer (1927, 312) quoted by Swenson (2003, 32).
45 This man was not Harold Edward Pickett, a gay rights activist whose papers from 1965 to 1988 are held in the New York Public Library.

current contraceptive methods based on more than 4000 patients he had seen in the previous six years. On his return, Haire invited Himes to accompany him on 29 October when he was due to give evidence to the Medical Committee of the National Birth-Rate Commission. He also accepted invitations to present his 'Contraceptive methods' lecture at two respected London teaching hospitals (St Mary's Hospital in Paddington and Westminster Hospital) and told Havelock Ellis on 12 September that 'we are progressing'. Haire invited Himes to hear his lecture at St Mary's on 10 November and he became ill the next day: this was followed by an operation and bad influenza.[46]

A group of south London health workers acknowledged Haire's pre-eminence when they launched the Peckham Health Centre in 1926. They wanted to separate health promotion from disease treatment and 'preferred this concept to that of Dr Norman Haire, who, together with Marie Stopes, was the best known advocate of contraception' (Lewis & Brookes 1983).

In just five years Haire's status had changed from penniless outsider to wealthy medical practitioner who was about to acquire a grand house and consolidate his success.

---

46 Details about this illness and an unspecified 1926 operation are contained in the case notes 'King's College Hospital, Medical Record for Norman Haire, Patient from 21 February to 3 April 1950' (HC – Box 5).

6

Moving up in the world

The 1920s were a 'tumultuous, revolutionary age'[1] and Ivor Montagu noticed a special feeling in the air and a 'widespread Jewish infatuation with communism among the intellectuals of his generation.'[2] This political passion was evident in Haire's 8 January 1927 response to GK Chesterton's article in *Lansbury's Labour Weekly*. Haire was tackling a formidable opponent: the 'colossal genius' who was also a newly converted Catholic. Haire quoted Chesterton's first paragraph as an attempt, 'with his usual literary skill', to distract readers' attention from the real issue by stating the case for birth control 'as none of its advocates would think of stating it' and then to 'demolish it with ease'. Chesterton said:

> It is rather like saying that cutting off King Charles' head was one of the most elegant of the Cavalier fashions in hair-dressing. It is like saying that decapitation is an advance in dentistry. It may or may not be right to cut off the King's head; it may or may not be right to cut off your own head when you have the toothache. But anybody ought to be able to see that if we once simplify things by head-cutting, we can do without hair-cutting; that it will be needless to practise dentistry on the dead or philanthropy on the unbegotten – or the unbegotten.

Haire pointed out that Chesterton's statement avoided the consideration that 'head-cutting' did not bear the same relation to hair-dressing or dentistry as birth control did for future generations' welfare. He asked whether Chesterton was 'so ignorant of dentistry as to be unaware that *if a patient's mouth is too small*' to accommodate the teeth, dentists usually removed some to protect the others. Haire, 'as an advocate of birth control', was 'grateful to Mr Chesterton for his

---

1 Orwell (1946, 3).
2 Riordan (2008, 517) quoting Litvinoff (1969, 158).

attempted analogy between teeth and children' and didn't believe 'any birth controller thought of it before'. He continued his parody by saying that Chesterton was 'an adroit controversialist' who carefully pointed out that birth controllers 'never say there are too many bankers, or suggest that city financiers should not have such large families' and that the 'Gloomy Dean' of St Paul's 'was not more gloomy about there being too many Dukes or too many Deans'. Haire said this was 'all very humorous and very sparkling' and made readers forget the very important fact that dukes, deans, bankers, financiers, the throng at Ascot, the diners at the Ritz 'do not usually have excessively large families'. Haire's writing had been witty and sparkling but it switched to a string of political platitudes as though there was a split between Haire's 'good' Dr Jekyll writing and his 'bad' Mr Hyde polemic (fortunately, his earnest prolixity was short-lived). *The Triad* in Sydney was so astonished by Haire's declaration that they reprinted his words from *Lansbury's* article in their March issue:

> I am a Socialist. I look forward to the time when the present ridiculous system of private ownership – apart from the personal things like a house, furniture, clothes, books, tools, etc – will have disappeared; when a man will be ambitious to leave his children, not a vast store of worldly wealth, but a good heredity, physical and mental. Mothers and children will, if necessary, be supported by the community instead of being dependent on the product of the labour of an individual. The community, which needs citizens, will recognise that the mother is doing a community-service by producing children, and will support her and them.

Lansbury's Labour Weekly was a twopenny newspaper published by George Lansbury, a British Labour pioneer, underdog-supporter, Marxist Socialist Democratic Federation organiser, East End member of parliament, suffragette ally, pacifist, imprisoned Labour mayor, anti-imperialist, the people's poor law guardian and republican and, according to historian AJP Taylor, 'the most lovable figure in modern politics.'[3] Taylor and the writer Tom Driberg had formed the two-person University of Oxford Communist Party and belonged to the

---

3 AJP Taylor quoted by Shepherd (2004).

university's Labour Club. Barbara Betts (subsequently Barbara Castle, a Labour politician who became a baroness) was a member of the Labour Club as a student in the 1920s and she reminisced about it and Haire's involvement:

> It was a lively body; the Red flag was quite often sung, there were social meetings, dramatic functions, films, dancing, party games, impersonations . . . and above all plenty of argument. The Club often worked closely with the city Labour Party, especially at elections. Much valued were its opportunities for meeting the opposite sex. With help from Norman Haire it went still further, and 'blazed the trial of sex knowledge'.

A 9 March 1927 editorial in Oxford University's student newsletter *Isis* quoted Castle as saying 'The most mentally proficient among us who bother about politics at all, possess distinct Socialist leanings.'[4]

Haire was trying to get his second book published and had chosen Havelock Ellis' publishers in Philadelphia, the FA Davis Company. Havelock Ellis sent them a letter introducing Haire and they agreed to publish *Hymen: or, the future of marriage*, however they rejected the first draft and Haire had to revise it. On 2 February 1927 Haire contacted Havelock Ellis with an apology for his two-month silence and explained that it was as a result of his illness with two severe attacks of influenza. The book was now being published by Kegan Paul but there had been further delays because their editor William Stallybrass had been away and had inferred that it would be better not to publish the book at all, even though Haire had accepted his suggested alterations and deletions. A week later Havelock Ellis discussed these book negotiations with one of his admirers, Winifred Henderson, saying Haire 'seems to go out of his way to stir up all the antagonisms he can', adding that he hoped Haire would not be offended by his letter about *Hymen*.[5] Ellis was foolish and disloyal to discuss this sensitive matter with her, particularly after Haire had warned him that Henderson was 'indiscreet'. Even worse: Ellis had told Margaret Sanger that early in his friendship with Henderson he had

---

4 *The history of the University of Oxford* (8, 1994, 399) quoting Castle.
5 Grosskurth (1985, 378, fn 42). The 'dangerous' quote is on p. 346.

discovered she was 'dangerous'. Three days after his letter to Henderson, Ellis sent Haire this advice: 'To persuade people you need to soothe, not stimulate, their prejudices. Also you frequently appeal to reason, as though that was the creative force in life, & not, at the most, a very slowly & imperfectly modifying influence in life'.

Although Havelock Ellis criticised Haire about antagonising, this is precisely what Ellis was doing when he sent a letter about Haire to an indiscreet, dangerous woman and, shortly afterwards, sent him fatherly advice. This was odd or malicious behaviour and the second part of his advice was particularly strange: if he felt it was wrong to 'appeal to reason', did he think it was right to appeal to emotion, the method which demagogues later adopted? Haire trusted Ellis and said that his criticism (not the publisher's call for changes) had *'clinched the matter'* because 'whether you like it or not you are one of my spiritual parents, and your word carries far more weight with me than my physical father's ever did.'

Ellis wrote again in May but Haire did not reply until July because he had been away a lot on the Continent and was in London planning for his birth control clinic. He was worried that *Hymen* was still 'unduly provocative' even though he had softened it a good deal.' He explained to Ellis that he found it difficult to compromise and considered this aspect of his temperament was one of his worst faults which he did his best to overcome. His success would have been impossible if he had shown weakness or compromised, but perhaps he presented this strength as a weakness to elicit a reassuring response. Havelock Ellis wrote on 1 October to congratulate him on the toned down book and hoped the agitation about it had not been serious and that his work in general continued to go well. In his reply Haire thanked his mentor and said he realised the book was still somewhat aggressive because he had 'not escaped that usual characteristic of people of Jewish ancestry – the inferiority complex' which he sometimes over-compensated for with aggression and he linked his rebelliousness to his relationship with his father. He said the book had been well received so far. *The Sunday Chronicle* demanded its suppression as immoral and the government threatened to ban it. As a result the first edition sold out within three days and a few days later a second edition was released. Haire said that on hearing this news, 'in my coarse fashion, I chortle!' Haire kept a statue of a full-bellied, chortling Buddha on his desk.

An inscribed copy of *Hymen* was presented to 'Emily BH Mudd, Haverford, Pa. by the author, England – August 1932.'[6] The recipient, her husband and friends had braved American regulations by establishing Pennsylvania's Maternal Health Center in 1927. She agreed to become the director's assistant because she was expecting her second child and an obscure law prohibited the jailing of pregnant women (Mudd 1998).

Although many of his letters to colleagues and friends seem to contain intimate details, Haire revealed very little about his private life. He waited 20 years to tell a *Hymen* anecdote during the broadcast of a radio debate; when asked if 'it would have been a loss to the world if he had not been born', he replied that his mother had come to England in 1927 when he was publishing a book on birth control. She lived there for six months and did not like him being concerned with such questions, but he convinced her and she said, 'Well, I think perhaps you are right after all. It is a pity I did not meet you a year or two before you were born'. Haire mentioned her frequent abortion attempts and, as a seven-year-old, he had discovered a 'paper-covered book on contraception' hidden in the top drawer of her wardrobe. One of his siblings called him 'an accident' so his parents must have made some attempts at contraception.

Unfortunately, Stopes' book *Married love* provided unreliable information and children joked in a skipping game:

> Jeannie, Jeannie, full of hopes
> Read a book by Marie Stopes
> Now to judge from her condition
> She must have read the wrong edition[7]

---

6 Haire's book is held in Harvard University's Arthur & Elizabeth Schlesinger Library on the History of Women. Available: pds.lib.harvard.edu/pds/view/2573684 [Accessed 20 January 2010].

7 Falcon-Lang (2008, 136) noted this was a dig at the advice Stopes gave in *Wise parenthood* which changed in successive print runs. The *BMJ* 10 March 1923.

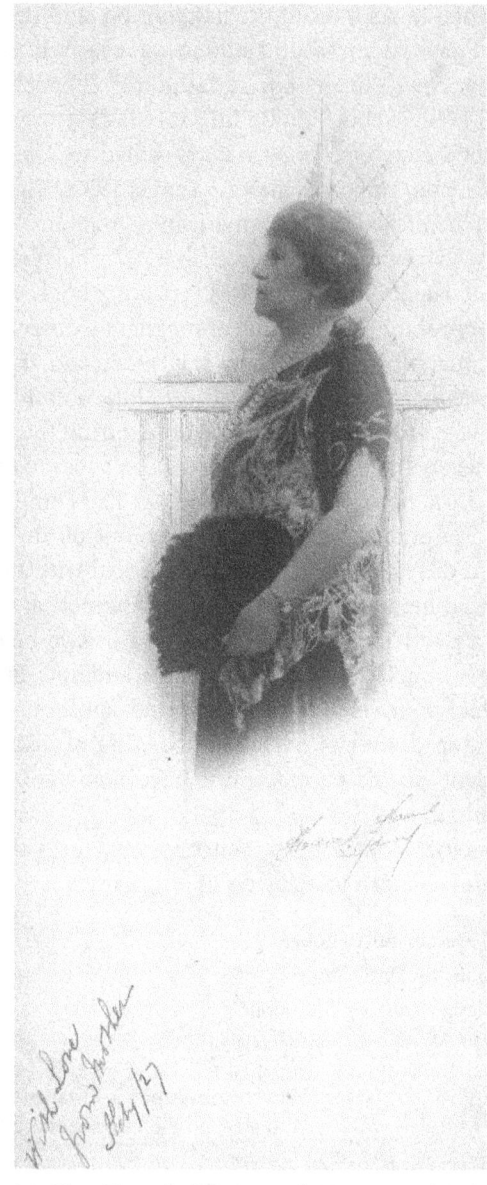

Figure 6.1. Clara Zions, holidaying with Norman in London, 1927.

The titillating title of Haire's book may have been an attempt to outsell Marie Stopes' 1918 bestseller. There is clarification in the full title – *Hymen: or, the future of marriage* – but it was usually shortened to *Hymen* which, spelt with a capital H, refers to the Greek god of marriage but spelt with a small h refers to the membrane covering the vagina. The book was published in London and New York and Haire sent an advance copy to Sebastian Sprott on 20 September in the hope that he would find it amusing although 'it was originally much better . . . the publisher insisted on the elimination of the frivolous bits – "no hint of levity" said he. So out they came.' This was sound advice because the book invoked controversy by rattling the bars of many securely caged taboos, particularly masturbation, disability and incest. Being outrageous *and* funny would have been intolerable.

Haire's book questioned the received wisdom and risked condemnation by claiming that a newspaper story about a deaf-mute couple with a large family of deaf-mute children should not have received readers' sympathy and financial support; instead the couple should now use contraception or be sterilised to prevent more such births. He criticised a journalist who had approvingly reported the lengthy jail sentence imposed by a judge in a long speech about the 'unspeakable crime' of an incestuous relationship between a widower of 48 and his consenting widowed daughter.

It was also courageous to compare the sex codes of the ancient Jews and Greeks and mention the frequency with which Greek mythological gods assumed animal shapes to 'mate with mortals' as an indication that for the ancient Greeks 'even bestiality was not regarded as revolting.'[8] Sanctimonious critics seized on Haire's comments about incest, bestiality and polygamy, which echoed words Samuel Butler had written in 1872[9],

---

noted: 'In the 9th edition she omitted a paragraph addressed to the "more careful women" on the "aesthetic" value of the gold pin (or wish bone) pessary, which appeared in the 7th, because she found that English doctors were not so familiar with contraceptive technique as American doctors'.

8 Masters considered bestiality 'a vice of clod-hoppers' which was also 'in fantasy at least, the pleasure of the most highly developed imaginations and the keenest esthetic sensibilities' (Masters 1962, 109).

9 Butler wrote *Erewhon* in 1872 and suggested in 1912 that any sexual practice

while ignoring his plea not for the *abolition* of sexual morality but for its *improvement*:

> Just as a piano needs tuning so that it may give the sweetest music, so I believe, our sexual morality needs readjustment – a little loosening here, and a little tightening there – if individual and communal life is to be as harmonious as possible. (*Hymen* 1927, 9)

His secular book prophesied that in future 'contraception will be universally practised by all normal people. The best advice on this subject will be obtained by all from doctors' although 'the methods of contraception most commonly used are untrustworthy and even harmful. There *are* trustworthy and harmless methods, but the public finds it difficult to learn them' either because of doctors' religious or social prejudices or because they lack contraception training and literally *cannot* help. Although parents carefully educate their children and supervise what they eat, they try to keep them ignorant about sex matters and this was 'a very insecure foundation on which to build a happy marriage' because it is 'better for a child to be brought up with only one parent than with two parents who are always quarrelling with each other.' These were self-evident truths to Haire, the ardent sexuality tuner.

William Inge, the Dean of St Pauls Cathedral, was called the 'Gloomy Dean' because of his pessimistic columns in the *London Evening Standard*. He supported birth control and eugenics and examined *Hymen* because Haire was 'known as an advanced thinker on these subjects.' He wanted to see how far the revolt against Christian standards had gone but he found Bertrand Russell's calls for reform in *Marriage and morals* 'even more provocative' and dismissed Haire's claims about high marital unhappiness because three-quarters of the 30 middle-class couples *he* knew had happy marriages. However, his anecdotal evidence ignored the possibility that these couples might have been *secretly* unhappy and he didn't address working-class marriages

---

in vogue long ago and far away could not be reprehensible. Graves and Hodge (1941, 89–90) thought it was a covert plea for both homosexuality and pre-marital promiscuity and said Butler was widely read in the 1920s.

but conceded that the 'record of the House of Lords and the idle rich in the matter of fidelity to the marriage vow is a very bad one' (Inge 1930, 350–52).

Winifred Holtby (1928, 73) mused that experts' advice was contradictory and she claimed that 'Dr Norman Haire would have boys and girls mate at sixteen'. She had misrepresented him by only giving the first part of his comment and omitting to say that he pointed out the adverse affect of chastity (physical or mental illness, masturbation or deviant sexuality) and suggested that adolescents should either marry young (with the option of easy divorce) or have 'pre-marital experiences' and use contraception. One discerning critic of books on marriage praised Haire for being 'as lucid as he is bold' and disparaged 'Mrs Sanger's earnest and somewhat nauseous preachment' (Shanks 1927, 430).

In November Haire gave Hirschfeld news about the proposal to ban *Hymen*, its subsequent sell-out sales and his publishers' plan to release a translation in Germany the following January. The 1928 *Book Review Digest* printed mixed reviews,[10] *The Times Literary Supplement* was neutral, saying that after his introduction about sex codes, sex taboos and attitudes towards prostitution and birth control, Haire had given his view of marriages of the future in which monogamy would be considered the ideal state but polygamy would also be legalised, children would be supported by the state, proper sex instruction would be given, and sterilisation of the unfit practised.

The New Triad liked his 'thoughtful and thought-stimulating little book' which did 'not mince matters' but dealt 'calmly and simply with aspects of sex' in a candid discussion of prostitution, trial marriages, concubinage, incest, and contraception. Haire took lifelong monogamy as the ideal, but discussed obstacles to early marriages, and believed that more individual freedom was inevitable in some matters along with more state control in others. He also showed that ideas of morality were a legacy from primitive religion and the reviewer concluded 'If

---

10   Other *Hymen* reviews include: *Nation* (5 September 1928, 232); *The Spectator* (24 September 1927, 472); *World Tomorrow* (September 1928, 376); *Booklist* (July 1928, 382); and *Boston Transcript* (28 April 1928, 2).

his vision of a eugenic state, partially regimented and controlled, is somewhat bleak, at all events it offers, beside an improvement of the stock, at least as great a chance of personal happiness for its members'.

The *British Medical Journal*'s reviewer (Haire or someone who shared his views) believed the thought-provoking book would only shock those who unquestioningly accepted conventional standards and had never tried to objectively examine life's problems. The reviewer praised the objective tone and Haire's well-reasoned arguments such as his response 'in answer to those who have so little faith in human nature as to imagine that if legal and religious prohibitions were withdrawn almost all men and women would fly to excess, the author declares that among the married and the unmarried sexual excess is far less common than sexual starvation. In his view excess is more often than not the direct reaction to and result of an antecedent starvation'.

The New York Herald Tribune was uncertain about Haire's view that morals should 'change as social necessities change' but suggested that readers accepting this view were in a 'position to follow him in his many intelligent suggestions for putting this venerable and still useful institution [marriage] on a more natural and healthy footing'. However, they felt that *Hymen* would not 'inspire a knight to do great deeds for his lady love'.

Sebastian Sprott had already published one of Haire's articles and was probably the unimpressed reviewer in *The Nation* on 5 September 1928 who was 'immunized' against so-called 'startling sex discussions' and felt the book had 'fallen short of its prophetic proclamations'.[11] If it was too tame for Sprott, it was too wild for the *St Louis* reviewer who was enraged by Haire's picture of a 'hideous (and we hope fantastic) picture of a godless future. A kick from a mule is stimulating in a sense, and so are some parts of *Hymen*, but it is not cheerful reading. If its prophecies come true, we should be tempted to embrace its predicted opportunity for State-aided euthanasia, and yet . . . the book repays perusal'.

---

11 *The Nation and Atheneum* was a radical liberal British political weekly newspaper which was formed from the merger of the *Athenaeum*, a long-established literary magazine and the newer *Nation*. It was purchased by a group led by John Maynard Keynes in 1923. In 1931 it was absorbed by the *New Statesman* which was known as the *New Statesman and Nation* until 1964.

The Medical Officer (10 October 1927) included this bizarre but anonymous response: 'Most of the author's suggestions as to sex education, birth control and sterilisation would increase human happiness. *But we are not made for happiness* [emphasis in original]. Rather we are made for greatness and self-control; the direction of our energies to good ends makes us great'. Haire scoffed at this Jeremiah's gloom and said, 'If I shared that philosophy, I should not practice at all. How could I attempt to relieve a patient's pain or suffering if I believed that, by so doing, I was increasing his chances of happiness, and so depriving him of a valuable opportunity of acquiring self control?'

Haire's empathy for his patients was paralleled by his generous support of friends. When Norman Himes wrote in June 1927 saying he wanted to meet Mr EW Lambert[12] and gain access to Lambert Limited's confidential figures on contraceptive sales for the past four decades, Haire was delighted to help 'My dear Himes'; he enclosed a copy of the letter of introduction he had sent Lambert and invited Himes 'to come around to look through my books'.

An opponent dismissed Haire's generosity as approval-seeking sycophancy. In reality Haire's generosity was inspired by altruism and his forthright manner often worked against his interests. For instance, he risked alienating Havelock Ellis the following month by challenging him for sending patients to a nurse who had 'sacrificed a great deal for her championship of Birth Control' but used the wrong size of Dutch pessaries and, as a result, women were becoming pregnant and turning to Haire for help. He said that he was not jealous and often sent patients to non-medical practitioners and also knew that many doctors were incompetent but he felt Ellis 'ought to know that this nurse has a considerable number of failures'. While some may have been caused by patient carelessness, he was convinced that some were due to the nurse's error of judgement. He was 'not hinting' that he should see these patients, because there were many suitably trained doctors and

---

12 Lambert Pharmacal Company's main product was Listerine. They merged to become the Warner-Lambert Pharmaceutical Co in 1955 and in 2000 they were taken over by Pfizer. Available: www.pfizer.com/about/history/pfizer_warner_lambert.jsp [Accessed 20 December 2009].

clinics which had a good deal of experience of fitting contraceptives. However, 'in the interest of the patients' he was 'suggesting that they would stand a better chance of getting really reliable advice if you sent them to some of these'. He hoped Ellis would not mind the suggestion but felt it was right to tell him of his experience of women who had been to this nurse. Haire meant Elizabeth Daniels, a nurse who had worked in local government but was dismissed in 1922 for the 'insubordination' of giving contraceptive advice. There was an outcry from her supporters and she went to Holland to learn about their contraceptive methods. When she returned to Britain she started her own clinic and trained other nurses.[13] Daniels did not like Haire's methods and complained to Norman Himes in September 1928 that Haire had fitted a 'much too small' Dutch cap – 'I have no failures and I know that others do'.

In the 1920s it took courage to defy the pronatalist norms by using contraception, and those progressive couples who did had their confidence shaken by disputes about the efficacy of various methods such as the public fight at the *Stopes v. Sutherland* trial over the Gold pin pessary. In two letters to *The Lancet*, on 16 July and 13 August 1927, Haire criticised Stopes' recommendation of Chinosol suppositories on the grounds that they were neither new, nor as satisfactory as quinine jellies and suppositories. She saw herself as the doyenne of the movement and took umbrage at real or imagined insults and bristled at any mention of the contributions made by other birth control pioneers.

Shortly after Haire's book was launched he travelled to Italy planning to see Dr Francisco Cavazzi in Bologna, who claimed to have got good 'rejuvenation' results with injections of testicular extract. On his return he lectured on Steinach's work to the Medical Practitioners' Union on 4 October 1927 and the South London Postgraduate Association on the 19th. Most excitingly of all, he told Hirschfeld on 24 November that St Thomas's Hospital Medical Society had invited him to lecture on contraceptive technique, reminding him that 'St Thomas's is one of our most important medical schools, and it was there that Havelock Ellis received his medical education'.

---

13 Soloway (1982, 282, 297, 302).

Cromer Welfare and Sunlight Centre.

Honorary Medical Director:
  Norman Haire, Ch.M., M.B.
Hon. Sec.: Hon. Mrs. Ivor Montagu
Hon. Treas.: Mrs. Eugene Bolton

59. CROMER STREET, W.C. 1.
(Off Gray's Inn Road—King's Cross End.)
Telephone   :   :   : Terminus 6130.

Antenatal, Infant Care and Sunlight Departments.

Birth Control instruction will be given, on request, by one of the medical staff, to any woman whose health or other circumstances render it advisable.

First visit any morning, Monday to Friday, between 10 and 1 o'clock.

NOTE: *This Centre is intended only for poor patients and no fees are charged.*

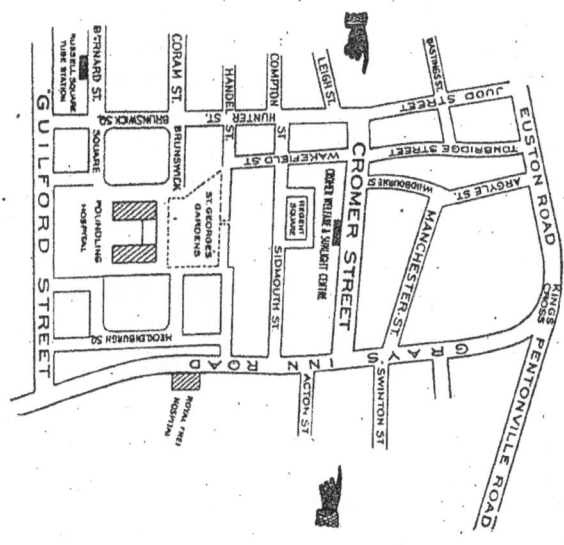

Figure 6.2. Flyer for Haire's inner-London Cromer Welfare and Sunlight Centre.

He was also launching his birth control clinic with funds from 'a grateful philanthropic patient' and he was about to move house. Factory workers used to jeer as the patients entered the League's clinic and, to avoid this, Haire chose a centrally located building at 59 Cromer Street, W1, near King's Cross Station, issued a map with directions, gave it a friendly, non-specific name and provided birth control as one of many services for mothers and babies. As a result he saw many women who were attending a health clinic for the first time.

Although Sanger was a trained nurse, her experiences in Holland convinced her that personal instruction was the best method, but she was also convinced that clinics should not be run by midwives, social workers or nurses because only doctors had the necessary gynaecological training and knowledge for the work (1938, 152). Not surprisingly, Haire had the same view and Sanger in her autobiography made another implicit criticism of nurse-run clinics in her comment that Marie Stopes' clinic 'proved popular, although instruction given by a midwife was limited to mothers who had at least one child' (1938, 296). No such restrictions applied in Haire's daringly advanced clinic where contraceptive advice was 'given, on request, by one of the medical staff, to any woman whose health or other circumstances render it advisable'.[14]

When the three-storey centre opened in October 1927, the Malthusian League,[15] despite their past quarrels with Haire over their clinic, generously announced the 'successful operation' of the 'Sunlight Centre' which 'is intended only for poor patients and no fees are charged.' There were antenatal, infant care and sunlight departments and they also taught contraceptive techniques to doctors 'for a small

---

14 In contrast, Sanger was advised in 1916 to 'avoid unnecessary antagonism' by asking prospective clinic patients to declare they were married and this was considered the norm: Family Planning Association of New South Wales services were restricted to married or engaged women until 1974 when the FPA (NSW) Board resolved that a spouse's consent was not needed for any clinic procedure.

15 In late 1927 the Malthusian League was disbanded with a stylish dinner because the Drysdales considered their work was done and they were no longer prepared to fund it (Ledbetter 1976, 229).

fee'. After reading about the centre in the League's *The New Generation*, Norman Himes sent Haire a congratulatory letter in January 1928 with a request, saying that he was 'preserving literature on all the important institutions dealing with birth control' and would see that selected American university libraries received copies of these papers which were very seldom kept. He asked Haire to send 'six copies of each of your leaflets, papers of explanation stating your purposes etc' and any future materials. Himes said flatteringly that the clinic would feature in his book on the work of the English clinics. Haire sent a card from the newly opened centre but said they had not yet produced any literature.

The centre was welcoming and well organised: a nurse lived on the top floor and, on four afternoons a week, two female doctors gave advice to mothers who could also bring their babies for treatment with 'artificial sunlight'. In March 1928 Haire told Havelock Ellis the good news about the clinic which had 'a huge number' of sunlight patients (inviting him to see this treatment) and a slow increase in the patients seeking contraception after they sent cards about the clinic to doctors in the London area. They used the sunlight lamp in an attempt to prevent rickets, a vitamin-D-deficiency disease that was prevalent in children in slum areas which stunted growth and caused narrowing of the pelvic bones and made childbirth dangerous. The clinic had a ground floor reception office, an area for prams (as the patients often had several children) and a large waiting room where patients could sit and play records or have tea, milk and snacks. Children were given toys to play with and volunteers minded them while the mothers saw the doctor.

Haire provided a friendly atmosphere and many patients came regularly and brought their friends who became 'enthusiastic propagandists' for their work. The waiting room was decorated with a mural and a slogan which gave a new happy ending to an old nursery rhyme and suggested the possibility of birth control:

> There was an old woman who lived in a shoe
> She had so many children she didn't know what to do
> Don't be like her. Ask the doctor for birth control advice.

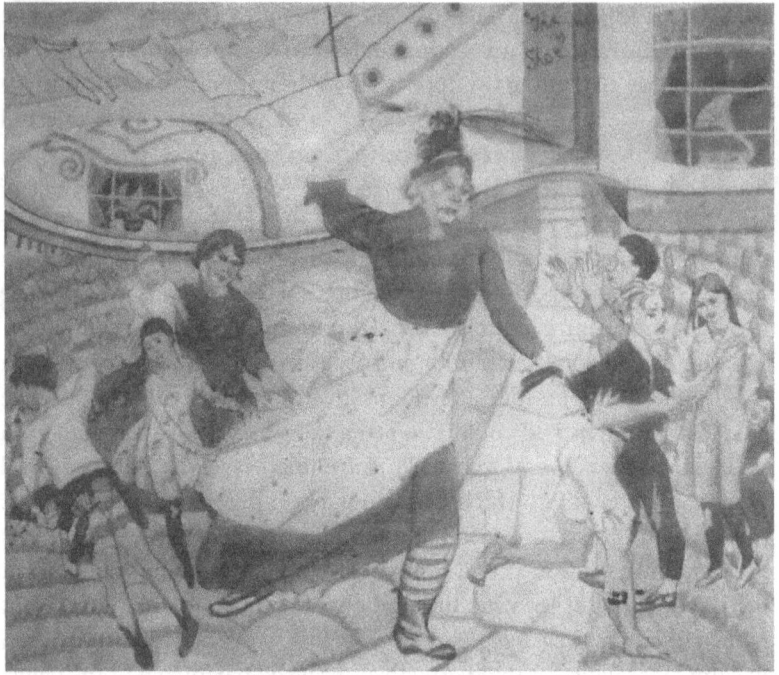

Figure 6.3. Old Mother Hubbard mural at the Cromer Welfare and Sunlight Centre. Haire Collection, Item 7.44.

Historian Peter Fryer quoted a pithier version the Malthusians had published in 1906 which moved into the realms of anti-family zealotry:[16]

> There was a young woman who lived in a shoe
> She had no children: She knew what to do!

Haire would have liked this explanation for the nursery rhyme's origins in *The annotated mother goose*: Parliament was the 'old woman' who lived in the 'shoe' of the British Isles, who 'didn't know what to do' with the 'many children' in its far-flung empire.[17] It was an apt analogy

---

16 Fryer (1965, 255–56). A similarly overenthusiastic slogan was proposed in the 1970s by Wendy McCarthy, the Education Officer of FPA New South Wales: 'Contraception on every conceivable occasion.' It was never used.

17 Baring-Gould (1967, 85–86).

which also applied to Haire who came from the antipodes, was unruly and knew exactly what to do. Haire wrote a thinly disguised begging letter in *The Times* on 7 August 1928[18] saying that his centre gave free treatment and did not receive any financial help from public authorities. Half of Haire's patients were referred by doctors in private practice or in hospitals, or from lunatic asylums after patients were discharged as 'cured', but this vital work was always threatened with the possibility of closure and Haire asked for Himes' help on 27 July because 'the need is urgent'. Himes said on 3 August he would see what he could do but the needs of his Boston centre were also great.

Ivan Crozier claimed (2001, 308) that 'Haire was known to be "gay-friendly", as well as providing abortions to the poorer classes at affordable rates, for instance at the Cromer Street Welfare Clinic'. Haire did not provide abortions there; he would have risked deregistration and jail and his pioneering clinic could have been closed, the whole birth control crusade put at risk if he *had* performed illegal abortions.[19] Nor could he risk being seen as 'gay-friendly'. The myth that Haire was an abortionist or had 'made a fortune from abortion clinics' was very persistent.[20]

Haire would have been committing professional suicide to take such risks and there was no need to because his rejuvenation patients were providing him with a very lucrative income. *The Triad*, an Australian magazine which media analyst Henry Mayer said was filled with 'not

---

18   Haire's letter about the Cromer Welfare and Sunlight Centre was in response to *The Lancet*'s 31 December 1927 report of the Society for the Provision of Birth Control Clinics, which ran nine clinics, in London (Walworth and Salford) and Birmingham, Cambridge, Glasgow, Manchester, Oxford and Wolverhampton, and saw 13,022 'new cases' and 17,228 'return cases'.

19   In *Sex talks* (1946, 161), Haire responded to accusations of hypocrisy for refusing to perform abortions while supporting law reform. He said it would be foolish to aid a few 'unfortunate girls' and which carried risks of imprisonment and 'bringing my work of enlightenment to a sudden end'.

20   Alexander (1989, 364, fn 63) thought the 'defamatory whisper' was in a letter from Joe Ackerley to William Plomer. Alexander told me that even if he 'could lay hands on the letter, it would prove nothing but that Ackerley had heard and believed some of the many stories about Haire'.

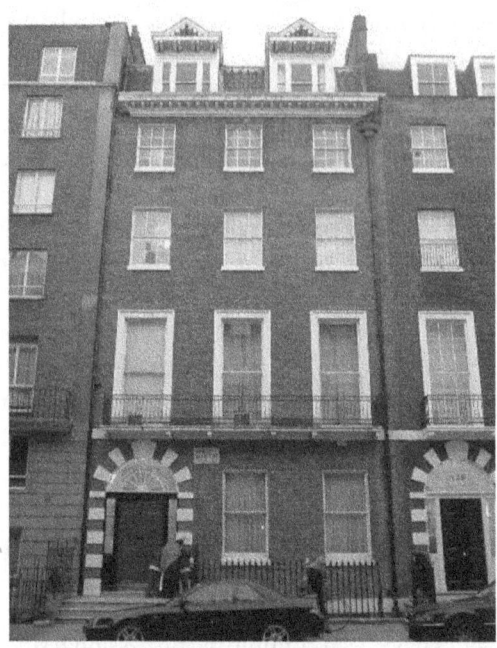

Figure 6.4. 127 Harley Street London where Haire lived and worked. John Wyndham took this photograph in November 2006. In Haire's time, his nameplate was the only one at the front door but in 2006 there were eight.

very inspiring articles [that] concentrated largely on style', commended Haire in January 1927 for 'successfully rejuvenating people by Steinach's methods'. In the May issue, Richard Davie praised Haire for doing 'great work in the cause of civilisation'. Haire, he wrote, was a 'vigorous and colourful man' who 'burned with a hard gem-like flame', bringing 'vigour and enthusiasm to Harley Street!' where he specialised in obstetrics, gynaecology and sex psychology and spent his life 'writing, organising, preaching' about birth control and eugenics. It had required great courage 'to dash around England defying prudes and prelates' by advocating birth control, to 'startle sentimental philanthropists in America' by saying that their activities were anti-social because they 'encouraged the unfit' and to support sterilisation. He obviously enjoyed the whirl of activity, the opposition, the controversies and the struggle to overcome indifference. Davie also admired Haire's 'quiet' voice and manner and his 'twinkling eyes' which he saw as the 'visible sparkling of vitality.' While Haire had quiet moments, he could also be boisterous, loud and earthy and, as a result of his voice training and acting experience, his words 'would be heard above all the others in theatre foyers and he was left off the invitation lists for art gallery openings' (Wallace Dawson 1998).

Haire, in his 20 September 1927 letter to Sebastian Sprott, mentioned 'some marvellous adventures in three countries' and then delivered his really exciting news: 'Just before Xmas I am moving to 127 Harley Street. I have bought the lease of a house[21] and spent my few remaining shekels in the purchase of some delightful lacquer. Three rooms are to be completely Chinese, including my bedroom which will be perfect harlotry!'

Haire had rented premises in several Harley Street locations since 1921 but now he was able to buy the lease of a six-storey home-office in this medical enclave in London's West End[22] which is so desirable that 'Harley Street' is an adjective, with 'Harley Street specialists' charging inflated 'Harley Street fees'. The lowliest inhabitants were suburban doctors who rented a room one afternoon a week but Haire now joined the high-ranking specialists whose front doors had only one brass plate or none.

He, like the house, presented a conventional exterior but inside the safety of this new sanctum he could be himself and indulge his taste for interior design. His choice of a Chinoiserie décor could have been to shock people, to assert his difference, to show he had travelled and appreciated Asian art or because he had heard about 'Queen Mary's Chinese Chippendale Room'[23] in Buckingham Palace and thought it

---

21 Letter from Haire to Sprott (1927) SP.

22 Harley Street is owned by Baroness Howard de Walden, 73, who is the fifth richest women in *The Sunday Times* Rich List 2010 after inheriting 92 acres of central London, now worth £1400 million; in 2008 the landlady, who is a devout Catholic, outlawed 'Lifestyle' abortion clinics in the street. In 1939 people paid around £10,000 for a 999-year lease for one of these Harley Street properties and probably £15,000 for one like Haire's with a lift.

23 Wendy Moonan (2008) gave details: In 1926 the artist Richard Jack painted

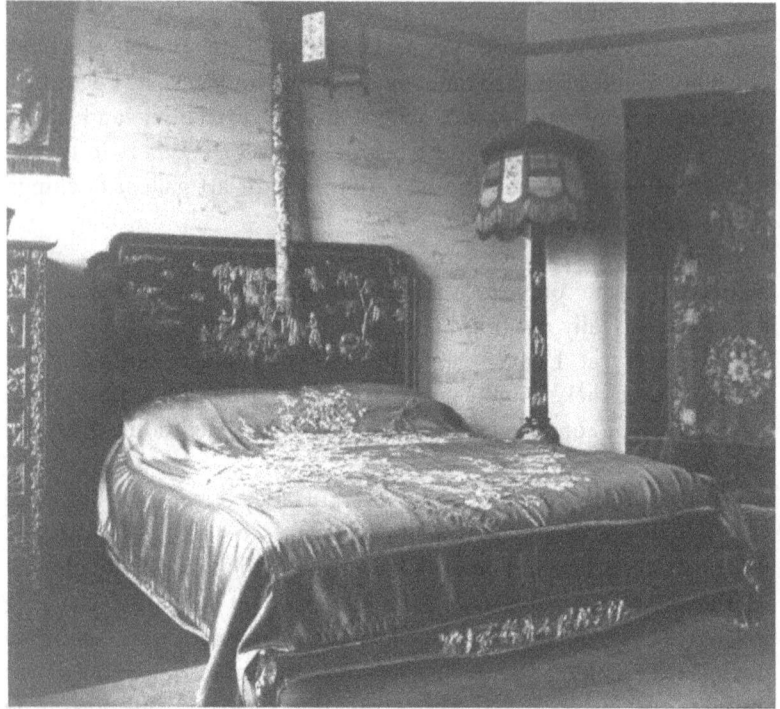

Figure 6.5. Haire's vast Chinese bed.

would be amusing to renew a once fashionable vogue.

His bedroom had a huge Chinese bed, 'big enough for three', and he sent photographs of it as a greeting or invitation to his friends.[24] Four decades after receiving one of these cards Hans Lehfeldt spoke about his friend's hospitality and the work Haire did at 127 Harley Street with its support staff of a butler, chauffeur, several maids and a Viennese cook plus secretaries and a nursing sister. Haire's patients were 'transported

---

'Queen Mary's Chinese Chippendale Room' in Buckingham Palace, an interior that combined Chinoiserie objects with Chinese antiques. The wallpaper was adapted from a Chinese silk pattern and the furniture was covered with vintage Chinese textiles. The combination was 'ravishing'.

24 Hans Lehfeldt showed members of the Hirschfeld Society this Christmas card Haire had sent him (Ralf Dose, 10 November 2000).

by wheelchair' in a lift to the top floor consulting rooms which had gynaecological instruments 'for carrying out sexological operations such as transplantation of glands and artificial insemination' (Lehfeldt 1991). He also had a garage for his Rolls Royce in the mews behind his house with accommodation above the garage for the chauffeur.

He was keen to show the house to his friends. One evening, Haire saw Havelock Ellis at a Film Society evening but, as usual, Haire slept through most of the film and snored so loudly that he'd had to apologise to the person next to him who sharply poked him in the ribs. He mentioned this on 9 March 1928 when he invited Havelock Ellis to visit 'any day except Wednesday', offering to 'send the car' to collect him and take him home. Havelock Ellis arranged to visit in July but had to cancel when he was confined to bed with a 'sharp attack of lumbago' and suggested it would be better if Haire called on him.

Ethel Mannin was impressed by her visit and in 1930 wrote about the consulting room's silver ceiling and wall hangings of 'exquisite Chinese embroideries on silk'. The dining room was even more exotic, with 'highly coloured dragons writhing like vorticism-gone-mad all over the ceiling'. There were silk tapestries and almond trees in blossom were painted on the drawing-room ceiling. It was 'all done superlatively well' and the bathroom was the only room to escape this decoration.

William Plomer (1958, 37–38) was sarcastic about the décor after he visited in 1935, noting that 'The door was opened by an uncommonly large and handsome butler' and after waiting briefly in a room of 'impersonal opulence' he was ushered into a coffin-like lift and 'fired off' to one of the upper floors. Haire greeted him and led him into a room which 'seemed hardly like a consulting room, unless he was a sorcerer as well as a sexologist'. It was 'furnished in bad Chinese made-for export style' and seemed like an opium den or 'the setting for a melodramatic film' with 'excessively carved furniture and screens, the joss sticks burning in a big porcelain vase before an image of Buddha, the bronze sconces in the form of dragons, from the mouths of which dangled the dried and spiky skins of globefish, enclosing electric lights'.

The house was beautifully furnished with a grand piano and it was 'absolutely the ultimate', according to a guest who said that one of Haire's

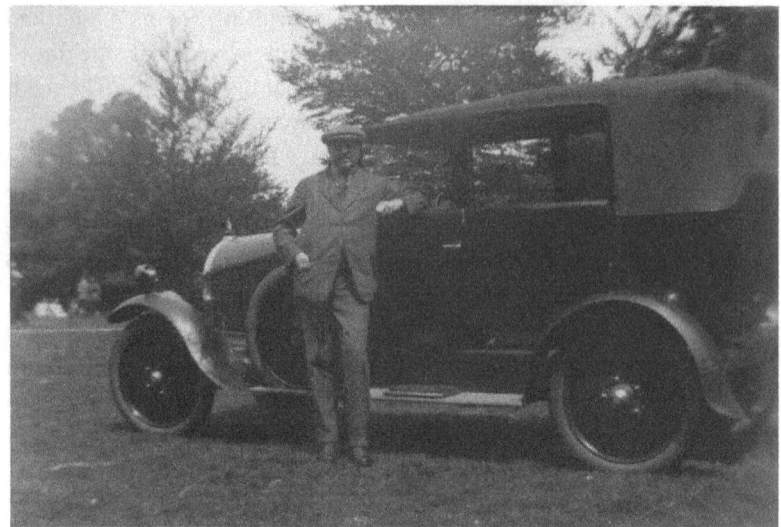

Figure 6.6. Norman posing beside his Rolls Royce – a chauffeur always drove.

soirées was attended by the Princess Royal. Haire complained that she had only commented 'what a pretty piano' (Fink 2002) but, even so, few hosts entertain royalty or can say they live next door to Lord Moran 'who is Winston Churchill's personal doctor and one of the leaders in the medical profession in Great Britain', and who caused a great stir in the House of Lords by giving statistics on the incidence of VD in the British Armies of Occupation.

In August 1939, a month before the war started, the *London Evening Standard* ran a profile of this street in which 'only great men like Lord Horder keep the house for themselves: perhaps run a country house too'. Haire was 'great' in this sense but the journalist was only interested in Haire's exotic décor:

> Probably the strangest rooms in the street are those at 127, occupied by Dr Norman Haire, the stoutly built advocate of a freer outlook on sex, who loves Oriental things, and from whose ceilings hang painted Chinese lanterns, glimmering on eastern pottery and paintings on the walls. (Barker 1939, 7)

Settled in his new premises, Haire was busily editing a new book to refute the claims made in *Medical views on birth control*, which was a compilation of well-known doctors' views, edited by Sir James Marchant, a Presbyterian minister and 'a distinguished and indefatigable opponent of birth control'. Haire had pleaded with Havelock Ellis to contribute an article to the book or to write a review but he did neither. Haire's requests were altruistic but he always felt Havelock Ellis regarded them as 'importunate'. In a medical history of contraception, the distinguished gynaecologist Sir John Peel (1964, 140) singled out Haire for praise and Marchant for censure: Haire's paper was 'the only one to rise above the level of mediocrity' in a special 1923 contraception issue of *The Practitioner*[25] while the book edited by Marchant – a symposium by nine eminent doctors published in 1926 – 'managed to achieve an even more uniform level of banality'. This was introduced by Sir Thomas Horder as 'the sort of scientific enquiry that the subject needs', but most of the writers opposed birth control and did not even adopt the very moderate position advocated by Lord Dawson. Peel said these two volumes (in 1923 and 1926) were fairly typical of much of the medical discussion of contraception during the 1920s.

Dr CP Blacker, a psychiatrist who became the Secretary of the Eugenics Society, expressed eugenic concerns about contraception in his book in 1926 so the objectivity of his review of Marchant's book in *The Lancet* on 28 May is surprising. He described the contributors as ranging from 'cautiousness to open opposition' and criticised the book because the questions patients ask their doctors remained 'not only unanswered but practically unraised. It can be taken as certain that this is very far from being the last word the medical profession will have to say on birth control'. He was right and Haire responded by editing *Some more medical views on birth control*, a collection of essays by ten 'moderate and well balanced advocates of Birth Control' including former British Medical Association (BMA) president Sir James Barr, Scottish surgeon Sir William Arbuthnot Lane, psychoanalyst MD (David) Eder, and

---

25 Haire sent it to Havelock Ellis on 27 April 1927 because, although it did not contain anything that would be new to him, it was 'an achievement to have got it published in a respectable journal like *The Practitioner*'.

birth control doctor Janie Hawthorne. The contributors were respected medical 'names': four doctors with experience in birth control clinics – Aletta Jacobs (Holland), Hannah Stone (America), Janie Hawthorne and himself (Britain); two well-known birth control advocates – Arbuthnot Lane and James Barr; and five who had not taken a prominent part in the debate – Aleck Bourne,[26] David Eder, Hamblin Smith (a criminologist), Charles R Goddard (in public health) and FAE Crew (a professor of biology and genetics).

Marchant's elderly contributors had little experience in contraceptive practice; Haire commented that Marchant did not 'accurately describe the goods he [had] to offer' because the medical profession had three views on birth control: those in favour, those against and those in the middle. Haire identified himself as a rationalist ('I attempt to base my philosophy of life on reason and not on superstition') and a hedonist ('I aim at achieving as much happiness as possible for others and for myself'). Although he scoffed about the supernatural, he deplored the intolerance expressed by advocates and opponents of contraception, saying that some birth control advocates heaped abuse on the Roman Catholic Church, while Roman Catholics often hurled extremely insulting epithets onto these advocates. He acknowledged Stopes' virtues[27] but not her claim to have received a spiritual revelation about birth control.

Halliday Sutherland also invoked religion to prove that contraception was physically harmful in his book *Birth control: a statement of Christian doctrine against the Neo-Malthusians,* and the Archbishop

---

26 Bourne, a Fellow of the Royal College of Obstetricians and Gynaecologists, became a hero in 1938 when he risked a 20-year jail term by informing police that he had performed an abortion on a 14-year-old rape victim. He was charged with procuring an abortion and acquitted in the *Rex v. Bourne* abortion trial that changed the case law on abortion in Britain, and, when news of Bourne's acquittal reached the *BMA* conference at Brighton, the 'doctors rose and cheered for minutes on end' (Simms 1975, 712, quoting London's *Evening Star* 20 July 1938).

27 Haire said Stopes was 'one of the most distinguished women of our age. Brilliantly clever, of world-wide repute as a palaeontologist, she, more than anyone else – except perhaps, Margaret Sanger – has made it possible for decent people to take part in an open discussion of Birth Control'.

of Canterbury wrote a preface for *Conception control* written by the distinguished gynaecologist Lady Florence Elizabeth Barrett. Haire commented: everyone would scoff if a dentist wrote a book 'after having received a revelation from the Deity on the subject of pyorrhoea', or a book on artificial sunlight had a preface from the Chief Rabbi, or a book had the title *Alcohol: a statement of Mohammedan doctrine against the froth-blowers*', yet 'nobody seems surprised by the analogous antics' of birth control opponents. He took issue with those who opposed contraception by rationalising that those most in need of it were so 'careless and thriftless' that they would not use it even if they knew about it. He found it amazing that Sir Arthur Newsholme (formerly Britain's Chief Medical Officer) took this view (Marchant 1926, 159) and Haire said that any doctor who worked at clinics for the poor could testify it was 'diametrically opposed to the facts'; the 'poor mothers' who visited his clinic were 'pathetically eager' to safeguard their health and their family's welfare by avoiding 'excessive motherhood.'

Noting that people who extolled the 'transcending joys' of large families were generally careful 'not to have their own quiver too full', Haire wrote, as one of 'those who *know* what being one of a large family means', to correct the myths made by 'those who only *theorize* about it'. Haire did not explicitly mention the link between class and the birthrate, although in 1917 H Scott Bennett, a socialist and the first notable Australian-born freethinker (Osborne 1979), examined this in *Birth control and the wage earner*. Bennett made the point that employers want cheap labour, military men want cannon fodder, politicians want voters, priests want parishioners and doctors want obstetric patients and they all commend 'rapid multiplication amongst the poorer classes' because 'Foxes think large families among the rabbits highly commendable', as Thomas Nixon Carver, Professor of Political Economy at Harvard, 'wisely and wittily remarked'. Perhaps Haire feared that a class analysis would alienate the conservative medical profession just as most Australian women in the 1890s did not want to harm their fight for the vote by supporting birth control.[28] This was

---

28 Brettena Symth bravely advocated votes for women and birth control and, to do so, had to form her breakaway Australian Women's Suffrage Society.

closest he came to discussing politics: 'Birth control is *not* a panacea for all evils; but ... no plan, without it, can hope to ameliorate the present miserable condition of a large proportion of humanity, or to achieve the increase of individual and racial health and happiness, towards which all but those of the meanest, or most perverted, intelligence must aim'.

Haire's chapter is the longest and most interesting one in the book but while some contributors may have found his revelations too personal, Sir William Arbuthnot Lane and Professor FAE Crew, Director of Animal Breeding at the University of Edinburgh, also raised contentious issues. Lane predicted that:

> The discovery of a thoroughly reliable preventative, or an abortifacient which will involve no risk to health or to life, will act like a bomb-shell, dissipating old ideas and customs, and altogether modifying and altering the lives and habits of the people ... the reign of cant and hypocrisy and the influence of Mother Grundy are going to cease abruptly, with probably an immense addition to the happiness, health and well-being of the community and the world in general.

Crew was similarly frank in his comments:

> I regard the sex relationship as a need, as a source of legitimate pleasure, as the most basic, the most beautiful, of functions ... Christianity, as often taught, condemns the joys of the body ... Certain Churches have taught that ... all matters of sexual intercourse are but carnal lusts to be ruthlessly condemned. The state of virginity ... even after marriage has been exalted; and it is held that copulation is polluting ... It is a matter of surprise really that the reproduction function has successfully withstood, not only the dysgenic forces of industrialism, but also the insistent condemnation of churchmen ... It is such teaching as this that has destroyed the innocence and the joy of sexual intercourse in Western civilization, and has endowed us with a legacy of repressions and morbidities, for it has prevented man gaining a knowledge of the sexual arts and has hidden from him any real appreciation of female sexual psychology ... In this teaching the old and the powerful have found an escape from their prison of deep-rooted jealousy of youth.

Crew suggested it would be easier to devise adequate contraception 'than to breed a race of asexual humans' and warned 'that the contraceptive should be chemical rather than mechanical', it should not offend and it 'should be used by the woman'. He concluded that the time would come when all churches would sanction contraception to make life on earth 'as magnificent as the postulated life hereafter'. Perhaps he had no fears about retribution from his university because his laboratory had just won a lucrative American grant to study the effectiveness of spermicides.[29]

I could not find any outraged responses to this strident censure of the harm done in the name of religion, where Crew's comments outdid Haire's. They were both candid about sex, and Haire once said that 'descriptions of coitus in sex books leave the reader informed on every point except why anyone should ever want to do what is described'.[30] Haire gave a sensible response to his critics' unreasonable and unrealistic demands for perfection in the matter of contraceptives when he said:

> They will apparently be satisfied with nothing less than an absolutely foolproof method, which can be used by a person without any intelligence yet yield 100% of success. It must not entail a visit to a doctor; the woman must be able to choose it herself without any special fitting; it must require no expense, no manipulation, no need for cleanliness, no care or trouble of any sort. It must under no conceivable circumstances be able to cause any harm.

He meant Stella Browne who complained about the lack of birth control methods which were 'generally applicable, non-injurious, aesthetically adequate, entirely safe, and cheap.' Haire commented in *Some more medical views of contraception* that no such utopian standards are required for glasses or false teeth and said it would be better to ask whether more harm was done by using contraception than by not using it.

---

29   Borell (1987) and Soloway (1995) gave details of the 1926 visit by Sanger and RL Dickinson to ask FAE Crew to develop a contraceptive research program; in 1929 he received a three-year American grant of $3000 to supervise Cecil Voge, a chemist who worked in his Edinburgh laboratory.
30   Craig (1963, 94) quoting Haire.

The Lancet gave a positive review of the book and three others on birth control on 14 July 1928, which is not surprising because the anonymous reviewer *was* Haire – the medical journal demanded anonymity but *The Saturday Review* did not and he had signed his name to similarly worded reviews the previous May. In the *Los Angeles Times* on 23 December, Lillian C Ford seemed to have paid little attention in her review because she called it 'a group of essays by celebrated European doctors on the subject of birth control, most of which are in its favour.' Ernest R Groves, an American sociology professor who had had to read a 'mutilated' version 'to protect it from censorship', regretted that the 'most valuable' sections on birth control methods were deleted. Rather than criticising the censors, he complained that the emasculated version was 'loosely constructed' with 'much repetition.' He regarded the most impressive thing about the book was its call for a 'thorough-going untrammelled, non-partisan investigation of common birth control practices and the discovery, if such information can be obtained, of their effect upon the body and the marriage relationship.' As the authors were each responsible for their own contributions, repetition was inevitable but, as Groves indicated, the book's call for a united approach was an important advance, even though the call remained unanswered for many years.

Haire reviewed Ludovici's book *The night-hoers, or the case against birth control and an alternative* in *The Saturday Review* on 5 May 1928 and, again, anonymously in *The Lancet* 'advising everybody', whether pro or contra, to read it because, 'in spite of its outstanding faults,' it was 'the best book against birth control.' Haire then considered *Parenthood: design or accident?* by 'Michael Fielding' (really Dr Maurice Newfield) and found it equally good, particularly the chapter on methods, which was 'sounder, more likely to be of practical value to the average married couple than anything I have seen in any other popular book of the sort'. He praised the author for calling 'a spade a spade' without being offensive or 'going into lyrical ecstasies', but he was annoyed because Newfield had hidden behind a pseudonym in fear that his medical colleagues or the General Medical Council might disapprove. Haire felt he was excessively cautious because there were many books *condemning* contraception by doctors who had used their own names and no action had been taken against them. He mentioned Dr Halliday Sutherland and Dame Mary Scharlieb, a gynaecologist who 'prophesied that "masturbation à deux" (contraception) would lead to degeneracy and effeminacy'.[31]

On 8 June 1928 *The Times* gave a report of the influential Animal Defence and Anti-Vivisection Society's public meeting to protest about the London visit by Serge Voronoff known in the press as the 'monkey-gland' doctor; they deplored his practice of grafting sex glands 'from live monkeys into men, women and children', calling it 'an offence against morality, hygiene and decency'. Haire was a conspicuous interloper in a 'sex starved' and 'peculiar looking' audience who 'nearly mobbed' him for casting a dissenting vote. In response to their claims that the testicle-donor's traits would transfer to the recipient, he scoffed 'nobody hesitates to eat milk or butter or beef for fear that they might come to resemble a cow' or feels that if a Boy Scout's donation of blood is used for an old lady she 'will develop a desire to go scouting'.[32]

The *British Medical Journal* wrote an editorial about Voronoff's 'gland grafting' on 24 March: a Surgeon Rear-Admiral was highly critical and Haire fought back, saying that the admiral had 'clearly written under a complete misapprehension of the nature of the various testicle-grafting operations'. He risked alienating the medical profession by writing that it was curious that British doctors seemed to know so little about the various rejuvenation operations which he said were widely practised elsewhere and 'those of us who have carried out the operations in a considerable number of cases are convinced that if one chooses one's cases wisely one often does get remarkable results. And it is important to emphasise the fact that the improvement which often follows the operation is not exclusively, or even predominantly, sexual'.

Haire travelled to Copenhagen in July to attend the congress where the World League for Sexual Reform (WLSR) was born, the 'child' of Magnus Hirschfeld. Atina Grossmann (1995, 38) described the delegates

---

31 Scharlieb, quoted in Rose (1992, 132, 255, fn 9).

32 Haire's article on rejuvenation appeared in *The Realist* (May 1929, 120–20), Macmillan's 'new journal of scientific humanism' which only lasted a year.

as 'a motley crew of sex reformers from around the world' – radicals and conservatives, professionals and lay workers – who presented 48 papers on birth control and sexual reform, emphasising law reform. However, in two concessions to international cooperation, it was silent about abortion and socialism. Haire agreed to be the Secretary of the WLSR's congress in London the following year.

Despite these responsibilities, he agreed when Norman Himes suggested he should make an American lecture tour. On 19 July he told Himes that he had hired an American manager and that he would probably make a three-month tour, a month after the congress. Himes sent a list of contacts on 3 August and suggested the manager should hire the Boston Symphony Hall (which seats 2600) and arrange for Haire to have a Harvard Union debate with 'some fool' because 'only a fool' would be unwise enough to 'oppose you'. Haire also asked for Sanger's help but the tour plans evaporated, which was just as well because for many months the congress was to dominate his life.

It wasn't all work and he spared time to have his caricature – shown on the cover – drawn by Edmond X Kapp, a troubled Jewish artist who illustrated the defining features of his famous sitters – an uplifted conductor's baton for Sir Adrian Boult, and the Duke of Windsor, dressed in top hat and gloves, fiddling with his bow tie. He identified Haire's chief passions – sexology, the theatre, and food – by showing him reading theatrically from a recipe with instructions for cracking eggs to make a 'sex omelette'. The curators of the Barber Collection at the University of Birmingham provided me with two drafts of this 1929 Haire sketch from their collection of 240 Kapp drawings (Wenley 2011). Yvonne Kapp, the artist's young first wife, gave these sad details about his life: as a German-speaking officer in the British army in World War I he had been sent to gather intelligence from a frontline foxhole and, when this was over-run, he survived for six weeks on tinned food until he was rescued. After the war he wanted to be an artist but two art schools rejected him on the ground that teaching would destroy his unique style. He quickly made his name but hated his sketches and called them 'stunt books of freak drawings' that commanded 'false prices and a press reputation with its false values'. He described the work as meretricious: 'clever, good-taste trash' (Kapp 2003, 123).

As well as posing for his portrait, Haire played a small part when Ivor Montagu directed a cast of his friends[33] in a 1928 silent slapstick movie called *Bluebottles* (British slang for police) which used innovative special effects. The stars were Charles Laughton and Elsa Lanchester and it was adapted from a story by HG Wells.[34] Montagu said Laughton looked 'gleefully murderous' and Haire, with his shirt tail hanging out of his trousers like a New York gangster,[35] 'carried away a body quite effectively'.

Haire was concerned about the issue of homosexuality and argued that it should be excluded from conferences because it might alienate mainstream audiences and impede sexual reform. On 24 November 1927, when 'Dr Leunbach of Copenhagen' issued a statement about the proposed activities of the new WLSR, Haire asked Hirschfeld whether they would cover all aspects of sexual life or only homosexuality. He thought it would be 'a pity' to limit itself to the latter and begged Hirschfeld to ask for definite details, as he intended to do, before giving his support. Hirschfeld was 'very much interested' and 'very grateful' for Haire's 'friendly letter' and hoped to be able to greet him '*very soon* as a member of the [WLSR's] organising committee'.

An ironic touch was provided by Wilfred Blunt (not the womaniser Wilfred Scawen Blunt but a blushing young man who sought help for his homosexuality) whose family doctor had referred him to 'our man in Harley Street'. The specialist 'could hardly disguise either his disappointment or his astonishment' to learn that the 29-year-old Blunt was a virgin and, while 'a long and costly' treatment was possible – £600 was mentioned – the doctor did not really recommend it because it was not guaranteed to help or be permanent. Blunt (1983, 209–10) learnt that he would probably have to learn to live with his disability,

---

33 Ivor Montagu was a socialist when he was at Cambridge University in 1924 and later became very active in the British Communist Party. He was a founder of the left-wing London Film Society and in the 1930s his wife Eileen was the Honorary Secretary of the Cromer Welfare and Sunlight Centre.

34 *Bluebottles* is one of six 1920s films re-released on video in 1996 by the British Film Institute. It is discussed by Montagu (1967, 20–21, 24).

35 The Shirt Tails were a 1840s New York gang who wore their shirts outside their pants and concealed weapons under their shirts (Asbury 2002, 20–21).

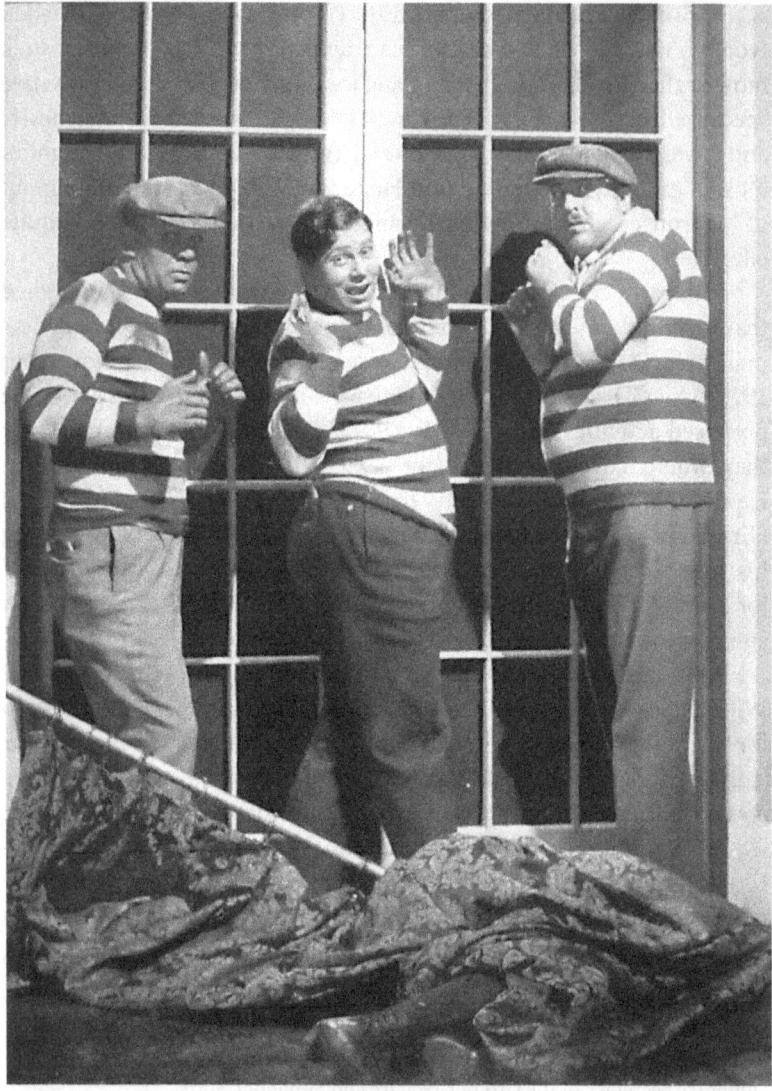

Figure 6.7. Still from Ivor Montagu's film *Bluebottles* (1928), Sergei Nolbandov (left), Joe Beckett (centre), Norman Haire (right), Elsa Lanchester (under curtain). Reproduced with permission of the Archive Trust of the Communist Party of Great Britain (1920–1991).

which, the specialist said, 'was not really odder, or rarer, than being left-handed, though far less socially acceptable. Perhaps more like being blind or deaf. Or, he added – rather charmingly, as if in an afterthought – a Jew (he was clearly one himself)'. If his specialist was Haire, Blunt had no idea he was also homosexual. An even stranger sequel concerned his brother, Sir Anthony Blunt, who was an art historian and Surveyor of the Queen's Pictures until he was unmasked as a Soviet spy. Although Anthony had been a practising homosexual for many years, Wilfred was not sure until, 'some time after the war', the middle-aged brothers 'exchanged confidences – curiously enough at a reception at Windsor Castle'. Such caution was required because 'until 1968, male homosexuals were treated not only as criminals by British law, but also as degenerates by the British public.'[36]

In his 8 November 1928 letter to Hirschfeld, Haire said he would be giving expert evidence the following day, with other protesters including Virginia and Leonard Woolf, Arnold Bennett and EM Forster,[37] in defence of Radcliffe Hall's *The well of loneliness* after the Public Prosecutor's decision to destroy all copies because it had discussed lesbianism. Havelock Ellis absented himself because his book *Sexual inversion* was 'convicted for obscenity' and his presence might aggravate the situation, and Bernard Shaw felt he was 'too immoral' to be a credible witness.[38] The editor of the *Sunday Express* said 'I would rather give a healthy boy or healthy girl a phial of prussic acid [cyanide] than this novel.' The writers who protested were not allowed to testify, the publisher was convicted and the remaining copies burned. Lesbianism was not against the law and attracted less censure than homosexuality

---

36   Blunt (1986, 249–50): 'Until 1968 the sexual act, even with a consenting adult in private, was a sexual offence'. Until 1861, sodomy had incurred the death penalty, though in the 19th century it was rarely carried out. It changed to 'penal servitude for life, or for not less than ten years', and remained so, theoretically, until 1968, when sex in private between two (not more) consenting males over the age of 21 was legalised in England and Wales. Scotland followed later and Northern Ireland in 1982.

37   The UK government's threat to ban books (including *Hymen: or, the future of marriage*) is quoted in *Virginia Woolf miscellany*, no 65, Spring 2004.

38   For details, see Tamagne (2004, vol 2, 155).

until the Radcliffe Hall case 'evoked a horrified public reaction' and 'exposed the contradictory assumption that knowledge of lesbian love was acceptable for an elect few but impermissible for the general public' (Rowbotham 2008, 446).

While these progressive individuals failed in this bid, they would soon pin their hopes on a newly formed body: the WLSR[39] which was founded by Magnus Hirschfeld and launched in Copenhagen on 3 July 1928. A year later, the WLSR congress in London received international acclaim and Haire helped to make this happen.

---

39 Dose (2003) gave details of the confusing WLSR congress numbering system: Hirschfeld called the 1921 congress the first so the four subsequent WLSR congresses became the second to fifth meetings. The League was born at the second congress in Copenhagen and launched in London at the third one.

7

ORGANISING THE 1929 CONGRESS

The congress was the major event in Haire's 1929 calendar but he had to juggle this with his correspondence, speeches and medical practice. On 18 February he contacted Norman Himes because he was unhappy about the American's review of his paper on contraceptive techniques at the 1926 International Congress for Sex Research in Berlin. Himes sent 'my dear Dr Haire' a placating reply; he had written the *New England Journal of Medicine* review on 3 January to alert American physicians to Haire's work and, although he described some statements as rather 'sweeping', he had also said it was 'first class' and 'should be read by every physician' describing Haire 'one of the best informed individuals' currently writing about contraception. Himes enclosed his damning review of James Cooper's book about contraception which must have pleased Haire who was 'not keen' on Cooper, the medical director of the American Birth Control League, because he was not as courteous as he would have wished and had a 'habit of forgetting to acknowledge his debts – not financial debts, but debts of *knowledge* transmitted to him'.

Haire thanked Himes for his reply and assured him that he felt no ill-will towards him because 'only fools are offended by criticism' and he must have assumed that it was safe to criticise the 'charming' RL Dickinson, the President of the American Gynecological Society. On his 1925 American tour, Haire had been impressed by Dickinson's description of the 'splendid work' at six leading hospitals in New York but, when he visited one of these hospitals, the staff knew nothing about a birth control clinic and Haire finally found the clinic's doctor who surreptitiously referred patients to his private practice and only saw six patients in six months. Haire liked Dickinson very much and admired his sincerity, vision and ideals but he felt that Dickinson was 'carried away by his own enthusiasm' and was 'not the man for details' with many of his achievements existing 'only in intention and in his imagination'. It is likely that Himes repeated this to Dickinson who was offended and from this date began to disparage Haire.

After starring in the Cambridge debate five years previously, Haire captivated the audience at Oxford University when he became the St John's Essay Society's most illustrious speaker. They often heard famous speakers such as Gilbert Murray but in 1929 they were dazzled by Haire whose three-hour and comprehensive exposition received 'intensive and appreciative attention' from an audience that was the largest in the Society's records. (*The history of the University of Oxford* vol. 8 1994, 99).

However, most of Haire's attention was focused on the congress and there were hundreds of well-wishers at the baptism of the newly formed WLSR[1] at its third congress in London from 8 to 14 September 1929. Haire played a vital role in its success and overcame huge obstacles with unflagging acumen, energy and skill, in collaboration with Dora Russell (née Black), a pacifist, progressive educator, prolific writer and a brave campaigner for birth control and sex reform who is now revered as a socialist feminist icon. She had had a privileged childhood and graduated with first class honours from Cambridge University in 1915. 'The very intellectual Miss Black' visited Russia shortly after the revolution and in the 1920s lived with Bertrand Russell in China. When she became pregnant, the philosopher who was 20 years her senior, divorced his first wife and, against her sexually liberated ideals, Dora married 'Bertie' in 1921.

She continued her writing and political activism and in 1923 went to court to defend a birth control pamphlet the police had seized and

---

1   Much of this information comes from the proceedings of the London congress (WLSR 1929), the Dora Russell Papers (DRP), the Margaret Sanger Papers (*MSP* – LC, MSP – NYU and MSP – Smith), the Institute for Sexual Science website Available: www.hirschfeld.in-berlin.de/institut/en/index1024_ie.html, the Magnus Hirschfeld Gesselschaft and the January 2003 issue of the *Journal of the History of Sexuality*. There was mirror image of the congress in Australia: the WLSR met in London from 8 to 14 September 1929 and, on 15 to 18 September 1929, the Australian Racial Hygiene Congress discussed similar topics in the rooms of the Royal Empire Society in Bligh Street Sydney. It was chaired by Sir Benjamin Fuller and Mrs Lillie Goodisson was the Organising Secretary. The RHA (NSW) published a 72-page report of the Congress which is listed at trove.nla.gov.au/work /21998922?versionId=26523352.

wanted to destroy as an obscene publication. It contained a diagram showing a woman how to insert a pessary and the court discussions centred on the finger in the illustration which 'might not be the finger of the woman concerned'. Such a thought had not crossed her mind; the emasculated pamphlet was permitted but it was of little use without the 'offensive' diagram. In 1924 she helped form the Workers' Birth Control Group[2] that adopted the slogan: 'It's four times as dangerous to bear a child as to work down a mine' (Russell 1983, 185).

Dora Russell and Norman Haire were delegates at Moll's 1926 International Congress for Sex Research in Berlin but Russell stressed that those on the left did not share the views of the sponsors. She and Haire were in sympathy with Moll's rival Magnus Hirschfeld and visited his Institute for Sexual Research where she marvelled at the institute's 'remarkable' records and the pictures on the stairway of homosexuals before and after treatment. This began a campaigning collaboration which lasted several years and worked well because both had theatrical flair, were fluent in German and French, and shared a passion for birth control and sexology. Ironically, the organiser of the 1926 congress was Albert Moll, a psychiatrist who claimed it was the world's first such *scientific* conference. This was a rebuff to his rival Magnus Hirschfeld who had opened the world's first Institute for Sexual Science in 1919 and whose 1921 International Meeting for Sexual Reform on a Sexological Basis deserved this credit.

Politics dogged the London congress from the start: on 19 October 1928 Haire told Russell that despite Havelock Ellis' fierce opposition to its being held in London, he was determined to 'go ahead quite enthusiastically in face of all opposition' although it would create much hostility, and they would 'be accused of all the perversions in Krafft Ebing'. A week later, the WLSR working committee gave their support and asked the pair to proceed because 'even a small and inglorious congress in London would be preferable to a bigger splash elsewhere.' Ellis wrote irritably to Margaret Sanger on New Year's Eve: 'I was

---

2 Russell (1977, 169, 173). Some other members of the group were Frida Laski, Joan Allen, Dorothy Thurtle, Leah L'Estrange Malone, Alice Hicks, Margaret Lloyd, Jenny Adamson, Stella Browne and Janet Chance.

consulted and was against its being held. But Haire has had his way. It will be, I expect, an All-Haire conference, which may be good for Haire, but perhaps not good for the cause'. His obstinacy was unkind and unwarranted. *Not* holding it would not have helped, just as you can't win a war by not fighting and, largely as a result of Haire's diplomacy, the congress attracted 500 delegates from 'almost every country in the civilized world.' Australian-style mockery of British reticence and the hijacking attempts by Havelock Ellis were implicit in Haire's speech of welcome: 'We English are so backward in respect of the free discussion of sexual problems, so notorious for sexual prudery and hypocrisy that the organisation of this congress was embarked on with great hesitation'.

Haire 'hated dealing with other people's money' so when he became the congress secretary he asked Dora Russell to be the treasurer. The two gifted organisers had to arrange publicity, attract speakers and delegates and find a venue. In November they rejected the BMA building although it would give a 'cachet of respectability' and then they considered the Friends Meeting House (wrong-sized rooms), the Little Theatre (too expensive), the Royal Academy of Dramatic Art (too dingy) and the London School of Economics. Haire decided that using LSE would not be possible after he had lunched with Bronislaw Malinowski, Professor of Anthropology at the LSE, who said the LSE's director (the economist and social reformer Sir William Beveridge) was 'madly conservative about sex' and that it would be counterproductive if he (Malinowski) or Harold Laski made an approach, and suggested their only chance of success would be if Dora Russell could get John Maynard Keynes to ask Beveridge.

They finally agreed to hire the imposing Wigmore Hall which has excellent acoustics and is an ultra-respectable, impressive yet intimate building, centrally located and close to transport. It was built in 1901 by the Bechstein Piano Company but the showrooms, concert hall and pianos in this 'enemy property' were 'arrested' in World War I.[3] The Hall's famous Arts and Crafts cupola over the stage, which shows humanity striving to reach the elevated realms of music, matched the WLSR's aims to uplift humanity, not by abolishing sexual morality, Haire said, but by

---

3 In 1916 Bechstein Hall was renamed the Wigmore Hall.

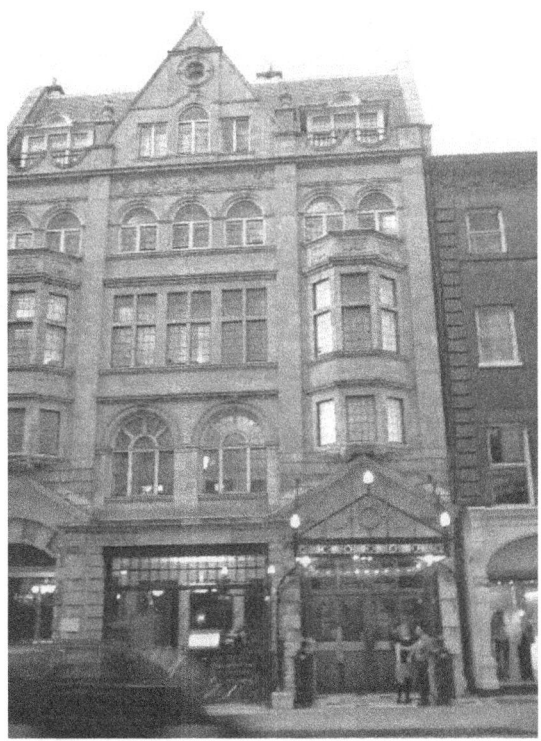

Figure 7.1. Wigmore Hall, London – the venue for the 1929 WLSR congress.

providing 'a new sexual ethic' which reflected 'scientific knowledge and social and economic circumstances' rather than an 'outworn' Biblical ethic which had been 'patched up' but had never been adequately or systematically revised.

In December 1928 Haire contacted notables from *Who's Who* and wrote to Sebastian Sprott urging him to join the WLSR and interest as his many of his friends as possible in the forthcoming congress (Haire to Sprott, 21 December 1928. SP). Within a month he received support from 'names' such as Clive Bell, Arnold Bennett, Alexander Carr-Saunders, Laurence Housman, Aldous Huxley, Ivor Montagu, JB Priestley, Lytton Strachey and Hugh Walpole.[4] By the first week in

---

4 Haire adopted the strategy of garnering high-level support, which Marie Stopes

January 1929, Haire and Russell had sent almost 1000 announcements that the WLSR would hold its next congress in London and they asked for support from intelligent people because sexual reforms were as important as economic or social reforms. Russell thought they needed help from a committee but Haire convinced her of the advantage of having volunteer helpers and a small executive because enthusiastic helpers worked well under direction but might become a hindrance if they became committee members. They followed his plan to become a two-person committee and choose people they knew and trusted as helpers.[5]

Robert Kerr, a socialist lawyer and editor of the Malthusian League's *The New Generation*, promised to give publicity if he and Stella Browne could give papers: his was 'The sexual rights of spinsters' and hers 'The right to abortion'. Haire sent Russell the news on 12 January, describing them as 'difficult people' who must not be allowed to cause strife. Their task as organisers was to take care not to offend helpers or those offering papers and to find a tactful way of escape, such as a time limit or slotting the paper into an inconspicuous position on the program. A week later Haire said he disliked Browne intensely but could not see how they could prevent her reading a paper: he reminded Russell it was 'Mr Kerr (not Dr and not Carr)', who suggested her paper. If handled tactfully, Browne and Kerr would give the congress publicity in *The New Generation* but if they felt offended they would attack the congress, or ignore it. He appreciated the importance of their proposed papers and ended his letter with the comment: 'I think that both abortion and the sexual problem for unmarried people will arouse just as much interest as Sex and Censorship'.

In her Stella Browne biography, Lesley A Hall (2011, 157) claimed this call for tactful management was evidence of 'Haire's Machiavellian paranoia', adding that 'there are no copies of Russell's responses' in her files. There is nothing sinister about this because Russell's files of the WLSR correspondence only contain the letters that Haire sent her and

---

had used so successfully in 1921, to overcome public reluctance.

5 Haire suggested these helpers: Miles and Dr Joan Malleson, Dr Douglas White, Dr Maurice Newfield, Captain E Broadwood and RB Kerr.

none of her replies. However, Russell appears to have tacitly approved of his plans to avoid strife because there was no mention of Browne or Kerr in his next letter, two days later. Haire thanked her for the 'names' and said it was 'splendid' that she managed to get endorsement from these notables; he hoped she could dine with him so they could discuss ways of securing publicity 'at length'. Haire had promised Julian Huxley he would ensure that if anyone offered papers on homosexuality none would be read and he had to find a tactful way to keep his promise.

Hall cited several of Stella Browne's contemporaries who said she was eccentric, highly neurotic or mad, and her habit of charting horoscopes was evidence of her irrationality. However, Hall gave no evidence to support her claim that Haire was paranoid, which is not surprising because he was a rationalist who wondered if some might find him 'too sane, normal and extroverted'. She criticised Haire for identifying and averting potential trouble. This deserved praise because his strategy demonstrated both his problem-solving skills and his careful attention to detail which ensured that the congress ran harmoniously and on track. Hall (2011, 118) described Haire as 'an Australian doctor who had come to England after the war and was determined to make himself a leading figure in the British sex reform movement'. She doesn't seem to like him.

When a 'food faddist' offered a paper, Haire sought Russell's advice on how to avoid accusations of autocratic decision-making. The Divorce Reform League's Rev. WF Geikie-Cobb agreed on 19 January to distribute 500 fliers as long as his own leaflets were distributed and, in order to get 'at the very least' 200 British delegates, they needed publicity in papers such as *The Spectator* and *The New Statesman* so Haire asked for Russell's help to 'wangle' this. They sent announcements to 8000 doctors because, Haire reasoned, 'the more money we get, the more publicity we can afford, and the greater will be the effect of the congress. The mere fact of being able to spend a lot of money on it will impress a lot of the people who are inclined to sit on the fence'. Psychiatrists had previously dominated the sexology field and the WLSR initially attracted a diverse group of professionals but Haire noticed a swing back towards medicine and commented to Russell on 27 January:

I don't know whether you will think I am biased, or stupid, in trying to get as many doctors in as possible. Nobody knows better than I do how stupid doctors are but they have very considerable value from the point of view of impressing the public. Also, if we can actually interest them, they can help very much in fostering a saner sexual outlook.

Haire went to Edinburgh on 25 January to try to get Professor Crew's support but Crew declined because he felt his participation in WLSR congress might ruin the one he was organising with Hirschfeld's rival Albert Moll. Haire promised to give Russell more details in confidence about this refusal and he continued to woo supporters and calm doubters. He took time off to debate whether 'the practice of contraception is unphysiological and a common cause of disease'; and, as the *British Medical Journal* reported on 23 February, Haire trounced his opponent Dr Halliday Sutherland by 24 votes to eight.

Dr Blacker sent a 'Strictly *Entre Nous*' warning to Julian Huxley on 18 February about 'Norman Haire's sexual reform congress':

> Before you have anything to do with it, read the complete statement of aims of the *Weltliga* [World League] as well as the watered-down version for British consumption. They come precious near advocating general free love. But we can discuss that when we meet.

Haire contacted Russell on 19 February after his trip to Berlin to see Moll. While there he had arranged to get help from other people, engaged a press cutting agent for the congress and asked Russell to send them a cheque for £2 and ask for a receipt. He warned her that Moll had been writing to friends in England 'abusing Hirschfeld' and suggesting that the WLSR was 'unduly interested in abnormalities'. He described Moll's suggestion as very astute but very unscrupulous because 'nothing else would have been so successful in frightening off English scientists'.

Haire's 79-year-old mother had died in Sydney on 20 February and, despite making him study medicine so he would be near her, she had had to travel to London to see him. Although he had worked closely with

Dora Russell for three years, he didn't tell her about his mother's death, instead showing her the letter he planned to send Julian Huxley to rebut Moll's allegations. Haire judged shrewdly that 'it would be bad tactics for us to meet this objection, except in cases where it is made. Where it *is* made, we must meet it most vigorously.' Haire sent Julian Huxley a long letter on 21 February to reassure him that homosexuality came 'within the purview of the League' and while it was '*one of* the special subjects for discussion' at an informal meeting of the League in 1921, 'It received very little attention at the Second Congress in Copenhagen', and would be totally excluded from the London congress. Haire said he had discussed this with Hirschfeld and Dora Russell before it was decided to hold the congress in England and they felt there were so many subjects of much greater general interest that they 'could find no room for sexual abnormalities'. All papers had had to fit in with the list of agreed subjects although Haire could not 'guarantee that everybody will speak and write as though no such word as "homosexuality" existed'. If Malinowski or Pitt-Rivers made some passing reference to homosexuality in a paper on anthropology, he 'would hardly be such a despot, or such a fool, as to forbid them to do so'. But he assured Huxley it would not be discussed and hoped that his detailed response would answer the doubts and questions of those who were in sympathy with the League but had hesitated to give it their support publicly. Haire pointed to the long list of supporters printed on the congress letterhead and said, 'You and I will be in quite respectable company'.

There was a flurry of exchanged letters and on 24 February CP Blacker warned his former teacher Julian Huxley that he had been very careful in all his comments about Stopes and Haire. He said enigmatically that he had 'verbally quoted' Haire's only remark about Stopes that did 'not verge upon the insulting' and in this way Blacker hoped to gratify them both. Although Bronislaw Malinowski and Julian Huxley planned to attend a rationalist dinner on 22 March, Malinowski thought they might not see each other so he wrote to Huxley who had passed on Haire's 21 February letter. Malinowski returned it to Huxley and added a note: 'I see from it and from several other sources that participation in the Congress will be absolutely on the right side of respectability. I think I shall be able to take your advice and send in my name.'[6]

The decision to exclude homosexuality from the congress was criticised by education reformer Cecil Reddie[7] in a pamphlet eulogising the BSSSP's first president, Edward Carpenter, who was openly homosexual – Reddie had hoped that the WLSR would follow Carpenter's lead. This exclusion was also condemned by lesbian feminist political activist and Melbourne University academic Sheila Jeffreys (1997, 186, 188) who praised the 1929 congress as 'the high point of sex reform in Britain' despite her belief that the WLSR's 'hidden agenda was the conscription of all women into intercourse with men.' Her claims of an anti-women conspiracy are just as ludicrous as claiming that the WLSR aimed to force all men to have sex with women and ignores the first of the League's ten liberal platform 'planks' which was to promote 'Political, economic and sexual equality of men and women'.

Haire returned from Paris on 2 April with news about Eugène Humbert, an anarchist Neo-Malthusian who had been jailed and, with his wife, had served another two years for spreading birth control propaganda. Haire told Russell that he was unsure whether Humbert had noble motives or 'was in it more for profit than *pour l'amour de Dieu*' but he conceded 'very likely some people say the same about me.'[8]

Haire paid the Medical Addressing company £5 to send letters to all 8000 doctors in London and sent Russell '*another* 8000 halfpenny

---

6 Malinowski did not attend the 1929 WLSR congress, probably because his book *The sexual life of savages in North-Western Melanesia* had irritated academic authorities and he wanted to wait until the fuss had subsided.

7 Sagarin (1975, 33) quoting Reddie.

8 David Glass (1936, 223-24) said that Humbert (the Secretary of the French Neo-Malthusian League) sold contraceptives and used the profit to fund his publications. He died in an air raid on the Amiens prison in 1944. Margaret Pyke, Secretary of the Family Planning Association, told the *BMJ* (1939, 308): '[A]n estimate of the abortion rate in France by M Eugène Humbert is 800 000 a year, as compared with 700 000 live births. This high rate is exactly what would be expected in a country where the practice of birth control is illegal'. Pyke was quoting figures in the survey Glass made for the Eugenics Society and published as *The struggle for population* in 1936.

stamps' and said that he, his secretary, his nursing assistant, a volunteer and a paid assistant were immersed in the congress but it was worth it. Their publicity received added cachet when it appeared in *The Lancet* on 20 April, not as a paid advertisement but as medical news: 'The Third International Congress of the World League for Sexual Reform would be held in London, under the presidency of Dr August Forel, Dr Havelock Ellis, and Dr Magnus Hirschfeld from 8 to 14 September'. The subjects for discussion were: marriage and divorce; birth control, abortion, and sterilisation; prevention of venereal disease and prostitution; sex and censorship; with a final day devoted to a miscellany of sexual reform papers. The congress was to be given in English, French, German and Esperanto and those wishing to read papers were asked to notify Dr Norman Haire, not later than 1 July. Readers were asked to send congress subscriptions and donations for preliminary expenses to the Hon. Treasurer, Mrs Dora Russell.

Haire saw *The Lancet*'s interest as a good sign that they were getting support from 'big names'. The *British Medical Journal* published a similar announcement on 27 April and the energetic pair continued to solicit donations from the rich and accept payment from exhibitors. When Israel Sieff, co-founder of the Marks & Spencer stores, promised his support, Haire paid a visit and asked Russell to write and ask him for 'a really good subscription'. She should say that a number of distinguished overseas Jewish sexologists would be coming and they wanted to receive them properly. They received some anonymous donations, £10 from both Sieff and HG Wells, and Haire asked if Russell would accept £5.5.0 from Bayer, the big German chemical people, to display their products. He added that there had been trade exhibits at the 1926 congress and he hoped to get six to ten exhibitors and use the money to subsidise a dinner for eminent people. They wanted to help Patrick Geddes, a pioneer urban planner, who could not afford to travel from Montepellier in France; on 29 January Haire had asked, 'Can't we touch Lord Melchett[9]

---

9 Alfred Mond, 1st Baron Melchett (1868–1930) was a British industrialist, politician, financier, Zionist and benefactor who in 1926 merged four companies into Imperial Chemical Industries (ICI). Haire had had a lunch meeting with him during the 1922 birth control conference.

or somebody so that we have money for such cases?' Haire listed other 'hard up' people they should not ask for money (including the elderly Aletta Jacobs and Professor VH Mottram[10]) and on 27 February provided the addresses of his 'sort-of-cousins' Madge Bolton and Julius Stamm asking Russell to 'write and touch' them, because his connection would make it difficult for him.[11] She should say they were expecting a number of scientists from Germany and wanted enough funds to entertain them decently and create a good impression; he said the very wealthy German-born Stamm was British by naturalisation and could 'help largely if you get on the right side of him'.

On 19 June Kegan Paul generously agreed to not charge for publishing the proceedings and also to donate royalty fees to the League. Haire told Russell the good news: 'Things have gone so marvellously that I feel that the Gods are preparing some horrible disappointment for us. It is really too good to be true'.

The next day he sent her the draft of another press announcement on the congress letterhead (which had to be frequently reprinted to accommodate its expanding list of supporters) and named the celebrity speakers from five European countries. The attendance fee was five shillings and all sessions were for WLSR members only; the membership cost £1.1.0. To add prestige and, in a sensible decision to protect Haire and Russell from criticism, the 22 June 1929 announcement was signed by the WLSR's key supporters.[12] Russell hoped Haire's 'excellent' letter would encourage 'ordinary' members because she didn't want the 'disappointment of only having distinguished people attending'. Haire gave her a plan of the hall on 28 June and proposed giving members booked seats so they would be easy to find. Haire asked the secretary

---

10 Patty Fisher, in her *Times* obituary for Mottram (1976, 16), called him a physiologist who specialised in nutrition and dietetics. He died at 93 and was an 'awe-inspiring' lecturer who wore 'bright blue shirts [in 1925!]'. Like Haire, he was amusing, wrote lucidly and was keenly interested in food.

11 Eugene Bolton and his wife Madge (née Isaacs) were members of the congress. *The Times* noted on 25 July 1925 that Bolton was the co-owner of a famous 17th-century painting by a Dutch artist.

12 The letter was signed by G Lowes Dickinson, JC Flügel, Julian Huxley, VH Mottram, AM Carr Saunders, CG Seligman and EA Westerman.

of the Labour Party at the London School of Economics to organise student volunteers and thought medical students might also help.

On 23 August Haire thanked Sanger for the news of her 'doings in Berlin' and said that if she gave him the date and details of her congress in Zurich he would do all he could to make it a success and would mention it at the London congress. He reminded her about sending a message for the congress and passed on a tip for hers: a lot of his friends in Paris had hired an English-speaking secretary and this might be a good plan for her. He had enjoyed their evening at the hotel and he looked forward to seeing her again when she was next in London, unless she could persuade a lecture agency to book him for a lecture tour before this. He would like to go if it could be arranged.

Two weeks before the congress opened, Haire still had not heard from Havelock Ellis and, in response to Haire's urgent telegram, Ellis delivered this devastating rebuff in a letter signed by '(Mrs) FL Cyon', his partner Françoise Lafitte-Cyon:

> He is much disturbed over the constant urgent demands reaching him concerning his participation in the Congress. He feels that it is time to take action and he has written to Dr Hirschfeld to propose the removal of his name from the League. This might simplify matters, he feels, and make it unnecessary for his name or portrait to be brought forward. He does not wish to be shown any more letters regarding the Congress until it is over, but sends his best wishes for its success.

Havelock Ellis had even more potential than Moll to scuttle the congress and Haire forwarded Russell this disturbing letter and his intended reply on 30 August, saying that he had telegraphed Hirschfeld to do nothing till he came to London. Ellis was behaving very badly but, to ensure that the congress would go ahead, Haire sent him a grovelling apology from which it is clear that Ellis sent a last-minute response. Haire's long reply to Lafitte-Cyon was to be delivered to Ellis after the congress. Haire expressed his 'unbounded' admiration and thanked him for the greeting and photographs; he apologised for his importunity in disturbing him but he had had to do his utmost as secretary of the congress to prevent anyone thinking Ellis 'was not in sympathy with it'.

He needed to persevere until he received a greeting and photograph, as it would have been a huge set-back for the League if Ellis withdrew his name, after once having given it, much worse than if he had never given it at all. Fortunately, the greeting and photographs would now prevent his absence being misinterpreted. Haire had found it very distasteful but it was a duty he could not have conscientiously avoided. It had also forced Haire to defy the father figure whose opinions he valued far more his real father's and that must have been very difficult.

Two days earlier, he had sent this cryptic note to 'Dear Ivor' Montagu:

> I have waited about four weeks for a reply about this carpet but as none has come I must now withdraw my offer. I have given him a very fair time to consider it. My own Chinese merchant had a look at it today and advised me not to take it at any price. He told me he is sure that it will not bring more than £10 in the European market. Shall I take it back to your place, and if so when?

It is quite extraordinary that Haire had time for such trivia when the future of the congress was in the balance. Was it just an offer to help a friend sell a carpet or was it a coded message? Montagu spoke several languages and this letter is in the archives of the Communist Party of Great Britain. He was later unmasked as one of two 'well-placed and highly influential' Soviet agents operating in a London spy ring.[13]

In his opening address Hirschfeld paid tribute to 'three great English men of science', William Bateson, Edward Carpenter and 'Havelock Ellis, who is fortunately still with us, though nowadays his work is done far from the hubbub of city demonstrations'. Phyllis Grosskurth mentioned the boycott in her biography of Havelock Ellis but dismissed it as a joke when she misquoted Hirschfeld:

---

13   West (2002, 117–34). Nigel West (real name Rupert Allason) is a British expert on KGB history whose 1999 book gave details of encrypted evidence identifying Montagu as a Soviet source, code-named 'Nobility', who worked with JBS Haldane, 'Intelligentsia'. Riordan (2008, 519, 529) noted that Britain's security services 'maintained a file on [Montagu] and suspected him of being a spy' and cited (West 2002) and the files – 'Ivor Montagu – British Communist film maker', (KV 2/598–601, National Archives).

Curiously enough, in 1929, at the Congress of the World League of Sexual Reform in London, Hirschfeld himself had to support the fiction and announced from the chair that Ellis was too ill to be present. But he still had to retreat to the country to escape the well-wishers who turned up at his door. 'I am very wild over that infernal Congress', he told Françoise. 'I think of withdrawing my name from the League. When people come there is nothing to do but to say I am away, my whereabouts uncertain, & that it is not known when I shall, if ever return, & that I may have committed suicide. Meanwhile they can be invited to write their damndest in the Visitors Book. I don't mean to see any of them'. And when the Congress was actually over, expecting another wave of invaders, he warned Françoise to be 'ready with pokers & shovels to beat them back'.[14]

Havelock Ellis was sulking because his efforts to sabotage the congress had failed. Despite this destructive attempt, Grosskurth did not criticise his petulance and Haire's relationship with him continued to be cordial. Havelock Ellis remained a nominal WLSR president but Margaret Sanger defected altogether, a month after sending a telegram expressing her 'great disappointment' in not being able to remain in London for the congress. She gave no reason and Haire pleaded with her to 'think it over well' because 'if you resign from an organisation after once having been on its international committee, you may give other people the impression that you definitely disapprove of it.' She replied that she had sent her resignation to Hirschfeld, explaining that she was 'arranging for Zurich', her 1930 Birth Control Conference. Historian Atina Grossman (1995, 39) believed her real reason was the fear that the 'WLSR's association with homosexuality, abortion and Communism would undermine her determined single-issue focus on contraception.'

Fortunately, outsiders were unaware of any conflict and the congress received positive media attention such as *The Times*, which published tributes on 9 September 1929 from those who were unable to attend: HG Wells acknowledged that Havelock Ellis' 'courage and persistence' had won 'much of their freedom of speech and thought in this essential

---

14 Grosskurth (1985, 379–80, fn 46 and 47) quoting from 18 August and 16 September 1929 letters in the BL's Lafitte Collection.

matter'; Hugh Walpole said that 'while we were flying and motoring faster and faster, our scientific and social views and rules about sex were of the 1880s'; Aldous Huxley was glad that there would be papers on literary censorship because 'it was time that the laws against the calling of familiar things and everyday actions by their correct and traditional names should be done away with'. *The Times* also quoted Haire's carefully worded plea for sexual tolerance:

> Those men and women whose sexual temperament diverges from the normal should neither marry nor have children. They should be allowed to live their own lives. Sex abnormality should not be overestimated, but, on the other hand, it should not be underestimated, and there should be no conspiracy of silence against it.

Dr August Forel, the WLSR's co-founder, president and 'your faithful comrade-in-arms' sent his good wishes and a short, simple statement because he was 'an old cripple' and could not attend: he believed that the future of sexual reform lay in 'eugenics and international world peace' which was needed to overcome the world's 'three chief devils' – 'war, capitalism and alcohol consumption.'[15] The 14 September issue of *The Lancet* quoted Russell's hope that the congress would bring publicity to the movement and her belief in the benefits of men and women freely discussing subjects of mutual concern. *The New York Times* chose a more adversarial headline for her talk on 9 September: 'Says women lead in sexual reform. Mrs Dora Russell tells World League meeting in London men are more reactionary' and the *Los Angeles Times* quoted Margaret Sanger's claim that 'the average marriage really hides slavery.' *The New York Times* also quoted Haire, 'one of the leading authorities on rejuvenation', who listed the League's worthy but unachievable aims:

> To establish sexual ethics and sociology on a scientific, biological and psychological basis instead of the present theological basis. There must be no conflict between the laws of nature and the laws of man, between science and ethics, between pure truth and true purity. The stronger our

---

15 Translation in Archive for sexology. Available: www2.huberlin.de/sexology/GESUND/ARCHIV/FOREL.HTM [Accessed 22 November 2008].

organisation and the greater our resources, the sooner we shall attain our object, which is freedom of humanity from the sexual persecution and sexual starvation which ignorance and intolerance have imposed upon it.

The New York Times published tributes from prominent Americans including Judge Ben Lindsey who proposed that young couples should have a childless trial marriage which could be ended by mutual consent and he emphasised why it was needed: 'There are 10,000,000 young men in the United States between the ages of 20 and 30 years of age. Only 4,000,000 of them are married, but the Church and the State are united in demanding that the other 6,000,000 be continent. Are they?'[16]

Sterilisation was topical because the British Parliament was considering whether all sterilisation should be prohibited because it maimed people[17] and 'sterilisation of the unfit' was fiercely debated, with *The Times* reporting that Dr Haire had proposed educating public opinion to ensure that the sterilisation of the 'unfit' would be voluntary if possible, but should be compulsory for people who were a menace to society. He said that laws regulating this had been introduced in some American states but while these had certain dangers and might be misapplied for political or economic causes, they were no more dangerous than segregating lunatics or jailing criminals.

The Times quoted Dr JH Leunbach, the Danish organiser of the 1928 WLSR congress, who called sterilisation the 'most important means available for race improvement' but complained about the taboos against it, saying that in Denmark a recent bill for sterilisation of certain classes of the unfit was limited to public institutions and needed the special permission of the Ministry of Justice. He said this

---

16 Haire advocated this in *Everyday sex problems* (1948, 11–12) and reminded readers they would not buy a car without looking inside or buy a house without seeing if it really suited them and urged them to take the same precautions when considering the long-term proposition of marriage.

17 The continuing confusion is shown in a 1966 letter by Professor Glanville Williams in *The Times* to refute a comment on planned parenthood, from the magazine *Which*, saying that 'male sterilization "might involve the doctor in prosecution for assault and battery, or for maiming"'; Williams responded: 'No criminal court has ever held voluntary sterilization to be unlawful, and it is impossible to believe that the judges would now take this step'.

illustrated the futility of legislation which he claimed hindered the progress of 'race hygiene'. In contrast, Dr David Eder took the liberal view that sterilisation would not get rid of the unfit and suggested that progress was 'attained best by minimum interference by experts in sexual relations, marriage, and procreation'. Although sterilisation, 'at the wish of the unfit', might be desirable, all compulsory legislation was undesirable – greater individual freedom was wanted, not greater legislative interference. Haire was called sterilisation's 'chief advocate' by *The Argus* on 12 September, which mentioned his Sydney origins and (incorrectly[18]) said he had been the 'chief' of Sydney's Royal Hospital for Women.

The Times, in its report of the papers on sex education and censorship, quoted Bertrand Russell who said that rational sex education would prevent pornographic literature causing harm and he deplored the fact that 'frankly salacious works evaded the law' while serious works were 'sacrificed to censorship'. The newspaper's reporter seemed puzzled by George Shaw's flippant comment that 'the only method of creating sex appeal was by clothes'. Shaw, whose pithy sayings include 'assassination is the extreme form of censorship', had the unique distinction of winning both the Nobel Prize for Literature and an Oscar.[19] His paper did not conceal his bleak conclusion that it was impossible to reach a consensus about the 'what and how' of reform, saying that 'everybody is a sex reformer':

> The Pope, for instance, is a prominent sex reformer; and the Austrian nudists are sexual reformers. If you had a general congress of [everyone] demanding sexual reform: nudists and Catholics, birth controllers and self-controllers, homosexuals and heterosexuals, monogamists, polygamists, and celibates, there would be some curious cross-party divisions. The Pope would find himself on nine points out of ten warmly

---

18 *Who's Who in Australia* (1950) listed him as 'formerly RMO (Resident Medical Officer) at Sydney's Royal Hospital for Women', although the 1939 and 1940 entries he provided for Britain's *The medical directory* listed him as 'Med. Supt. Roy. Hosp. Wom. Paddington, & Newcastle Hospital, NSW'.

19 George Bernard Shaw won the Nobel Prize in 1925 for his contribution to literature and an Oscar in 1938 for his work on the film *Pygmalion*.

in sympathy with Dr Marie Stopes. And it is quite possible that the most fanatic nudists and the most fanatical homosexualists might [strongly object] to polygamy and divorce. All of them would probably disagree on such questions as the age of consent.

The *British Medical Journal* gave a two-page report of the congress: Marie Stopes had opened the discussion, Dr CV Drysdale summarised the chief advantages of contraceptives, Dr Hans Lehfeldt said contraceptives should be reliable, innocuous, cheap, unobtrusive and simple but this ideal had not yet been found, and Dr Haire said that during the past ten years he had taught contraceptive technique to over 7000 persons and had at first believed the rubber occlusive pessary used with lactic acid jelly was the most effective method, but was now convinced that the Gräfenberg ring was superior for some patients.

The papers must have been totally absorbing because, although the congress was held during a record-making heatwave of 88° Fahrenheit (31° Celsius), no one mentioned the heat.[20] Dora Russell reminisced about it 40 years later and praised Norman Haire and Jack Flügel, her two 'delightful colleagues', who had worked with her in the preparations. Haire had introduced her to Jack and Ingeborg Flügel and she soon became their close friend. Jack wrote a psychoanalytical study of the family and his translations helped alert English-speakers to Freud. In his address at London's first mass rally of the Men's Dress Reform Party, Flügel urged people to wear 'better and brighter clothes'.[21] Haire welcomed this opportunity to display his rationalism. Figure 7.2 shows Haire in 'rational' knickerbockers and sandals (an expensive symbol of anti-affluence[22]) outside Oak Cottage where Ethel Mannin lived in Wimbledon.

Russell continued the story, saying that 'Norman, though often criticised, was a very loyal friend'[23] and 'intensely sincere' in his views

---

20 *The Times* (9 and 10 September 1929) reported an 88° heatwave in London.
21 Flügel quoted by Burman (1995, 275).
22 Nicholson (2002, 141) said sandals were specially made and expensive but 'sandal-wearing communicated libertarian ideals, a preference for beauty, health and comfort over respectability and a rejection of materialism'.
23 Russell (1977, 217). She said on page 252, when Haire heard rumours of the

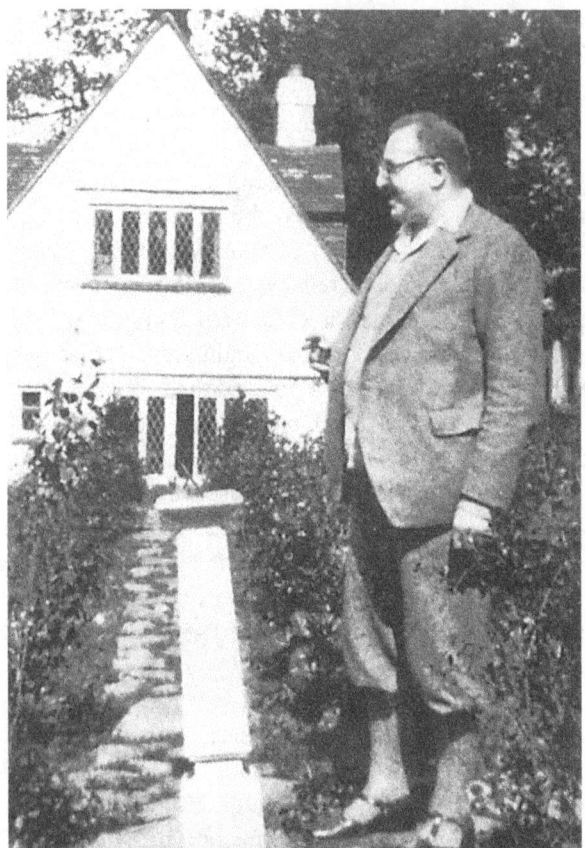

Figure 7.2. Haire in 'rational' knickerbockers and sandals.

about sex. She described his 'infectious, bouncing vigour' which 'came over well in his address of welcome to the Congress'. She and he were pessimistic at first but they had enlisted 'names' and then the list of supporters snowballed. Flügel, in his address of welcome in Esperanto,[24] said that sex affected all aspects of life – individual, family,

---

Russell's divorce, 'he tried to dissuade Bertie'.

24 Flügel (1929) translated by Kep Enderby. Flügel said sex-related problems were 'among the most important, and at the same time most difficult, that present themselves to modern humanity'.

social, economic, national, even peace and world civilisation. There was a very large International Committee in which she, Haire, and Jerdan represented Britain. Every European country except Portugal was represented as well as Argentina, Australia, Canada, Chile, Egypt, Iceland, India, Liberia, the Malay States, New Zealand and the United States. Alexandra Kollontai, who believed in free love and became the world's first female ambassador, sent a message from Russia. Laurence Housman, Ivor Montagu, George Ives, Desmond McCarthy and Bertrand Russell gave papers on censorship in literature, theatre and cinema and Bernard Shaw 'drove home his telling points under the guise of entertaining nonsense'. He claimed expertise in sex as a playwright, since 'the theatre is continually occupied with sex appeal', and just 'as a costermonger has to do with turnips; and a costermonger's opinion on turnips is worth having'.

She mentioned the subterfuge they needed to show a Russian film about abortion. Initially, they had considered an offer by one of Haire's cousins, the head of a British cinema chain, to provide ushers and free use of a theatre near Oxford Circus any week-morning or any night from a quarter past eleven. However, because the film would not pass the censor, Haire and Russell arranged a private showing in a studio at the end of a supporter's garden and issued special tickets. There were moments of burlesque when the press pestered them and even shadowed them on the day of the film, forcing them to take evasive action by 'leaping in and out of cars amid much giggling'. The audience appreciated the film though they did not see the full version but the one which had been cut by German censors. Dr Martha Ruben-Wolf introduced the screening and thanked the 'courage and determination' of Russell and Haire and the hospitality of the owner of the garden studio. The expurgated version was meant to be an awful warning and only showed a woman's abortion-related death and omitted the part showing skilled abortions. Ruben-Wolf said that in Russia no pregnant woman could be punished for having an abortion, only midwives, or unskilled persons, or doctors if the abortion was done carelessly, or if excessive fees were charged. She had seen the full version of the six-year old film in a small Russian town where it had played 150 times to attentive audiences.

Despite their differences, Stella Browne paid Haire a great compliment in her congress evaluation for Sanger's *Critic and guide*. Her first impression had been 'one of energy, enthusiasm and a wealth of courageous and accomplished individual speeches' which proved the injustice of traditional moral codes and their inability to meet present and future needs. She was struck by the internationalism of the movement and the varied progress in each country; the leaders were Germany, Austria, Scandinavia and Russia; 'Latin civilisations were very poorly represented' and Britain and the United States 'showed up well and contributed some memorable papers'. When the League's British Committee (Haire and Russell) first announced that the congress would be held in London, 'they were greeted in many quarters by expressions of shocked surprise and gloomy expectations of failure' but 'fortunately they did not allow themselves to be intimidated'. They received so much 'interest and support' they were able 'to take the Wigmore Hall for a whole week'. Sessions were very well arranged and, although there was inadequate discussion of the papers, this was partly compensated by the very wide publicity given by the London and provincial press and in leading German newspapers.

Browne noted Magnus Hirschfeld's memorable opening address which dealt with the need for an overview of sexual science and the implementation of a systematic social policy based on science and justice. Sexology had acquired the dignity of an independent science in about 1900 he said, and mentioned three books which had made the most significant contribution.[25] In 1913, when he attended the International Medical Congress in London, the session had been interrupted by the cry 'votes for women!' and now female voters were 'striving to mould future laws'. Browne praised Hirschfeld's 'geniality, true internationalism and unsurpassed knowledge of the persons and phases of our movement' which had made the congress a 'propagandist and social success'. Generously, Browne said, 'the same is true of the Secretary to the congress, Dr Norman Haire, on whom fell both the bulk

---

25 Hirschfeld (WLSR 1929, xii): these were *Studies in the psychology of sex*, by Havelock Ellis, *The sexual question*, by August Forel, and the *Sexual life of our time*, by Iwan Bloch.

of the initial organising work and the superintendence of the congress itself. He was indefatigable, and most tactful, and in his speeches forcible and lucid'. She called it 'an encouraging and memorable historical landmark' which had stimulated American debate.

In her 1977 autobiography Russell said the 1929 congress resolutions passed on marriage and divorce, sex and censorship, sex education, birth control, abortion, prostitution and venereal disease were the basis for a tolerant and humane society. Although some had not been fully recognised, the delegates had, in Hirschfeld's words, 'broken through the conspiracy of silence'.

Afterwards Haire felt 'like a corpse' and apologised to Russell: 'I don't think I have expressed to you my appreciation of how you worked all through, but especially during the last fortnight.' The stress had taken its toll on Russell, and Haire wrote to her again on 6 October to see if she had recovered or 'crocked up', adding that his secretary was sick and off work and 'Jerdan has lost about a stone and a half and is suicidal at the moment. Never again!' Two days *before* he made this resolution not to take on any more big projects, he had already broken this pledge (and would break it again in 1934) when, at the urging of a congress delegate, he started to plan an American lecture tour. His temptress was Ernestine Evans, a high-profile literary agent for the American firm JP Lippincott who had published books by Havelock Ellis. Haire asked Sanger if she could find out whether her friend Juliet Rublee, or Addie Kahn (the wife of a wealthy financier), might financially back him for an American tour. She promised to 'keep her ears open for such and will cinch it for you' but once again it was an empty promise.

Haire had invited congress delegates to inspect his birth control clinic and Stopes retaliated a month later by claiming that he did not treat poor patients. Haire responded that he *did* see 'the destitute poor' – several thousand of them in the last eight years. Haire saw about 40 women an afternoon and worked three afternoons a week. He was providing free treatment at his Cromer Welfare and Sunlight Centre near Kings Cross. The financial burden became overwhelming and, on 24 October, Haire sent Stopes 'a despairing appeal for help' and asked if she knew a source of research or funding to save his centre.

This appeal coincided with the publication in 1929 of a study of the first 1000 patients to visit the North Kensington Women's Welfare Clinic which was prepared by Norman Himes and his wife Vera, who had spent 15 months in Britain examining birth control clinics for working-class patients. Their report began with a historical overview from 1877 when the 'able lawyer Charles Bradlaugh and the energetic and eloquent Annie Besant' were prosecuted for publishing the Knowlton pamphlet; to 1921 when Lord Dawson endorsed birth control and, as a consequence, Britain was 'inundated with a flood of literature, some of it useful, most of it trashy and perhaps even harmful' (Himes & Himes 1929, 579–80).

The Himes thanked the North Kensington clinic officials for allowing them to inspect their files, noting pointedly that London's two largest clinics, the Walworth Women's Welfare Centre and Dr Stopes' clinic, had never permitted this. They were unfair to ignore the clinics associated with Haire and Stopes and, because Haire and the Malthusian League had severed their ties with the Walworth Centre, the decision to withhold information would have been made by the new operators. Stopes had published a report on her first 5000 patients in 1925 and Haire first began publishing his results in 1922. Having done so, they might not have felt the need for external scrutiny or else they may have feared that the North Kensington Clinic, 'which had received substantial recognition from the beginning', would outperform them. This must have riled Haire and overshadowed the praise he received for the congress.

Unfortunately, wider problems were looming: the world's economy was deteriorating and Haire suffered from this and other setbacks.

8

The darkening years

George Orwell found the 1930s 'stagnant', Gertrude Stein said 'there was no future any more', Patrick White believed 'there was nothing in Australia and no prospect of it' and a British feminist complained about a 'boring obsession with sex.'[1] WLSR members did not share her view and their hopes, which had been buoyed by the September 1929 congress, were dashed in October by the start of the Great Depression.[2]

A suicide on 9 January 1930 was a portent and Haire noted in the WLSR congress proceedings that publication had been delayed by the death of Ernest Jerdan, the Assistant Honorary Secretary. He had been translating foreign papers and collaborating on the editing but 'died suddenly before the work had been completed'. Haire paid 'tribute to the splendid service he rendered to the League before, and at, the congress in 1929. We in England shall find it hard to fill his place'.

Ernest Jerdan was Australian, a law graduate from the University of Sydney and in the 1920s he had been a Teachers' College lecturer, a co-editor of a short-lived literary magazine[3] and a tutor for the Workers' Educational Association of New South Wales (WEA). He admired both the irrational occultist Aleister Crowley and the ultra-rational Bertrand Russell and thought Russell's *Free thought and official propaganda* was 'almost the perfect lecture'. Jerdan was part of Sydney's bohemia in the 1920s and featured in a nostalgic 1959 'epistle' that artist Ray Lindsay sent to his brother Jack in London; history professor Peter Spearritt

---

1 Orwell (1941, 148); White, quoted by Marr (1992, 113); and the feminist Helena Swanwick is quoted by Kiernan (1998, 74).

2 The impact on Haire is shown in his November 1930 note to Havelock Ellis: 'I have been without a car for about two years, but I have just ordered one again and expect to get it by the middle of November (BL. Add 70540, f. 56).

3 It was called *The New Outlook* and was published by the University of Sydney's Public Questions society from April 1922 to December 1932.

called it 'one of the wittiest and bitchiest letters ever written from this city'. Jerdan had published some of Jack Lindsay's early writing and the brothers called him 'Tinny', an abbreviation of an archaic Australian term for a tin-bummed, or lucky person, who is impervious to kicks. Ray described him as 'a fair, nebulous-looking young chap who had had quite a brilliant academic career' but was 'rather vague and sexless'. Jerdan had been a tutor at Jack's WEA camp on Sydney's Tambourine Bay (now Longueville) and married a 'warm and likeable' student and for her sake he suffered the 'indignity of adult circumcision when he converted to Judaism'.[4] Jack said he had failed to consummate the marriage but had 'indignantly denied the imputation of impotence'. Jack could not decide if Jerdan was 'a sociologist interested in literature or a literary man interested in sociology' but Jack was always depressed when he discussed books with him because he found it hard to argue against Jerdan's 'bright well-informed, sane and absolutely-tinny outlook'.

Nine months before his death, Jerdan sent Dora Russell a charmingly normal apology because 'the combined effects of vaccination cum tonsillitis' had prevented him from coming to stay at the Russell's Beacon Hill School on the West Sussex Downs:

> It is curious how many times I have been coming down to the school and have not. There have always been excellent reasons but I think we must suspect that our old friend the unconscious is up to something. And I fancy I know what it is. It is a sort of fear (almost) of meeting Bertrand Russell (not that it follows I necessarily would if I did come down). One is a little awe struck of the possibility of meeting the deity face to face. I remember that the first night I met you I was conscious of something of the sort – you were His Wife (though partly I resented his having a wife!). Please do not imagine that I am generally speaking so coy and flapperish; I am I think a reasonably intelligent person with a very good opinion of myself. But it happens that BR has occupied quite a unique part in my life and I can still recall quite vividly the afternoon (in 1914) when I was working in the summer house at Mosmans Bay Australia and my friend

---

4   Arnold (1983, 55). Dr Patrick Buckridge sent me Ray Lindsay's 1959 Epistle. There are more details about Jerdan in Buckridge (1994, 103–04).

suddenly arrived and in a characteristic fashion said 'My God listen to this' and steadily went on reading for two hours ... from the Philosophical Essays which he had just discovered. Neither of us had heard of B.R. before that. Something was lit up in me that day which I hope has never gone out. So you see the possibility of actually 'seeing Shelley plain'[5] and he perhaps 'stopping and speaking to me' is for me a rather prepare-to-meet-your-God sort of ordeal. I feel fairly certain that this is the factor behind my repeated shoving off of the visit . . . However I am most anxious to see the school (and of course really to see him) and by the grace of God I no doubt shall, one day.

He apologised for his long letter but felt his conduct had been curious and 'required some explanation' and she sent this witty reassurance:

> I have no doubt that the unconscious would boggle at meeting a god with whooping cough. As regarding gods having wives, Mr Russell asks me to say that since he belongs to the Pagan variety he feels he is entitled to that privilege. We both want you very much to come down. I do not really think the delay is your fault; it is quite as much due to the difficulties of keeping so large a family free from infectious diseases in such a bad year. I will let you know as soon as Mr Russell is considered safe, as he wants to meet you very much.

Haire, who had been thin and delicate as a child, spoke of meeting Jerdan when he was a 'little fat boy' three or four years his junior at Fort Street School; he was the star pupil of the German class and a very talented university student. When they met again at Sydney University's Dramatic Society at the end of 1914 he found Jerdan's company 'very congenial' and they met six more times before Norman graduated in early 1915 and then their paths diverged. Jerdan, who planned to marry, contacted Haire in London and asked him to be a sponsor when he converted to Judaism but Haire had opposed the marriage because he

---

5   A reference to Robert Browning's poem 'Memorabilia' which begins:
      Ah, did you once see Shelley plain,
      And did he stop and speak to you,
      And did you speak to him again?

was too young and might not be 'sexually normal', perhaps alluding to Jerdan's 'youthful enthusiastic friendship' with Nathian Robinovitz[6] which suggested either homo- or bi-sexuality and would explain his ease with Haire without the need for a relationship.

Haire had once written to ask how his marriage had turned out. They resumed their friendship when Jerdan came to London. They soon 'became quite intimate', collaborating on a German translation in 1926 and, in Christmas 1927, Jerdan moved in with Haire. He planned to study medicine and Haire offered him free accommodation for the six-year course and 'did as much for him as if he had been his own brother'. 'Some day' he would be repaid and meanwhile Haire found him pupils to coach, introduced him to key people and got him a commission for a book on psychoanalysis which he never finished. Jerdan wanted to be psychoanalysed as the first step to becoming a psychoanalyst and Haire introduced him to the psychoanalysis pioneer David Eder and Jerdan had analysis with Eder 'fairly regularly'.

Jerdan earned about £5 to £7 a week with prospects of regular payments for translations; things were going well and Haire said they never quarrelled, although there had been one or two differences of opinion because Jerdan was cavalier about money and would give his last penny to a friend and was similarly generous with Haire's possessions. Once, when Jerdan was away, Haire found a strange man breakfasting in his kitchen and ordered him to leave. Jerdan said later, 'Oh well, you offered me a room and food, and as I wasn't using it for a fortnight I thought A might as well have it'. He thought Haire was peculiar for making a fuss and felt it showed his 'exaggerated sense of property'.

Haire told Stopes on 24 October 1929 that he had planned to unwind after the congress by going to the south of France but instead he addressed 4000 people. It was 'rather an ordeal' since it was the first time he had lectured in French and he also fielded questions from the audience. He returned to find Jerdan 'rather depressed' and in November Jerdan began to talk about suicide. Haire consulted Eder who said that Jerdan *had* been periodically suicidal even before he left Sydney but was

---

6 Arnold (1983, 22). Robinovitz later moved to Melbourne, changed his name to Norman Robb and ran an avant-garde bookshop under that name.

much better and there was no cause for alarm. Jerdan had abandoned his medical studies and his medical work at Middlesex Hospital and his translations had deteriorated badly. At Christmas he seemed depressed but not suicidal and Haire took a week's holiday. On his return, Jerdan complained that he was sleeping badly because of the noise from the Frigidaire. Considering the refrigerator was in the basement kitchen and his room was on an upper floor, there would have been little noise from it but his complaint shows his distressed state.

Haire saw Jerdan briefly on the day he died; he wanted Jerdan's help in the afternoon but he had gone out. As Jerdan planned to spend the weekend with Ethel Mannin, Haire was not concerned until she contacted him the next morning. He had not visited her but must have had a key to another friend's house in Brighton and went there knowing it was empty. That afternoon, the Brighton police phoned to say he that had gassed himself. Jerdan left a note for 'My dear Wauchope':

> The one essential thing for a successful suicide is that one should be immune from interruption for a sufficiently long time. Your empty house offered a heaven sent opportunity & I hope you will forgive me that I availed myself of it. You will find £28 in notes in my pocket which will perhaps recompense you to some extent for the trouble & inconvenience I am causing you. Don't let the Police do you out of a penny of it. Whether the coroner finds that I was sane or insane I do not care, but I would like to make it quite clear that nobody & nothing is responsible for this except that I am utterly sick of life & have decided to end it.

He left a note on the kitchen door warning his friend to keep his children out of the room because he would (he hoped) be dead inside. At the inquest the next day, Haire tastelessly wore one of Jerdan's silk scarfs and asked Mannin if she recognised it and, when she did, he admonished her for being sentimental, adding that 'it was a very good scarf; what was I supposed to do with it – put it in the dustbin?' Understandably, she found 'his rationality could be monstrous'. The coroner found Jerdan 'brilliant but over-strung'; the £50 in Jerdan's bank account almost covered the costs of the funeral and Haire paid Jerdan's debts. There was no religious ceremony and, after scattering his ashes, his friends reproached themselves and Haire blamed himself for not realising Jerdan's true condition and treating him as 'super-normal' and Mannin pondered whether he had been 'super-human or sub-human'.

Haire's secretary, Ruby Lockie, said his first response on hearing the news had been to dissolve into tears: he was shocked, unhappy and could not sleep for weeks, telling Hirschfeld, 'I didn't know how deep the friendship was until he died.' Jerdan had lived in his house for two years and Haire considered him 'part of the furniture', something which belonged in his everyday life; Dora Russell felt she should have insisted on the visit because 'the country and the sight of the children's happiness would have been good for his nerves' and Hirschfeld regretted the 'loss for our movement'.

Ethel Mannin and Jerdan had been lovers for six months and she 'believed in' Jerdan's analyst David Eder 'as some people believe in God'. In 1930 she wrote a thinly disguised account of Jerdan's death, acknowledging that some would say she should not have written it and others would accuse her of dramatising her emotions and using a tragic experience as 'copy'; they were right and her 'outspoken' *Confessions and impressions* produced 'a crop of libel writs'.[7] She claimed to have given Jerdan 'all the happiness he had ever had in his thirty odd years' and said this was not 'egotistical vanity' but 'quite simply true'. She had not noticed Jerdan's mental state and her biographer suggested why: 'fuelled by drink' she found herself in strange company and 'in strange beds' but she had 'sobered up' after the suicide. 'At that black period' Mannin was trapped in a never-ending 'black tunnel' when Haire alone could make her laugh and she vowed to value his friendship all her life because:

> He has the real kindness of the really intelligent person. He does not just sit around and say how sorry he is; he does something about it. Perhaps

---

7 Mannin's biographer was Robert Huxter (1992, 83, 86). Mannin's vignettes also angered Evelyn Waugh who believed she had 'made free' with the names of several of his friends (*The Times*, 26 July 1933, 4). She even featured in a Miles Franklin award-winning novel (Stivens, 1970, 74) as a guest 'sodden with drink and Marxism' at a Norman Haire party.

that is why whenever there is a crisis in my queer life I may be observed indulging in an orgy of theatre-going with Norman Haire.

Her gratitude quickly vanished and in 1971 she dismissed his friendship 'as a cover-up for his homosexuality'; she had told Haire that their frequent theatre-going made one of his cousins think they were having an affair and he was amused and encouraged the idea. She did not empathise with his need for this ruse but was disgusted and vainly resented the idea that people thought she had 'such a Caliban' as a lover.

There was a long delay before Rachael Jerdan in Sydney was informed about her estranged husband's death and she was grief-stricken by the news. Haire had mistakenly believed that they were divorced and had asked his solicitor Lionel Dare to write to Jerdan's relatives in the hope that this formality might reduce the shock. Dare did not send the letter.[8] Mrs Jerdan sent Haire a series of searching questions and in July 1930 Haire sent her the first of four frank replies in the belief that this approach would help her to face reality and get over her grief.

These extracts from his own grieving outpourings are hard to follow because they are drafts of the letters he sent and her replies are missing. Jerdan told Haire of his 'violent feeling of repulsion' towards his wife and considered her the 'evil genius of his life' although 'his attitude later softened'. Jerdan claimed he had never been in love but had married her to prevent her committing suicide and had often thought of killing her by pushing her over the cliffs at Sydney's South Head. Haire found him 'brilliant but unstable' and in the words of Omar Khayyam, one of 'the

---

8 Haire might have overlooked Dare's forgetfulness because he was funny: in the 1940s, members of a gastronomic club were dining at a high-class Sydney restaurant and ordered an Irish stew as a joke. 'Lionel Dare, a prominent divorce lawyer', took on the role of chief food critic, pacing up and down while composing his thoughts as though he was about speak in court. He launched into a detailed criticism, saying it was not a real Irish stew because it contained carrots! The irate manager evicted the group and told them to never come back. From Joseph Glasscott's *A table of delights: the first fifty years of the wine and food society of NSW (1939–1989)*. Available: www.wineandfood.org.au/NSWnsw/nswhistory.htm [Accessed 1 May 2008]. The *Macquarie dictionary of cookery*'s Irish stew does not contain carrots.

luckless pots He marred in the making' due to 'poisoning of the germ plasm caused by his father's alcoholism.'

In February 1929 Jerdan had been 'transformed' by his liaison with Mannin and he looked radiantly happy until he 'began to lose his gaiety' in July. Haire attributed this to the demands of the congress, even though 'he did very little until the week of the congress when he rallied and was marvellously helpful'. Haire said Jerdan's paper, 'Sex and shame', was one of the best. Jerdan believed that 'all our difficulties are due to sex being the forbidden subject' because, as Ernest Jones noted, 'sexual topics are as carefully avoided in medical schools as they are in girls' schools'. He alluded to the failure of psychoanalysis to help him and to the shipwreck which traumatised his wife:[9] 'at present psychoanalysis has no better conception of the normal than a person who has successfully come through a shipwreck. It may later know one who has never put to sea!' The chief enemy to sexual reform 'is located in ourselves and must be dealt with there' and Jerdan stressed his belief that 'in the fight for sexual happiness, it is those among us who are without shame who will cast the most effective, if not the first, stone'.

Haire's sister, who had been in London on a visit, was returning to Sydney and delivered Jerdan's possessions to his widow – a watch, a pair of gold cuff links and a typewriter. Haire could not find his silver cigarette case and did not include a painting by Elioth Gruner. He thought Mrs Jerdan might like to donate it to Dr Eder who was very fond of Jerdan and because Jerdan owed him a good deal of money for his analysis. Haire was sure Eder would appreciate the painting but said he would only give it with her permission.[10] Gruner's *Morning light*

---

9   In the 1940s Betty Shwabsky (1999) taught with Rachael Jerdan who never spoke of her husband's suicide and was 'very neurotic'. After Rachel had been shipwrecked, she refused to travel by boat or any form of public transport. Rachael was the daughter of Rabbi Mandelbaum and taught Latin at the William Street Girls High School near the Australian Museum.

10 The painting's fate is unknown. In August 2005 I contacted the Manuscript Librarians at the Art Gallery of NSW who checked Elioth Gruner's letters in the papers of Sir Hans Heysen from 1925 to 1930 and letters in the Elioth Gruner Papers but neither contained references to Jerdan, nor was Phillip Brackenreg (from the Artarmon Galleries, NSW) able to find anything when he looked

had won the Wynne Prize for Australian landscape painting in 1916 and these troubled men may have been friends or lovers; Jack Lindsay (1960, 121) described Gruner as a desperately unhappy man who 'could not achieve a settled love-relationship and remained at an uneasy bisexuality'.

Haire apologised for his unsympathetic response to one of Mrs Jerdan's letters in which she accused him of not complying with her request to have Jerdan's letters; he said some were 'of the most intimate nature possible' and were from people she did not know. The uncensored thoughts Haire sent Mrs Jerdan seem shocking but it was also hard for him because it was 'impossible or at least terribly difficult, to discuss such matters by correspondence'. He wished they 'were able to have a talk about him' but she was afraid of the sea and would not travel. In his final letter to her in December 1930, Haire disagreed with her negative views about Mannin's book and agreed it was a matter of taste but said his standards were probably more like Mannin's than hers. He understood that 'the triangle (or perhaps I should say polygon) being what it was' she was unlikely to see Mannin 'through rose coloured spectacles'. Perhaps Haire was part of the polygon.

He said Mrs Jerdan seemed to 'admire neurosis!' and felt she was patronising Mannin by saying she was 'too sane, too normal, too much the extrovert'. He agreed that Jerdan had sometimes admired the 'blessed fools of the world' and thought this probably led to the disaster. Haire considered it was an unhealthy taste but they were unlikely to agree about Mannin's book and she would probably say that he was also too sane, normal and extroverted. He admitted he was unqualified to make a psychological judgement and that classifications were imperfect but then stated that Jerdan had 'dementia praecox' (an old term for schizophrenia); perhaps Jerdan suffered from manic depression (bipolar disorder).

Haire's antidote to grief was activity and on 22 February 1930 he asked Hirschfeld for information about Peter Martin Lampel whose play *Revolte im Erziehungshaus* (*Revolt in a reformatory*) concerned boys who had been abused in an all-male institution and resorted

---

through a Gruner log-book of sales.

to homosexuality.[11] Haire wanted to know what had happened to Lampel and asked Hirschfeld to forward his letter to him because play rehearsals would start on 10 March and the producer wanted Haire to play the minister of religion which he found 'very amusing' and they needed Lampel's photograph and biographical details. Ralf Dose explained the context to me in 2006: Lampel was a 'political crackpot' who had 'drifted from the extreme left to the extreme right and back'. He became a 'shooting star' with his first play but the second (about illegal preparations for a gas war in Germany) became a political scandal and was banned in late 1929 after a single performance. Lampel was living at Hirschfeld's Institute when he was arrested after the police had read a book in which he had foolishly confessed to murdering a right-wing political opponent. On his release from jail, Lampel became a communist fellow-traveller and had gone into hiding, so Haire asked Hirschfeld to forward his letter. He was later jailed by the Nazis under the German Criminal Code's anti-homosexual paragraph 175.[12] Although Hirschfeld congratulated Haire on the play's success on 18 March, Haire seems not to have acted in it.[13]

Dora Russell was pregnant and minding sick children when she received a chatty letter from Haire on 29 April asking her, when things became less hectic, to send him a copy of the congress resolutions because there were many versions in Jerdan's files and this was delaying work on the proceedings. Haire was sorry that she could not attend the WLSR's Vienna congress in September and asked if she was sending a paper. He had addressed a 'meeting of lower middle class people in the very Red commune of St Denis' (a heavily industrialised community ten miles north of Paris) and in Paris he had had 'great fun' when he addressed Berty Albrecht's society where members demanded full details

---

11   The play led to educational reform and Joseph Fishman, an American prison inspector, explored the topic in his 1935 book which Haire included in 'The international library of sexology and psychology' series.

12   Paragraph 175 was a provision of the German Code to make homosexual acts between males a crime. In 1935 the Nazis increased the scope and penalties under this law and thousands died in concentration camps.

13   When Lampel's play was performed at London's Gate Theatre, *The Times* on 29 May 1933 listed Haire as translating it from the German.

about the WLSR and British birth control methods. Albrecht had close ties with British radicals and started the WLSR's journal *Le problème sexuel* to promote birth control and abortion (Gruber & Graves 1998, 306). Haire's news was mixed on 25 August: the proceedings were at the printers but very few English people would attend the congress; he and his secretary Ruby Lockie were going and, perhaps as an inducement to Dora Russell, he said that Roy Randall[14] (one of her lovers) would probably go.

Haire and Hirschfeld became co-presidents of the League at the Vienna congress and Havelock Ellis continued as the honorary president. Although Ellis had unkindly predicted that the 1929 congress would be an 'all-Haire Congress', Haire had been promoting the WLSR congress, not himself. He showed an extraordinary lack of ego in his 21 September report to Havelock Ellis about the WLSR's 1930 Vienna congress, which he *hadn't* organised, when he said it was 'a distinct advance over the previous ones. In Copenhagen in 1928 we had about 100 congress members; in London about 500; and here about 1000.' But there were problems with the Vienna congress which Haire's 29 March 1932 letter to Hirschfeld identified: if a proper agreement had been drawn up in Vienna, and a stenographer had taken verbatim notes which were signed by all present, it would have avoided any doubt about what was decided and prevented a lot of quarrelling. However, Haire showed great restraint by not pointing this out to Havelock Ellis and he was also diffident about his own success a year later when he mentioned he would give an address on birth control in German at a public meeting in Berlin on 21 November 1931. During the past year or two, he had increased his lectures in French and German and found that his early stage training was most useful. He took great pleasure from giving a successful lecture and supposed that it satisfied his 'exhibitionistic component'.

Haire did not boast when Moll's Second International Congress for Sex Research (ICSR) was ignored by the press apart from a paid advertisement in *The Times* on 31 July 1930 saying it would be held

---

14 Randall had given a paper at WLSR (1929, 254–67) called 'The individual aspects of prostitution among the English middle class'.

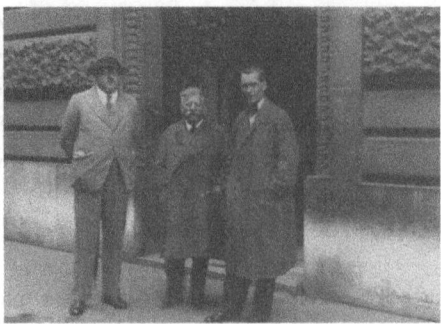

Figure 8.1. Norman Haire, Magnus Hirschfeld and Karl Giese at a WLSR congress.

from 3 August to 9 August, was 'purely for scientific research' and that the congress president was Professor FAE Crew from Edinburgh University (Greenwood 1931). After praising Moll's 'well-grounded and clear-sighted critique of eugenics' at the ICSR's first congress, Ralf Dose (2003, 10) noted that there were no papers on sex reform in their second, and the study of sexuality 'returned to its animal origins'. The ICSR focused on research while the WLSR drew its members from lay organisations and focused on reform.

There was rivalry between the two organisations and this shows in the letter Crew sent to Julian Huxley 'about this [ICSR] Congress business'; unless Crew heeded the advice of Moll and his group in Berlin he would have to 'drop the idea of getting the Congress to this country'. He found the Moll–Hirschfeld disagreement 'absurd' – Moll would not let the congress be held in London if there was any association between Hirschfeld and himself. Crew supported Haire's stance and the 1929 WLSR congress but 'as president of this other show' he had had 'to avoid difficulties that are the peculiar pleasures of Moll and his antagonists' and found it 'all very silly'.

Haire gave a paper on the Gräfenberg ring at the 1929 congress and Margaret Sanger invited Haire and Gräfenberg to present their findings at her Birth Control Conference in Zurich. He had learnt to be more cautious and now advised people not to place too much importance on statistics and urged them to agree on the definition of 'failure', which, he felt, 'should be reserved for cases in which a given contraception

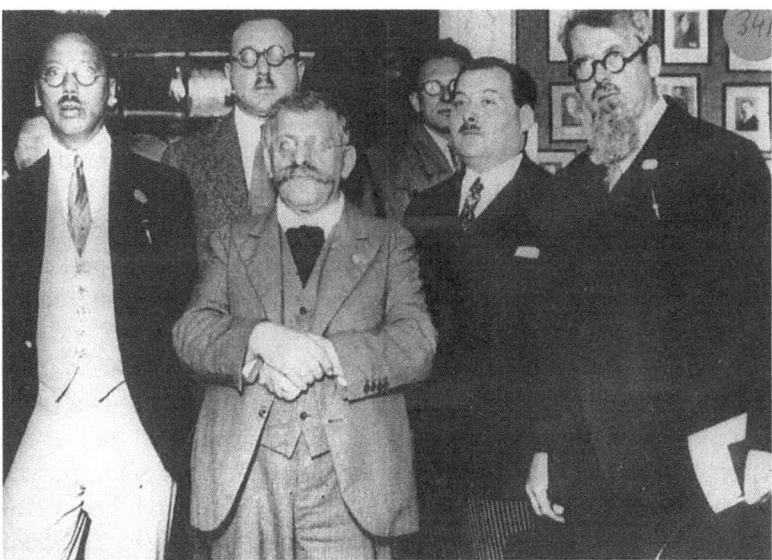

Figure 8.2. 1930 WLSR congress. The WLSR principals are (from the left) Dr JH Leunbach from Copenhagen, Norman Haire, Magnus Hirschfeld, Pierre Vachet from Paris and Dr Josef K Friedjung from Vienna.

when used has failed to prevent contraception' (Haire in Sanger & Stone 1931, 219–20). He warned delegates that statistics were based on data obtained from patients who may or may not be telling the truth or their memory may be faulty. In addition, when patients said they used a method which failed, there was no way of knowing if they had used it consistently. When Haire began to publish his results in 1922 and 1923, he was 'very sanguine about statistics' but the longer he worked in this field, the less confidence he had in their reliability.

In old age Jessie Street reminisced about her 1930 visit to London when she had attended a birth control meeting. There she met Haire who reminded her that they had been to university together in Sydney. Street also attended the Birth Control Conference in Zurich and, not surprisingly, found Sanger the most outstanding personality there, but she also praised Haire, saying that he 'was also very well known and made a valuable contribution'. She mentioned his Australian habit of taking off his coat and working in his shirt and waistcoat with his braces showing and said it was 'not done' in the best foreign circles. There is a photograph taken at the 1930 banquet of the WLSR congress in Vienna, in which he stands out as a rationally dressed rebel in an open-necked shirt, amid a sea of black ties and dinner-jackets.[15] Although Haire was a member of the Men's Dress Reform Party, he had ignored their honorary secretary's advice to not wear braces or a waistcoat, 'so that a man might remove his jacket on a hot day and still retain his good looks and his fair name!'[16] However, in a photograph of the main speakers at the Vienna congress, Haire is in the back row wearing a conventional shirt and tie in figure 8.2.[17]

On 16 October 1930 Haire received news from Hirschfeld about another suicide, that of 'our dear friend Peter Schmidt' at the age of 38. On his Berlin visit the previous year, Haire and Schmidt met several times and lunched at Wannsee, a lakeside picnic spot. Schmidt, who specialised in prolonging the lives of others, shot himself because he did not think life was worth living. In his self-help book *Don't be tired!*, Schmidt called fatigue a 'world epidemic, beneath the burden of which the greater part of humanity is daily groaning more loudly'. He was manic-depressive.[18] Bad news was mounting. Haire had been ill with pneumonia and this explained why he had not answered a letter from Dr Henry Gillett who denounced contraception and praised couples who achieve 'power and love by dedicating their lives to God'. Haire declined to discuss the matter with him because their standpoints were so different: 'when a man begins to talk God to me, I stop arguing with him; he is not open to reason'.

When an abbreviated version of Haire's 1930 WLSR Vienna congress paper was published by the International Medical Group for

---

15 Ralf Dose (February 2002) gave me this photograph from the Magnus Hirschfeld Society collection which is from Paul Krische's files.

16 Burman (1995, 127–78) quoting AC Jordan.

17 Available: www2.hu-berlin.de/sexology/GESUND/ARCHIV/WLSR.HTM [Accessed 22 July 2011].

18 His death was reported in *The Washington Post*, 7 October 1930. Schmidt's world fatigue quote (1930, 10, 139) is in Sengoopta (2006, 106–07).

the Investigation of Contraception,[19] the group's chair, CP Blacker, was guarded about Haire's evaluation of 100 cases over 11 years of experience with the Gräfenberg ring, and called for 'a much larger and more detailed analysis'. Haire reported on 400 cases at the Gynaecological congress in Frankfurt in 1931 and said he found '70% of the cases were completely satisfactory' but five years later he found the method 'very disappointing' because it did not offer complete protection, thus removing 'the great advantage' it had seemed to offer (Haire 1936, 151). There *were* problems of infection and expulsion but a modified form of this IUD with a plastic component achieved medical respectability and revolutionised contraception in the 1960s,[20] although there have been similar problems with some newer versions. Haire pointed out in the *British Medical Journal* that although some doctors had unknowingly inserted the ring into pregnant women, it had not caused any abortions. Blacker felt this suggested 'that women may conceal the fact they are pregnant, and ask to be fitted with a Gräfenberg Ring in the hope that the insertion of the ring will terminate the pregnancy.' Later Haire inserted the ring during menstruation to be 'absolutely sure' the patient was not pregnant.

In the 1930s some British birth control associations had amalgamated as the National Birth Control Association[21] which, in conjunction with the Birth Control Investigation Committee (formed by staff at the North Kensington and Cambridge clinics), held a conference in May 1932. The *British Medical Journal* published details on 4 June and Dr Enid Charles, from the Department of Social Biology at the London School

---

19 *International Medical Group for the Investigation of Contraception*, third issue, 1930, 40–43. The *BMJ*, 24 March 1928, said it was the 'offspring' of the Geneva 1927 World Population Conference and was a group of medical practitioners who aimed to co-ordinate biochemical, physiological, and statistical research about contraception and disseminate it globally.

20 Haseltine (1963, A3), Thiery (1997) and Chesler (1993, 356).

21 A birth control centre was established in London in 1928; it became the Birth Control International Information Centre, then merged with the National Birth Control Association and changed names in 1938 to become the Family Planning Association. Available: www.nyu.edu/projects/sanger/secure/aboutms/organization_bciic.html [Accessed 20 September 2010].

of Economics, using three sets of statistical data, ranked the success of contraceptive methods as 98 percent for condoms with other measures; 82 percent for condoms alone; 66 percent for *coitus interruptus* and 54 percent for quinine alone. The final session considered Gräfenberg rings which were 'applied extensively' in Haire's Cromer Welfare and Sunlight Centre but were not used in any Society for the Provision of Birth Control Clinics (which began as the Malthusian League's Walworth Clinic). Dr Helena Wright listed the contraindications for its use – fibroids, heavy menstrual bleeding or unhealthy pelvic conditions – and warned patients of the increased likelihood of dangerous vaginal or intrauterine infection which, in this pre-penicillin era, was a very grave risk. Haire stated in the *British Medical Journal* on 18 January 1930 that if the risk of complications 'is too great to compensate for the advantages of the method, it must be abandoned.'

After the WLSR's 1930 congress, Haire kept urging Hirschfeld to set a date for the next one. This was particularly difficult to arrange as Hirschfeld had left the Institute in December 1930 on a world tour and he never returned to Berlin. Hirschfeld completed his trip in January 1932 after lecturing in America, Hawaii, Japan, China, India (where he caught malaria) and Egypt (where he was hospitalised in Cairo). The WLSR committee considered Moscow but the Russians did not respond to a dozen letters and clearly could not organise the congress, so a venue was eventually selected in Brno, Czechoslovakia. They had also considered Madrid and Paris but Hirschfeld suggested July or August and these dates were rejected by Pierre Vachet, the French WLSR committee member, because everyone would be away on holidays. Curiously, Karl Giese, in his 26 May 1931 letter to Haire, sent his congratulations because he had just heard from Hirschfeld that the WLSR meeting in Karlsbad[22] had been satisfactory. It was unsatisfactory from Haire and Leunbach's viewpoint because they found their meeting with the publisher of the first issues of *SEXUS* (the WLSR's quarterly magazine) very disappointing. Moreover, it was *not* a WLSR meeting but the inaugural meeting of the International Federation of Socialist

---

22 Karlsbad (Carlsbad in English) is in the Czech Republic and is now called Karlovy Vary.

The darkening years

Doctors[23] and the group photograph of this Karlsbad meeting[24] held on 23 to 25 May 1931 shows Haire in baggy pants and knee-length Fairisle socks sitting in the front row beside nine formally dressed delegates with 100 delegates standing in rows behind.

I gave a copy of the photograph to Ralf Dose and he thanked me for this 'worthy addition' to the Magnus Hirschfeld Society's collection, and commented that 'the list again shows clearly how close the WLSR were to socialist ideas because there are so many names which appear in both organisations'. He said that most members of the Federation of Socialist Doctors were left-wing social democrats and communists and, at their first meeting, the two British delegates complained that the discussion was more about abortion than socialism. Havelock Ellis had a different complaint and informed a member of the British Society for the Study of Sex Psychology, in a 3 January 1932 letter, that it was unfortunate that Hirschfeld's Institute and the WLSR had become 'so largely homosexualised' (Grosskurth, 1980: 379). He was forgetting the fact that both had been founded by homosexuals.

Haire was also editing Wilhelm Bölsche's *Love-life in nature: the story of the evolution of love* (1931), a massive book translated from German, which a reviewer in *The International Journal of Psychoanalysis* (1932) described as a meandering, quasi-poetical description of animal and human love life which was unlikely to suit English taste.

Marie Stopes had a long memory for grudges and she complained to Haire in 1931about things he had written in 1926; she expected to be given credit as the doyenne of birth control and objected because he had said *The Lancet* 'led the way' in 1922 by sending a representative to the birth control conference in London and by his mentioning of the special 1923 contraception issue of *The Practitioner*. She would have missed the Australian humour in Haire's facetious 'apology' on 16 February:

> I am so fully aware of the extent to which your propagandist activities have contributed to the advance of the Birth Control movement in this

---

23 After 1933 they moved to Prague and in 1938 to Paris (Callesen 2001, 60).

24 Lotte Fink's daughter Ruth Latukefu gave me a copy of the photograph and a letter about the 1931 convention written by Professor Stephan Leibfried, University of Bremen, Germany on 1 February 1982.

country, that I am perhaps inclined to regard this point as one which is to be taken for granted, and do not therefore mention you every time, as one would mention some other person who has made one or two little contributions, to the progress of the movement. I think that this is the explanation, not only in my case, but in the case of many other people whom you may think to be deliberately failing to acknowledge your services in one place or another. One does not mention Lister, every time one discusses antiseptics, and it is much the same sort of thing with regard to Birth Control.

Haire wrote to Stopes again on 5 August to congratulate her on the new edition of her book *Contraception*. He also wished her a happy holiday and said he was going by car to Italy 'to get some practice in Italian'.

He continued to plead with Hirschfeld to fix a date for the next WSLR congress and reminded him on 28 December that 'the League is your child' and asked him to say that he agreed to hold the congress at the end of September and would attend. It would be foolish to let it be still-born because the preparations were rushed with insufficient time to do things properly; they must let their committee member Pierre Vachet in France know at once; there was no more time for discussion and Hirschfeld should telegraph either September or June to fix the date. He begged him not to attend the Eugenics congress in New York the following August because his presence was essential at the WLSR congress. Haire said the economic position in England was very bad and people were unable to pay doctors' fees, adding a very British-style comment 'still we keep cheerful'.

One cheerless consequence of the recession was an increase in the abortion rate, and Haire argued that it would be better to make abortion legal because, as the abortion law reformer Stella Browne said, 'Not abortion, but forced motherhood is the crime' and it was 'women's right to freedom of choice'.[25] Haire, in *The Week-End Review* on 31 October 1931, encouraged contraception rather than abortion because the saying 'prevention is better than curette' had more than wit

---

25 Haire quote (WLSR 1929, 110); Stella Browne (WLSR 1929, 181).

to commend it. Haire, in *The Lancet* on 26 December, described a new method for the interruption of pregnancy by introducing an antiseptic paste into the uterus which usually caused a miscarriage within 48 hours. The method was described by Dr JH Leunbach at the WLSR congress in 1929 and Haire said that in his own experience, gained 'over a considerable period', it was better than all former methods and very much better for pregnancies over eight weeks.[26] It would have been a career-ending admission to write, and for medicine's ultra-respectable *The Lancet* to print, unless lawyers were confident that the police would not classify this as illegal abortion.

In January 1932 most of the WLSR difficulties seemed to be resolved and a Paris congress was planned for 22 June. Haire invited Hirschfeld's associate Karl Giese to stay for a week in London after the congress and requested (and was sent) an English version of the Hirschfeld Institute's psycho-biological patient questionnaire [*Fragebogen*]. However, they had forgotten a 1920 French law which forbade the advocacy of birth control. Haire discussed this with Vachet and told Hirschfeld on 2 March that unless the congress was for doctors only and held in complete privacy, everyone would be arrested and the foreigners would be deported. Vachet thought that the left might win France's elections in May or June and they might permit the congress to be held. Planning by mail was difficult and the well-organised Haire also had to cope with Hirschfeld, the League's dithering president, who on 29 March proposed holding the congress in Holland in July. Haire pointed out that there was now too little time to prepare for it and, as he had confinements booked from May to August, he would be unable to attend. In exasperation, he told Hirschfeld on 11 April that it was now impossible to hold the congress in Paris that year, although, if he had agreed to hold it in September as it had been suggested, it could have been arranged. Haire argued that it would be better to have no congress than a small, unsuccessful one in Paris, and it was cancelled.

---

26 Haire later distanced himself (1936, 172–73), saying the technique began 'in Germany some six or seven years ago' but no drug or combination of drugs will interrupt pregnancy without danger to the health of the mother; he also warned about the German paste in *BMJ* on 20 March 1937.

Haire complained to Dora Russell that the WLSR had 'been moribund since the 1929 congress'; very few members had renewed their subscriptions in Britain and they were unlikely to do so unless the WLSR offered something in return. On 8 March 1932 he suggested they should hold meetings, starting on 22 April with a 'respectable' lecture in the London School of Hygiene by Dr Georg Groddeck, a German pioneer of psychosocial medicine, with a more risky one on abortion to follow. He estimated that, as the lecture theatre held 280, a shilling admission charge should earn about £20, enough for an unpaid lecturer. Haire told Hirschfeld on 29 March that he had held a large reception in his house for the German lecturer and hoped to hold monthly WLSR lectures.

On his return from the Brno congress, Haire reported that delegates' interest in abortion had 'eclipsed all the other problems set down for discussion' and, as a result, the British section of the WLSR chose this topic for the 3 November meeting because the time seemed ripe for discussion.[27] Haire stressed the need to reform Britain's 'iniquitous' laws which denied poor women access to safe abortions and caused a 'constant stream of pregnant women of the richer classes' to visit Europe for terminations. In Russia, where abortion was legal, 'mortality had fallen to practically zero' with 'even those doctors of anti-Bolshevist tendency' acknowledging the success of these abortion clinics. Haire was a skilled speaker who kept his audience's attention by combining facts with personal anecdotes; this time he spoke about his cousin and the wife of his barber, who at the hands of the same well-known abortion doctor, had septic miscarriages which had left them permanently damaged and unwell. This was the preface to his message that, for healthy women, competently performed abortions were as safe as any other operation. He emphasised his point with a parable: if removing tonsils was illegal and people were forced to try and remove them with hooks, skewers, hatpins and crochet needles, or could only have them removed by dirty old women or drunken

---

27 Haire's paper was 'On revision of abortion laws', *Anthropos* 1934. [BL – Add 58567. ff 60, 61]. Speakers included Berty Albrecht (Paris), Stella Browne, Janet Chance, Dora Russell and Dr Norman Haire.

or incompetent surgeons clandestinely, these operations would also be fraught with great danger. *The New Generation* (December 1932: 137–38) provided an overview of the speeches. Haire urged those who were fighting to change the present law 'to avoid breaking it in secret' and said the constant stream of women to have abortions abroad were 'some of Britain's invisible exports'. Their distinguished French visitor Berty Albrecht gave her speech on the anthropology of abortion in perfect English, describing it as 'no more a rigid entity than marriage or inheritance' and our views and laws should keep pace with civilisation's intelligence and conscience. Janet Chance, one of the pioneering socialist-feminist crusaders for abortion law reform, said that those who opposed reform did so, not from any tender care for the unborn or the quality of the race, but 'in the superstitions of Sinai and the demands of the God of Battles'. Dora Russell said that ten years earlier Stella Browne had brought her into the struggle to get contraception accepted and had always stressed the need to fight for abortion as well. Haire also paid tribute to the work Stella Browne had done since 1915 to legalise abortion and declared himself 'a convert to her view and to the lesson of the Russian experiment' and she in turn thanked Haire and Russell for their courteous tributes. She felt the movement was 'well launched' but warned members not to be too optimistic or too moderate; 'if we demand *much*, we might get something; if we asked *little*, we should certainly receive less' and urged them to ask that *the woman should decide, in the early months of pregnancy* because 'quick and safe relief from unwelcome parenthood would help men and women to greater mutual understanding, enjoyment, and tenderness'.

Haire said he refused 'from ten to twenty' abortion requests each week because no doctor with any common sense, who could earn an honest living without breaking the law, would take the risk – if convicted, he would be jailed, his name removed from the medical register and he would never work as a doctor again. 'Only a fool or a saint would run this risk' but his patients were 'usually very surprised, disappointed, and resentful' by his refusal and expected that, because he wrote and spoke in favour of changing the law, he would willingly break it. He found this hard to understand because 'it should be obvious' to anyone that such a doctor would be the last person who could afford to break the law and that he must regard every applicant for abortion as a possible *agent provocateur*.[28] In every case when a doctor interrupted a pregnancy, he should ask himself could he justify this operation to the satisfaction of the authorities and, unless he was sure that he could, he should refuse (Haire 1934, 47–48). He even had a card printed:

> As there exists in the minds of a large number of people a confusion between contraception (prevention of conception) and abortion (interruption of an already existing pregnancy), it is necessary to point out that in this country the latter is illegal, except where the continuation of the pregnancy endangers the life or health of the mother. Mr Norman Haire has no moral objection to abortion as such, but cannot transgress against the law. He cannot undertake the interruption of an already existing pregnancy except on unmistakable medical grounds.

There are two versions of Haire's meeting, or meetings, with Aleister Crowley, a drug addict and prolific writer of bad poetry, who claimed to be 'The Beast from the Book of Revelation'. Haire found him repulsive and 'thoroughly evil' and called him a predatory 'polymorph pervert' to be 'sedulously avoided'. Rumours he had heard about Crowley were confirmed by Leila Waddell, an Australian violinist and Crowley's mistress and 'High Priestess', and this intensified Haire's distaste. While Haire was studying and lecturing at Hirschfeld's Institute in early 1932, Crowley was also living in Berlin and asked to meet Haire who replied with an emphatic 'No'. In London, Crowley again asked for a meeting and Haire refused again but this did not deter Crowley. Twenty years later, Haire wrote about this unwelcome visit, saying that in the middle of 1932, while he was in bed recovering from a severe attack of rheumatic fever, Crowley had called at his house one night, pretending to be an old friend and was shown up to his bedroom. Crowley, he said,

---

28 Haire warned Hirschfeld on 27 January 1933 about a case where police used *agents provocateurs*, in a raid on a house where transvestite dances were held, and arrested 50 people. Three were charged with keeping a house for the purposes of giving immoral exhibitions, and the others for frequenting the house. The majority were to face charges in court.

was 'drooling, drink-sodden, and raddled' and his conversation was 'feeble and silly-lecherous' like 'an old ham-actor who had fallen on evil days'. Haire, who was surprised to find him such a tenth-rate ineffectual figure of evil, quickly got rid of him and said he never saw or heard from him again (*JSE*, 4 February–March 1952, 156).

Crowley's biographer John Symonds (1989) said that Crowley first met Haire in Berlin on the first day of 1932 and then in London on 18 July 1932 where, Crowley noted in his journal, they had 'a most amusing and interesting talk' from 10 pm to 1 am. Symonds said that Haire was good at 'telling dirty stories' and describing his patients' bizarre sexual practices and that Haire and Kenneth Tynan had shared Crowley's 'millennial expectations [of] complete sexual freedom'. Symonds was wrong about Haire's expectations – his life was constrained because he was homosexual and this was then a crime. The theatre critic Kenneth Tynan was a more fortunate libertarian who engaged in sexual Olympics and spankings with enthusiastic partners (Billington 2001) but the millennium had *not* arrived; when Tynan said 'fuck' in a 1965 debate on late night BBC television, the morals crusader Mary Whitehouse wrote to the Queen saying he 'ought to have his bottom smacked.'

Haire was still convalescing from rheumatic fever in early June when he gave two very important presentations in perfect French as the co-president of the WLSR. As the WLSR's French representative Pierre Vachet predicted, France's May 1932 elections gave the left their greatest parliamentary victory since the war (Jackson 1987, 145). Haire spoke in Paris on 24 June 1932 to France's new President and one of his senior ministers and then on 27 June at a private meeting of the French sexological societies. A record of his speeches survived because Haire sent them, bound together in a 19-page pamphlet, *La réforme sexuele,* to Ivor Montagu who kept them (Haire 1932).

In his short 24 June speech at the Sorbonne, 'Doctor Norman Haire of London' addressed the President of the Republic, the Minister for Public Health and members of the Association of Sexological Studies, the Scientific Sexology Society, the Society of Criminal Health and the Society of Mental Health. He welcomed the formation of these new French sexological societies (one was led by Berty Albrecht who would later die a heroine of the French Resistance) and said that these societies marked France's official entry into the scientific domain struggling for the good of humanity. He was in sympathy with their aims and wanted to help them find a 'happy formula' for a code which both their radical and conservative members would find acceptable. He warned that this would require long and detailed work and, when they announced the results of their research and tried to implement reforms, they would discover a curious phenomenon: if they said that the earth was flat, people would attack their scientific thinking and if they said that influenza was caused by solar spots or cured by a green umbrella, people would doubt their medical ability, but none would claim 'you hit your mother, or are part of the white slave trade, or have ten wives and twenty mistresses, or that you sleep with a camel'. However, if they said that prostitution should be regulated (or abolished or made free) or if they said that contraception should be permitted (or punished by the guillotine) everyone would accuse them of being Bluebeard, the Marquis de Sade, a child of Sodom or a fallen angel. He said that people pass objective judgements about a scientific problem, without emotion or animosity, but, in the sexual domain, people expressing conclusions are prey to accusations of the most violent and vile sort; he knew from his own experience and he wished them well and, speaking from the heart, exhorted them to 'have courage, more courage and *always* courage'.

In his 27 June address to the private meeting of French sexological societies, Haire stressed how impossible it was to grapple with sexual problems objectively and that, if the things he said made them 'feel angry, indignant or disgusted', they should remember that it was not their intellect which reacted but their emotions. If anyone was shocked by what he was about to say, they should 'consult a psychoanalyst who will discover hidden complexes' which prevented them considering sexual questions objectively. He was concerned with physical and mental health and not the 'soul' because he based his philosophy on reason and not superstition and wanted to see healthy and happy people in this life. He said attitudes about sexual problems were 'terribly muddle-headed and wrong' and caused unnecessary suffering and that only those specially trained or sympathetic people who listened realised just how widespread the problem was. Usually such confidences were only shared with 'sympathetic, tolerant and unprejudiced' people who were more likely to understand the sufferer's outlook if they had also experienced some such unhappiness. Morality, particularly sex morality, was a matter of custom which changed over time and varied from country to country and from class to class – 'What is truth on one side of the Pyrenees is a lie on the other', to quote the French philosopher Blaise Pascal. Haire gave examples of these differences: abortion was legal in Turkey and the Soviet Union but illegal in Europe; in France teaching methods of birth control or using them was forbidden by law; in America it was legal to teach birth control but illegal to instruct people to use them. In England, Holland and other countries, the law permitted the promotion, instruction and use of birth control. In France, homosexuality between adults was considered a private matter and not punished by the law, whereas in England, America and Germany male homosexuality was considered a crime but lesbianism was permitted. He concluded by saying that his proposals were ideas not dogma and ended on an ironic, partly boastful note: he was 'English' and his experience was mostly based on sexual life in England – although he had 'done research on five continents and in 20 different countries', he did not claim to have special knowledge of life in France.

Two months after his two stunning performances in Paris, Haire told Hirschfeld that, because his post-rheumatic fever pulse was still 'far too fast' he was going to the south of France for two weeks to recuperate and would then go by car (via Vienna and Budapest), arriving in the ancient city of Brunn (Brno) on 19 September, the day before the congress. He described himself as the fat man with the camera in 'Bruean' [sic], Czechoslovakia, in the photograph (figure 8.5) he sent his brother Bert.

The Chicago Daily Tribune gave a brief report saying the conference aimed for 'political and economic sexual equality of the sexes' and also noted two American speakers: Dr Hannah Stone would speak about the Birth Control Clinic of New York, and Dr Abraham Stone would lecture on 'Sexual disharmony'.

It was the last WLSR congress; others were planned for Moscow and Chicago but Stalin's rise made Moscow impossible and the Depression

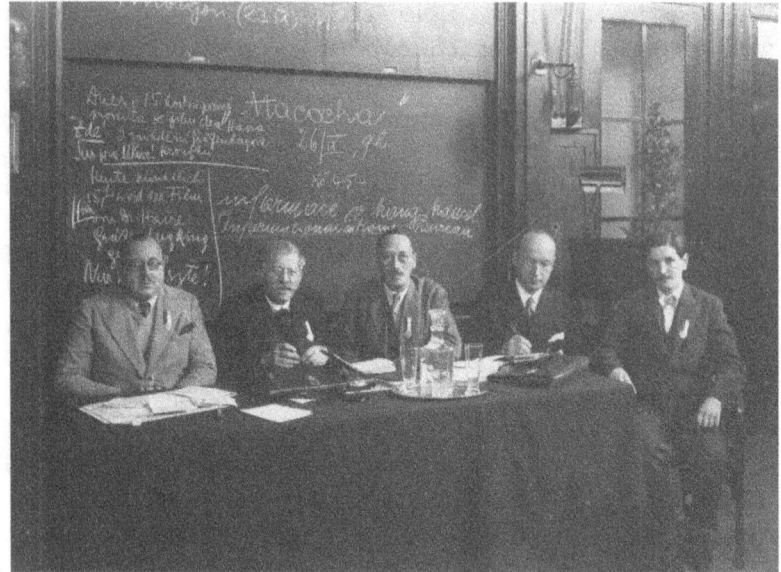

Figure 8.3. Presiding table at the last WLSR congress in Brno, 1932. From the left: Norman Haire, Magnus Hirschfeld, JH Leunbach, Antonin Trýb from Brno University and Josef Weisskopf who organised the congress. Note: The blackboard lists Haire's lecture for physicians only about the Gräfenberg ring.

ruled Chicago out. The WLSR claimed 190,000 members worldwide when it was disbanded in 1935.[29]

Ironically, considering Haire was kept under close surveillance from 1940 on suspicion of being a secret communist, in 1935 he had pleaded for the WLSR to remain apolitical. He was opposed by JH Leunbach, a Committee member of the Danish WLSR, who was greatly influenced by the psychiatrist Wilhelm Reich (who was in exile in Denmark) and believed the League could do nothing important unless

---

29 Dose (2003, 3) quoted statistics: in 1930 the WLSR had 182 individual members and the rest of the 190,000 members belonged to organisations. Both figures are valid and the higher one was not mere puffery: the WLSR had organisations which were members but unfortunately, there is no official members list. Dose believed the WLSR was right to count the corporate members because they belonged to groups which shared the WLSR's views and political aims.

it allied itself with the class struggle (Neill 1945, 21 quoting Reich). Three factors made the WLSR fail: Hitler's rise, Hirschfeld's death and the group's internecine struggles. There was considerable overlap between the WLSR participants and those at Sanger's two meetings (the World Population Congress in Geneva in 1927 and the Seventh International Birth Control Conference in Zurich in September 1930). History professor Anita Grossman (1995, 41, 43) compared the WLSR's Vienna congress and Sanger's Zurich conference: in Vienna the socialist city government funded a lavish banquet and arranged 'crowd-pleasing' exhibits, while in Zurich many speakers stressed the widespread 'sexual misery'. Ironically, the Zurich conference was *not* the end for the birth control movement but it *was* for the WLSR whose Vienna congress was a defiant display before death.

Shortly after the WLSR's 1929 congress in London, John Lane's The Bodley Head press began 'The international library of sexology and psychology' series of low-cost English reprints; Haire was their editor and received one percent for all the titles in the series. Surprisingly, on 7 August 1929 Haire rejected a book proposal from Magnus Hirschfeld, telling the publisher that it was the first time he had ever read a book by Hirschfeld which he had not liked. The co-author of the book (in English, *The erotic world*) was psychiatrist Dr Berndt Götz but Haire said he recognised the style and was sure it was written by Götz alone (it was later published in Dresden by these co-authors). Hirschfeld was a close friend and for this reason Haire asked the publisher to keep his report confidential.

Haire was usually very astute but he made a politically unwise suggestion in January 1932 when he recommended inclusion of a book by Dr Annie Reich, the wife of Wilhelm Reich. He said it was a simply written, skilful mix of Freud's theories and a condemnation of capitalism, describing children's hidden sexual lives and telling parents how to deal with these needs. He recommended it very strongly and said they should sell it for two shillings or two and sixpence; he could point out in the preface that 'while many people may disagree with the politics, it would be interesting for English readers to see the Communistic attitude towards sexual education, in Germany.' Haire

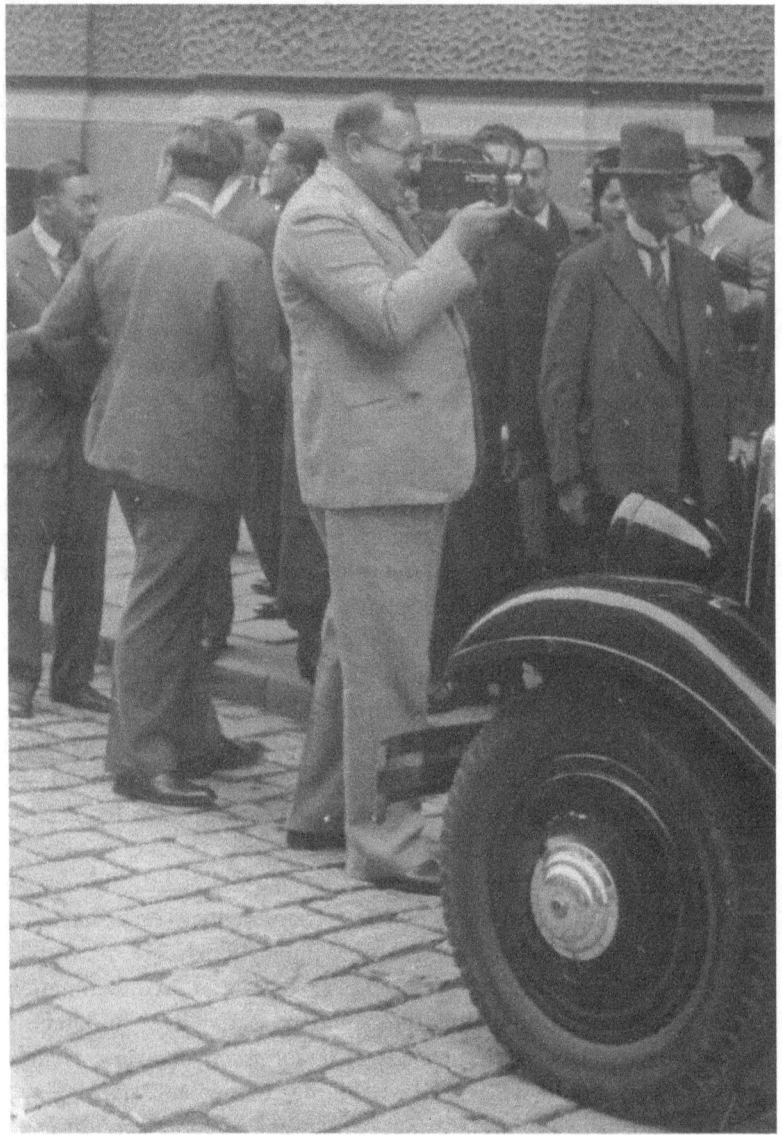

Figure 8.4. Haire with his movie camera at the Brno congress.

wrote to The Bodley Head's Ronald Boswell on 10 January, saying he was disappointed that they would not publish it. On 8 November he also failed to persuade Allen Lane and their decision was personal not political: the publishing house was sliding into chaos and Lane was frequently 'going to "vice-parties" and cavorting with Ethel Mannin and her bohemian friends in the gin-soaked pleasances of the Thames Valley' (Lambert 1987, 250–52). In May 1932 Allen Lane asked Haire, in his role as general editor of 'The international library of sexology and psychology' series, to approach Havelock Ellis and propose that his works be published in the series. Haire knew he had had an unfortunate experience when the first volume of the *Studies in the psychology of sex* received a hostile reception in Britain which made him vow to publish all future work in America but, given 'the universal recognition' of his eminence, Haire hoped that he might reconsider. Haire asked him again in August but Havelock Ellis did not accept the proposal to reprint his *Studies in the psychology of sex* although some of his other writing was published in Britain.

The series did include *Man and woman in marriage* by CBS Evans, an American gynaecologist, although Haire suggested to Allen Lane that 'it might be wise' to get legal advice because the book might be prosecuted for obscenity. Haire wrote a lukewarm preface saying that he disliked the book's Americanisms and the way it mixed 'science with sentiment and religion' but, because it contained so much of importance, he had decided to include it in the series. In the book's promotion Haire was called 'the eminent gynaecologist' and, fearing this might anger Britain's General Medical Council, he wrote a legalistic letter to the *British Medical Journal* on 5 August 1933 which included a denial of 'all foreknowledge or responsibility' for the publisher's 'error of taste'. However, his letter is not in their files of 1922 to 1951 correspondence with him, and Haire's relationship with Allen & Unwin survived this public criticism.

In March 1933 Haire told Norman Himes he had written an 'extensive article about contraception' for Alfred Harmsworth's very popular *Concise home doctor: encyclopaedia of good health*.[30] He may also have contributed an article on contraception to the *Encyclopaedia of health* which Sir William Arbuthnot Lane edited[31] but nothing came of David Eder's plans for him to do some articles in his proposed encyclopaedia. Haire was informed by Margaret Sanger that the editor wanted him to contribute but when no invitation came, Haire asked Havelock Ellis on 9 March 1928 if he would mind asking Sanger to remind Arbuthnot Lane because he 'very much' wanted to contribute. He also wrote the introduction to Niels Hoyer's *Man into woman*, an account of the surgical procedures by which Einar Wegener, a well-known Danish painter, became the world's first transsexual but had soon died after additional surgery. Haire warned that until more was known about sexual physiology it would be unwise to perform such operations even at the patient's request. He said with psychological treatment the painter might have led a reasonably happy life instead of embarking on the painful and dangerous operations which proved fatal. Interest in sex change operations soared when Bronx-born George Jorgensen 'went abroad and came back a broad' – as Christine Jorgensen (Reis 2001, 385). Haire was speaking from personal experience when he said years later that, after sensational press reports about alleged sex change operations, 'well-known sexologists' were deluged with letters from persons who wanted the operation (*JSE* April – 1950, 200).

The hardships of the Depression were not as bad for Haire as they were for many others although he went without a car for two years and his patients could not pay their bills. However the restrictions to civil liberties which started in this period became worse as the decade progressed. The high hopes for sexual reform were to be shattered.

---

30 The Amalgamated Press was established by Alfred Harmsworth (later Viscount Northcliffe), described by *Encyclopaedia Britannica* (1965, 16, 616) as 'the most successful newspaper publisher in the history of the British press and the creator of popular journalism'. Haire's article was on pages 395–96 of *The concise home doctor*, published in 1932 by a subsidiary company.

31 British Books Ltd published it in their 'Golden health library' series and it was advertised in *Good Health: Organ of the Good Health League* (March 1933, 17).

9

Escalating troubles

Man into woman aroused curiosity in Britain but another book caused outrage even though old taboos were dying, people were discussing the dangers of sexual ignorance, laws were becoming more liberal, many countries had set up birth control centres and even 'religionists' were acknowledging the need for sex education. The book, which Haire included in his series, was a translation of *Sex life and sex ethics* by René Guyon, a French-born judge on Thailand's Supreme Court.

Guyon was also a sexual philosopher who approved of Haire's rejection of conventional sexual morality and had sent him the manuscript in 1930. Haire described it as 'one of the most important contributions to sexological literature' and suggested the publisher should call it 'Sexual acts and sexual ethics' or perhaps 'Sex acts and sex ethics*'* because William Stallybrass, the paunchy principal of Oxford's Brasenose College, had told him that 'sex' was a less offensive word than 'sexual'. Stallybrass argued that it was 'a good thing to keep all old traditions, especially the bad ones', but ignored this advice by arriving at the college ball with the Lord Chief Justice, Baron Goddard on his arm.[1]

The publisher preferred *Sex life and sex ethic*s but to Haire that seemed too far from the subject and he suggested 'Sex ethics' or 'Sex conduct and sex ethics'. The publisher insisted on their safe title, perhaps because the book included incest, homosexuality, fetishism and necrophilia. Guyon's book, and its sequel *Sexual freedom*, formed 'the doctrine of sexual legitimacy and sexual freedom' in which all things were acceptable unless they harmed others. To him, the prohibitions imposed by church-based moralists were the root of all neuroses and he called chastity the 'veritable triumph of neurosis' and said that enforced abstinence was as illogical as training a person to forgo food. His views

---

1 *Time*, 13 October 1947. He was William Sonnenschein until his father changed his name to Stallybrass in 1917 when King George V changed his.

are still being evaluated[2] but in the 1930s Alec Craig worried that if sex reform took this path it would 'meet with early extinction at the hands of reactionaries'. He also regarded Guyon's dismissal of 'individualised love' as nostalgia for primitive conditions and felt his proposals – that the 'new morality' should be for all age groups and was of no concern to the law – would give license to libertines whose actions would damage communities and vulnerable individuals (Craig 1934, 134–39). Haire helped to promote the books because 'However little acceptance his views may find, M Guyon's exposition of them is so clear, so concise, so logical and so courageous, that the book should prove valuable to all students of Sexology, no matter to what school of morals they belong'.

Haire sent Hirschfeld an explicit warning in December 1932 because whenever French people heard his name mentioned they always replied, 'Oh, of course, he is homosexual'. To protect his friend, Haire always replied that he had no reason to think he was homosexual and that it would be as stupid to reach this conclusion because he wrote about homosexuality as it would be to suppose that he was a transvestite, exhibitionist or sadist because he wrote about these subjects. Haire emphasised that 'the impression *does exist* in Paris' and it was his 'duty as a friend and grateful pupil' to tell him before he decided to live there because 'a lot of enemies' would 'make themselves unpleasant', particularly if he was accompanied by either of his young secretaries, Karl Giese or Tao Li. Haire suggested Spain would be cheaper, conditions there were more favourable to their world view and he would get help from the League's Spanish branch.

This letter could indicate that Haire's caution was so ingrained that he would deny the reality of Hirschfeld's transvestism and homosexuality, or that he had to write the letter in code to prevent it being intercepted. Haire sent Hirschfeld two press clippings for his amusement: the announcement that Princess Alice, Countess of Athlone, would be the patron of a Malthusian Ball and a brochure for this event which was held at the Dorchester Hotel on 22 March 1933. It was in aid of the global work done in London by Sanger's Birth Control International Centre and in May *The Birth Control Review* reported that the ball had made history as

---

2 See Haeberle (1983, 159–72) and Etzioni and Baris (July 2005, 224–26).

the first time the British Royal Family had allowed the use of its name in connection with the birth control movement; it attracted wide publicity and was graced by hundreds of influential 'writers, scientists, clergy, educators, medical men and women, military and naval officers, actors, actresses' as well as politicians and representatives from 'every church' and the 'best-known families in England.'[3] Haire said that this indicated just how respectable birth control had become in Britain. When there was no response, Haire worried about Hirschfeld and his institute and sent a prescient letter on 24 March saying they were 'all very shocked at the political persecution in Germany'. To him it seemed 'even worse than the outbreak of the Great War'. He 'always regarded Germany as *the* home of civilisation', and now all his ideas about it were shattered. 'It really seems as if life is not worth living at all'.

He was anxious to hear how Hirschfeld was, mentioned that he had had a series of bad colds and had lost his voice in a bad case of laryngitis and was going to Spain for a motoring trip in April to try and recover. Haire did not let ill health hinder him; on 28 March he apologised to Dora Russell for missing her school's play night because he had had to operate on a woman who was gravely ill after a nurse had tried to abort her with slippery elm twigs. He invited Russell to dine at his house after an April WLSR lecture by the Conservative politician Bob Boothby (later Baron Boothby). Haire had also asked 'just a dozen or so' other politician friends to supper and told Russell he was anxious about the next day's lecture on the Gräfenberg ring to the Federation of Progressive Societies.[4] It was to have been accompanied by slides and a film: Haire had received written permission to show them, and all the tickets had been sold. However, at the last moment 'the humbuggers!' (the Federation) had withdrawn their permission and he expected pandemonium would follow with everyone wanting their money back.

---

3 Graves and Hodge (1941, 95–96) mistakenly mentioned a ball held in 1924: 'A large and successful Birth-Control Ball was held at the Hammersmith Palais de Danse'. Lesley Hall (2009) wrote, 'This is one of the several places where Graves and Hodges' rather informal approach (which approaches sloppiness at times) let them down'.

4 He gave this 'physicians only' lecture at the 1932 WLSR congress, and the 9 January 1932 *BMJ* advertised another for the Paddington Medical Society.

However, sometimes pleasant unexpected things happened, such as the honour of having his name mentioned in WH Auden's poem 'A Happy New Year':[5]

> Doctors attended behind each chair,
> Behind the men was Sir Thomas Horder,
> Behind the women Dr Norman Haire

His poem has distilled the essence of the way society operated in those years when the Establishment's Lord Horder upheld the male status quo and Haire, as a maverick advocate of contraception and sexual reform, supported women's liberation.

Haire kept a diary of his January to April 1933 trip to Spain and Portugal and listed the cost of hotels, garages, petrol, oil for the car, rubber goods, shaves, tips, food and cigarettes (he smoked a pipe and Player's ultra-masculine Navy Cut cigarettes). He sailed from Folkestone in Kent to Boulogne where the landing charge and tip came to 72.50 francs and he shouted a companion identified as 'Sawyer' a 14-franc dinner, making a note that he had given him 100 so he was owed 86 francs. In Spain he gave 'La Sawyer' 150 pesetas and another 50 when he got a letter of credit for £25 (equal to 100 pesetas). This was generous considering a brothel and whore had cost five pesetas each and a cushion and seat at a bullfight was only half a peseta. During this sexologist's holiday Haire gave several lectures – in Spanish – on birth control at the University of Madrid[6] and had been astounded by the high rate of venereal diseases in these countries.

When he returned, there was a letter from Himes who expected to send the first volume of his *Medical history of contraception* to the publisher by August. It began as his Harvard PhD thesis which was an overview of ancient and modern methods of birth control and it had

---

5 WH Auden's poem appeared in Leonard and Virginia Woolf's *New country: prose and poetry by the authors of New Signatures* (1933, 199). Reproduced with the permission of Curtis Brown Ltd.

6 Haire asked Havelock Ellis to show him the second issue of the Spanish *SEXUS* and any other cutting dealing with the *Jornadas Eugenicas* (his lecture there) and their interview with him (Haire to Ellis, 21 June 1933 – HC – 3.16)].

a bibliography of 2000 references in the first volume alone. Himes' seminal work was published in 1936 as a single 521-page book but he doubted if there would ever be a new edition of his *Guide* which 'alas' sold very poorly.[7]

There was a tantalising advertisement in the *British Medical Journal* on 6 May 1933 for a Symposium on Birth Control by the London Jewish Hospital Medical Society in the inner London area of Stepney Green. The two speakers were Haire and Dr Enid Charles; she was the author of *The practice of birth control: an analysis of the birth-control experiences of nine-hundred women* and in 1934 her controversial book, *The twilight of parenthood: a biological study of the decline of population growth*, challenged the eugenic views of that time. I could not find details of the 1933 symposium because archivists at the Royal London Hospital Archives and Museum had no relevant records and suggested contacting the London Jewish Hospital Medical Society but their archivist did not respond to my requests.

In Germany, the Nazi campaign intensified in May 1933 and, after confiscating Marxist, communist, pacifist, Jewish and other 'un-German' books from libraries and private owners, Goebbels officiated at the notorious 10 May book burnings in Berlin's Opera Place. Stormtroopers and Nazi youths burnt about 20,000 books from Hirschfeld's Institute for Sexual Research and the Humboldt University and made abusive speeches about their authors: psychologists and sexologists such as Freud, Hirschfeld and Havelock Ellis, moderate liberals such as Haire and Sanger, and those who were long dead such as Richard Krafft-Ebing, EH Kisch, Iwan Bloch and August Forel. The following day *The Times*' Berlin correspondent listed the books burnt, including the complete works of Karl Marx and Lenin along with Anglo-Saxon authors such as Upton Sinclair, Ernest Hemingway and Jack London. The reporter observed 'The destruction of books on sex by Dr Magnus Hirschfeld and other books classified as "obscene" or "trash" will cause no regret to the great majority of Germans'.

---

7 In *The International Journal of Psychoanalysis*, 14, 1933, an anonymous reviewer of Himes' 46-page work, *A guide to birth control literature* 1931, 'queried the wisdom of omitting reference to the writings of Havelock Ellis, HG Wells, Bertrand Russell, Dean Inge and Lord Dawson of Penn' and others.

Haire wrote two letters on 19 May; in the first he told Karl Giese that he had received a letter from 'Papa' (Hirschfeld) who had gone to Paris and he reassured Karl that he would not disclose Hirschfeld's address. Haire said they were 'stupefied' by what had happened in Germany, and particularly by what happened at the institute and asked if they had expected a raid when 'the Jew-baiting began'. Did they have time to remove and hide, or destroy, any books and papers that they did not want to fall into Nazi hands? Papa had asked Leunbach and Haire to see him in Paris as soon as possible and he supposed they would decide on the future of the League and perhaps open a headquarters in Copenhagen as Leunbach suggested.

Haire sent the second letter to Hirschfeld, expressing his shock at the mayhem in Germany and reassuring him that WLSR members would do their utmost for those in jail but he warned that while the British condemned Hitler's treatment of the Jews, many were less concerned about his anti-communist actions. Haire wrote again on 10 June, sending his 'best regards' to 'our Dutch friend' (Haire's partner Willem Van de Hagt) but apologised that he could not provide Hirschfeld with accommodation. In September Haire warned Hirschfeld not to say he was 'coming to England for a consultation' because the BMA, fearing an influx of German doctors, had asked hospitals not to take them as students, and had requested the Home Office to refuse them entry. He should say he was coming on holiday and be careful to avoid taking paid work because he would risk deportation if he earned any money in Britain.

A month after the book burnings, WLSR members were stunned by the death of Dr Hildegart Rodriguez, the brilliant 19-year-old secretary of the WLSR's Spanish branch and a socialist whose activities as a writer and lecturer helped to popularise sexology. Havelock Ellis had been in 'constant friendly correspondence' with her for two years and she 'took his breath away'. Ellis enthused about her wonderful radiance to Sanger, saying that his 'Spanish lawyer girl seems quite one of the wonders of the world!'; he called her mother one of his 'New Mothers' and attributed the girl's virtuosity to her upbringing and celebrated them both in the June 1933 issue of *The Adelphi*, finding to his horror that his article on

'The Red Virgin' coincided with her murder – shot dead on 9 June by her mother in sexual frenzy.[8] In court the mother said that a prominent Englishman – she meant the 67-year-old HG Wells – offered to take the girl to England but she would not let her go alone. Haire was terribly upset but 'not altogether surprised' because the *ménage* had been very odd and Madrid was rife with conflicting rumours. He invited Havelock Ellis to discuss it over dinner and he accepted the invitation; on 14 June Haire asked if he had any special food requirements. The prospect of seeing Haire's film of the two women must have been irresistible (Grosskurth 1985, 434). Haire often invited him to visit his London home but the old man usually refused, although they dined together quite often in a Soho restaurant (Grosskurth 1985, 377). The reclusive Havelock Ellis, who lived out of London, was selective in the invitations he accepted and did not like going out at night.

In September 1933 Ellis agreed when Haire proposed to 'motor down to his house' in Haslemere, Surrey and make a special film. Afterwards Ellis told Sanger about the pictures Haire took with his movie camera when he and Françoise Lafitte-Cyon walked around the garden. She was 27 years younger than her partner and she liked Haire finding him 'engagingly simple and childlike, in spite of the qualities which make so many people detest him'. Ellis added, 'he is tremendously active and professionally prosperous, as well as in writing and editing sex books'.

As the year ended Haire told Hirschfeld that he had not been well and needed a holiday but he had been kept in London because he had three confinements scheduled and a planned series of ten sexology lectures. In October, November and December he delivered these lectures for the Promethean Society,[9] a short-lived organisation of young radicals who

---

8   Haire (BL Add 70542. 16 May 1933, f. 64 [really 16 June]) informed HE that a final-year medical student, who was present at the post-mortem operation, said there were two bullet wounds in the head, one in the left breast and one *au sexe*. So it evidently was a 'sexual crime'. See also Sinclair (2003) and *Margaret Sanger Papers Project Newsletter*, 30, Spring 2002.

9   Like Shelley, who saw Prometheus as the champion of human liberty, the Promethean Society dreamed of creating a glorious revolutionary future. *The Socialist Review: A Monthly Review of Modern Thought* (1933, 56) announced Haire's lectures as 'A new experiment in adult education'.

discussed politics, sexology, philosophy and art and published a journal called *Twentieth Century* (Hynes 1977, 83). Haire told Dora Russell that the lecture course at the London School of Hygiene and Tropical Medicine cost ten shillings and had been fully booked, with about 50 people having to be turned away. He suggested it would be good to repeat them for the WLSR and, if there was any deficit, he would make it up but he expected they would make about £50 profit.

He said he had considered going to Egypt but could not get a good cabin on the boat so went to Sanger's American conference instead. However, it is hard to believe that his participation as a key conference speaker was such a spur-of-the-moment decision. On 3 January 1934 *The Times* reported his departure for the United States on the *Aquitania* and that he would be away from London for about six weeks. Margaret Sanger announced in *The Washington Post* on 7 January that he and Dr Cecil Voge would attend the American Conference on Birth Control in Washington, describing them as 'two of the British Empire's leading birth control advocates'. By making this announcement she was acknowledging that Haire's importance was equal to that of Dr Voge who, with Edinburgh's Professor Crew, had Sanger's support and American funds to find the 'perfect contraceptive' (Soloway 1995, 650).

Time described the birth controllers' Washington march for 'their annual harangue' of 'unheeding Congressmen' at the White House, saying they were led by Margaret Sanger 'in green' and Mrs Thomas Norval Hepburn (mother of six including actress Katharine Hepburn) 'in black', in their fourth bid to overturn the ban on contraceptive information. Their chief opponent was Charles Coughlin, a Roman Catholic priest and demagogue whose weekly anti-Semitic, pro-Nazi radio broadcasts were heard by millions.[10] *The Washington Post* reported on 19 January that the packed parliamentary chamber had jeered when Father Coughlin claimed that Negroes and Poles were 'out-begetting the Anglo-Saxon and Celtic races' and again when he depicted birth control as being 'criminal for Catholics and dangerous for the nation.' On 29 January *Time* quoted 'London's Norman Haire' who said that 'Father

---

10 On 20 November 1938, two weeks after *Kristallnacht*, Father Coughlin delivered an anti-Semitic radio address in which he defended Nazi violence.

ESCALATING TROUBLES

Coughlin doesn't care how much the children suffer on earth, so long as they are prepared to pick up their little harps and sing Hallelujah'. Sanger thanked Haire for his 'splendid presentation' in New York, which had made the symposium a success. Haire invited her to his New York farewell 'at home' and said that he planned to return in late October for a business tour, unlike his previous lectures 'for the love of God!' He told Ellis that he 'saw a good deal of the sexual life of New York', so fatigue might have prompted him to confide in Sanger on 30 January:

> I think that will be my last conference. Conferences are for the young. We older people (I was 42 last week) can do more by reporting our results at other meetings, unhampered by the shortage of time which is inevitable at conferences, or by publishing them in full detail instead.

He had a habit of making such resolutions and ignoring them. Nor did he make the American tour in late October but went to Italy instead.

Curiously, Haire's activities were reported in Sydney by George Southern, a psychologist, physical educationalist, body builder and alleged paedophile[11] who wrote a passionately confused book called *Making morality: a broadside attack on morality, likely to make wowsers yell and thinkers think*. When it was banned, he proudly published and printed it himself sending copies to experts including Australian naturalist David G Stead, Havelock Ellis, Julian Huxley and Bronislaw Malinowski. He asked if they thought the book was obscene or indecent, should it be banned, would it have a good or bad effect on public thinking and was it in harmony with scientific thought (Southern 1934, 6). He incorporated their replies into his book, including one by Dr William J Robinson, an American contraception crusader who responded on 22 January 1934:

> The same ideas in a much more radical manner are expressed in René Guyon's *Sex life and sex ethics*, which has an introduction by Norman Haire, who, by the way, is in my rooms to-night and having dinner with me.

---

11   Lisa Featherstone, the 2005 CH Currey Memorial Fellow, examined Southern's Papers (Mitchell Library at MSS 7173) and made this claim in her 19 June 2006 presentation to the State Library of NSW.

Havelock Ellis was astounded by the questions and asked, 'But what is Australia coming to! It is terrible indeed to hear of the restrictions that have been placed on liberty of thought and literature in Australia' where he had spent 'the happiest years' of his early life and received inspiration for his 'life-work in the psychology of sex.' He told Southern that when he was there Australians would not have tolerated these restrictions. He had hoped that Australia would help to lead the world and had never imagined that 'so beautiful a land would merely raise a race of slaves'. During his teenage Australian sojourn, no one had challenged his freedom but it would have been very different if Ellis had stayed in Australia and began to write or speak about sexuality as an adult; in the most notorious example, William Chidley's beliefs on diet, dress and sexuality led to his forced detention in Sydney's Callan Park Mental Hospital from 1912 until his death in 1916 (Edwards & Hall, 1980). He was a patient when Haire worked there and Haire found him 'quite odd' but 'not dangerous'. However, he had been considered 'sufficiently insane to be a public nuisance' because he walked around Sydney streets in a very thin silk garment discussing love and at one time had been the chief attraction on Sunday afternoons in the Domain (Haire to Havelock Ellis, 11 April 1928 – HC 3.16).

Havelock Ellis criticised Southern's book on some issues and said that many readers 'would not agree that Communism (or Fascism either) is needed to speed up the process of Sexual Reform'. Southern failed to establish a WLSR branch in Sydney[12] and remained Australia's only member, despite writing to 14 'eminent and broadminded' Sydney people, selected from a list Haire had given him. Some sent good wishes and one woman said she 'dared not' have her name publicly associated with the League, 'lest all the parents of the innocent (?) girls under her care be shocked out of their skins.' Southern lamented Australia's lack of Norman Haires, Julian Huxleys, HG Wells, Bernard Shaws and

---

12 See Racial Hygiene Association papers, 7 June 1932. After his WLSR proposal, opinion was divided on whether Southern should be asked to resign. He had been elected to the RHA's Executive on 20 July 1931.

Bertrand Russells but he did have one supporter, 'a Socialist' who was 'a very able and fearless journalist'. This was probably Mervyn Skipper.[13]

The Times announced on 9 February 1934 that Mr Norman Haire had returned from the United States by the *Ile de France* and was back at 127 Harley Street. Three days later, he gave his first London lecture on 'The elements of sexology' on behalf of the WLSR. All three of these series of seven-week courses were advertised in *The Times* and each course cost ten shillings and six pence.[14] Haire also told Norman Himes he was tired of giving free lectures and Himes replied that he was 'through with lecturing for the love of God or the love of anyone else'. Haire said in his two Glasgow lectures people were sitting on window-sills and many were turned away, but, despite the success of the lectures the fee had not quite covered his expenses.

After Marie Stopes snubbed him at one of the meetings, he guessed the source of her unfriendliness when she wrote to complain that he had made 'misrepresentations' and 'interrogatory' remarks about her and her work. He replied that he had no idea what she meant and patiently explained the situation in a long, peace-making response: he thought the remarks were either made by intentional mischief-makers or else by people who admired her so ardently that any criticism of her views seemed like sacrilege, adding that 'we all have "fans" of that sort'. When audience members asked questions such as 'Is Marie Stopes right when she says . . .', he always replied that he disagreed with her on certain points but accompanied this by acknowledging the magnificent work she had done for the birth control movement in this country.

'Up till 1928' Haire said that he had been incensed by her criticisms of him and his work and by the unflattering remarks that many of their mutual friends said she made about him. Then Haire had decided that hostility was stupid because they 'were both far too *big* to have a silly

---

13 Mervyn Skipper was an art critic and edited *Pandemonium*. For censorship of Southern's book, see *Pandemonium* (6), July 1934; articles by Southern are in issues 4, 6, 7 and 8. See also Tregenza (1965, 32–35, 92).

14 *The Times*, 20 January 1934, 8; and 7 April 1934,1. The first lectures were on Tuesday evenings from 13 February to 27 March 1934, in Transport House, Westminster, and the second series on Wednesday evenings at the London School of Hygiene, from 10 April to 22 May.

little personal quarrel'. And so he took the first step in Copenhagen by praising the work Stopes and her husband had done for birth control. In 1929 he invited her to read a paper at the WLSR congress, which she accepted. Since then he had taken every opportunity to praise her splendid work and he had done this not only in Britain but in America, France, Spain, Germany, Austria and Czechoslovakia. People still told him that she made unfriendly remarks about him and it sometimes made him sad, but he always hoped that the reports were untrue. He asked her, if she heard any more rumours, to ask the person who reported them to give 'details of place, time, and nature of the misrepresentations or disparaging remarks' and to let him know more precisely what these objections were. He ended, 'We both have enemies enough to fight in the Anti-Birth-Control camp without engaging in quarrels or misunderstandings between ourselves'. Stopes kept Haire's letter in her correspondence files and added two hand-written comments: 'No ref to all the really big things I have done!' and 'No ans'. Her wish for more flattery, and her decision to ignore his attempt at reconciliation, reflects well on Haire and very poorly on her. She saw herself as the queen bee of birth control and was herself stung when people did not pay her the homage she felt she deserved.[15]

Haire boasted to Hirschfeld about his forthcoming lectures 'for *clergymen*!!!' and sent Havelock Ellis details of the lectures on 29 May; there were 'about three hundred at each of the first and second courses, about two hundred at the third, and about one hundred in the special course for clergymen'. It was 'quite a new departure' for Britain and he was very gratified by the lectures' popularity. The Bodley Head was to publish them later in the year. Reader pressure prompted Allen & Unwin to ask Haire in 1936 if they were to have 'the pleasure of publishing it for you?' but the lectures were not published.

However, The Bodley Head published a book by an Australian-born sexologist, Robert Storer, despite Haire's caution in May that he thought publishing one of his books would lower the tone of the series and publishing three would be very unwise.[16] There must have been a

---

15   Haire to Stopes 14 March, 1934. BL. Add 58567, ff 63–64.
16   John Lane published one of Storer's books in 1934 and three others were

feud because Haire told the publishers to ignore anything Storer alleged that he had said and to wait until he spoke to them directly in a meeting. In 1933 Storer had been charged for trying to sell his sexual survey book to a Sydney policeman and the case made history when, for the first time, expert witnesses were allowed to testify and the judge decided the book was not obscene.[17] Haire's caution *was* justified, however, because Storer was struck off the British Medical Register in 1935 and he was later jailed.[18]

In May 1934 Haire sent Havelock Ellis another cautious invitation saying that several times he had wanted to phone or write to ask him to see the film he had taken of the couple in their garden but he knew how much Ellis hated being disturbed. He said, 'the film came out very well' and again offered to send 'the car' (his chauffeur-driven Rolls) However, the differences in the electrical system made it impossible to show it at Havelock Ellis' house and a variety of causes prevented him from ever seeing it. He was an old man who did not like going out to dinner so he is unlikely to have accepted Haire's 9 July 1934 invitation to dine with Joseph Lewis, the American freethinker and crusader for atheism, who was about to visit London. The previous year Haire wrote to Havelock Ellis about another visiting American, William J Fielding, the author of 'very good popular books on sex' who was very anxious to meet him. Haire described Fielding as a very pleasant and sympathetic person and advised him to write to Havelock Ellis himself although he held out little hope.

Haire told Ellis that he had 'very thoroughly revised' *The encyclopaedia of sexual knowledge* and was 'vain enough' to think that the parts he wrote, or re-wrote, were the best, although there was much he would have preferred to leave out. Paul Ferris discussed it in his book *Sex and the British* (1970, 179) and called it 'soft core

---

published by J Bale, Sons & Danielson Ltd in 1934 and 1935.

17 Coleman (1963, 81–82); Wyndham (2003, 90).

18 On 8 June 1935 the *BMJ* reported that Storer was struck off the British Medical Register for advertising his Cavendish Institute of Pathology; he was also struck off the Australian register. He was arrested in September 1938 (in a car with a 15-year-old boy) and sentenced to 12 months in jail.

pornography in disguise' which had escaped censorship because it was presented as an educational work but readers' hopes for titillation had made it a bestseller. Haire had warned the publisher on 9 July that their 'rather sensational' advertising for the book was not suitable for English taste but they insisted and were fined £10 and £3.3.0 costs for sending 'indecent matter' through the post. Haire wrote to the *British Medical Journal* on 21 July to correct the 'false impression' in their report, explaining he had been unable to present the facts in court because he was attending an obstetric case in Scotland.

It is possible to piece together this Scottish 'case' from two different sources – Haire himself (who mistakenly thought his case was anonymous) and a birth notice in *The Times*. In June Haire told Hirschfeld he was going to stay at Strathallan Castle in Perthshire to confine a woman whose sterility he had cured and, on 5 July 1934 *The Times* announced the birth of a daughter at the castle to Irene, wife of Sir James Denby Roberts.[19] Haire discussed this in *Everyday sex problems* to show that 'even a millionaire would have difficulty in equaling the facilities available at a good obstetric hospital'. He said he had traveled from London to Scotland twice, spending three weeks each time at the castle. The owner provided all the necessary utensils and linen from a list that Haire had sent him but the lighting was so poor that the castle servants had to fetch an electric light from the owner's private ice-rink and install it in the bedroom to provide adequate lighting for the confinement. Haire was accompanied by an anesthetist and two nurses who had to sterilise the instruments on a portable kerosene stove which was quite inadequate and they had to go down two flights of stairs to the basement kitchen for boiling water. Haire said how serious it would have been if there had been any serious complications.

Haire had many interests and, like the Hungarian-born polymath Arthur Koestler who in the 1930s had to work as a hack writer, from the 1930s to the 1950s Haire edited three mildly salacious encyclopaedias on sex that were translated into several languages and provided a bonanza for the publishers, who were reputed to have made £15,000 from the

---

19 The Roberts had married in 1927 and the sterility treatment Haire provided must have succeeded because they had two more children.

first book in France alone (Koestler 1969, 271). Haire did not benefit from this; he was paid a lump sum, received no royalties and had no financial interest in the book sales. He probably lost money because he had to give court evidence in 1951 when a bookseller was prosecuted for selling these 'obscene' books.[20] The 'essentially innocent – if somewhat reckless' bookseller was sentenced to 12 months' imprisonment and his company had to pay £200 costs even though *The encyclopaedia of sexual knowledge* had been freely on sale for years.

Koestler (1969, 261) wrote a chapter 'Introducing Dr Costler' in his autobiography *The invisible writing* and complained about not earning much as 'A Costler, MD', the half-hearted disguise he used for the three books he wrote between 1934 and 1939 in 'intervals between various imprisonments'. At the invitation of his publisher cousins (Willy and Ferenc Aldor), Koestler and two others produced *The encyclopaedia of sexual knowledge* 'in about six to eight weeks' from about a dozen standard reference books the publisher provided, including van de Velde's 1926 bestseller *Ideal marriage* which had already made the Aldors rich. Koestler complained that his 'rogue cousin' Ferenc Aldor did not pay him royalties and had threatened to disclose Dr Costler's identity 'to the world public': this was unreasonable because Koestler had been paid a flat fee of 3000 francs (Scammell 2009, 106) and he should have chosen an obscure name if wanted to hide his identity. When he claimed that *The encyclopaedia of sexual knowledge* was his only book to 'meet with a unanimously friendly reception', Koestler ignored criticism and only quoted the flattering book jacket reviews.

Haire also relished such hyperbole and quoted Sir John Hammerton who *Time* described as a statesman and the 'husky' editor of *War illustrated*. 'Mr Haire', he said, was 'as prominent and as great an authority on sex education as any single individual in the medical world'; his 'wide and very deep experience in this difficult branch of knowledge enables him to estimate accurately the difficulties that confront him, and to tackle those difficulties without being mealy-mouthed' and his writing

---

20   Haire in 'Prosecutions for obscenity', *JSE*, February–March 1951, 157; and Alec Craig, reported in *The Eugenics Review*, 64(4), 241.

would present readers 'with some of the most valuable and stimulating chapters' in *The enclyclopaedia of sexual knowledge.*

It sold 50,000 copies in 1930s Britain and sold over 5000 copies in several updated editions until the late 1950s (Dose 2003, 13) but it is now largely forgotten (Craig 1963, 104). This suited Robert Dalby whose 2005 book was criticised in the *British Medical Journal* on 21 January 2006 for 'greatly distorting the research findings' about circumcision. An example of this is a paragraph that Dalby quoted from *The encyclopaedia* which, he claimed, showed that Haire had a 'hostile attitude towards the foreskin.' Haire was the editor of this section and the paragraph about balanitis (inflammation of the penis head) did not paint a 'lurid' picture but suggested simple treatment: 'strict cleanliness and care in keeping the parts dry.' Dalby altered this to read 'Norman Haire wrote that either scrupulous cleanliness or circumcision was needed.' Similarly, radical feminist Margaret Jackson objected to a passage she attributed to Haire in the encyclopaedia's chapter on 'Frigidity in woman'. It had asserted that there was a constant struggle between a man and woman within marriage because the woman refused to submit and that she could not have an orgasm because she rebelled against being conquered. Haire was a hedonist not a misogynist and he did not write this; as his editor's notes show, this chapter was compiled from van de Velde's marriage manual and Wilhelm Stekel's book on frigidity.

Responses to *The encyclopaedia* ranged from admiration to outrage. Some disliked the 'new sphere of sexology' which Havelock Ellis described as still being 'the youngest, and the Cinderella, of various branches of medicine'; it is still seeking legitimacy (*Sexologies* 2009). When Dr Alan Guttmacher reviewed *The encyclopaedia* for the *Journal of Contraception* in January 1937, it was ironic because, despite being American, he did not like the 'juicy title' or the term 'sexologist' and called it 'a neologism without the benefit of benediction by the *Oxford Dictionary*' – less surprisingly, a British reviewer also objected to the term 'sexology.'[21] Guttmacher admired 'the intrinsic merit' of some

---

21 A reviewer in *The Times Literary Supplement* (10 April 1937, 268) found Craig's *The banned books of England* 'well documented and (subject to the use of words like 'sexology', which may grate on the purist) well written'.

parts and the book's approach to topics, although the section on 'procreation' showed 'an amazing absence of scientific critique.' This was not surprising because it was written by Dr Levy-Lenz who specialised in sex-change operations.[22] Guttmacher praised the author of another section [Haire] for 'wisely' denying that the '"Safe Period" is safe'. He regretted that Haire's chapter on 'The prevention of conception' was omitted and ridiculed the disclaimer that, as the chapter 'written for the English edition might possibly have come in conflict with the United States laws concerning transmission of contraceptive information through the mails', the American publishers had substituted another which contained 'views and opinions with which Dr Haire is in strong disagreement and is not to be considered as representing Dr Haire's viewpoint'.

Guttmacher applauded, 'Good for Dr Haire, even though his views are not expressed we feel quite sure that they would be more like our own than the anonymous American scribe'. He liked the chapter on sexual aberrations best of all for pointing out, first, that mild aberrations are normal for most people and only become pathological if they became 'overshadowing and uncontrollable' and, second, that such 'bypaths of normal sex play' are not perversions at all if done in couples' own rooms. However, he found it 'a spotty collection' that was only suitable for a student 'who can separate the wheat from the chaff'.

Despite his opposition to censorship, Alec Craig expressed his doubts in a letter to Norman Himes in October 1941, saying that Britain's Eugenics Society had asked him to review *The encyclopaedia of sexual knowledge*, Volume II by Drs A Willy, L Vander, O Fischer and others (London, Francis Aldor, [no date]). He thought it was a reprint of an American publication but in wartime London the British Museum was closed and he could not confirm this. He said the review copy was 'not a very attractive affair' but he did not want to do the book or the authors an injustice. He asked Himes if he knew the standing of the American edition of the authors, noting that a previous volume had been issued by the same publishers in 1934 under the general editorship of Norman

---

22 Dr Levy-Lenz with Dr Felix Abraham performed the world's first sex-change operation in 1931 at Hirschfeld's Institute in Berlin.

Haire. He said this had had a rather more scholarly appearance but he found 'more than a suggestion of the bogus about both volumes'.

Himes cautiously confirmed Craig's suspicions but said it was difficult to answer questions about *The encyclopaedia of sexual knowledge*, Volume II, because he had been too busy to do any library research. Although he had not inspected the book carefully, he thought it was 'not very high grade scientifically' but conceded that he had insufficient knowledge to even give a preliminary opinion; perhaps they should judge the book on its own internal merits? He had never heard of the authors so he had assumed that the book was English because if it had an American origin he would have known about them if they had any standing.

The third book, *The encyclopaedia of sex practice*, was originally published in French in 1933. This time the authors were Drs Norman Haire, A Willy, L Vander, O Fischer, R Lothar, T Reitter and others, edited by Norman Haire. Koestler said it was jointly written by Manes Sperber, a Jewish psychotherapist, and Fritz Kuenkel, who helped teachers and parents deal with difficult children. Koestler said he was in a concentration camp when the book went to press and that, without his knowledge, the publisher had 'rehashed' the first book's physiological chapters and added several new ones. They also added 32 colour plates. 'A Willy' may have been the phallic-sounding pseudonym of the book's publisher Willy Aldor[23] who chose it to help sell the book to an audience interested in titillation not science. Koestler continued to carp about it, perhaps because 'A Costler, MD' was left off the list of authors and in 1969 he disparaged it as 'a confused, repetitive and irresponsible compilation' edited by Norman Haire. Koestler was being too harsh – it was perfectly good in parts and Haire as editor vetted the contributions and added corrections if he did not agree; one contributor had claimed that 'infants who masturbate are an exception' and he commented in a footnote that it was more true to say 'infants who do not masturbate

---

23 Ralf Dose suggested 'A Willy' might have been Henry Gauthier-Villiers, the *nom de plume* of a French writer and rake who worked in his family's publishing firm and directed a stable of ghostwriters whose articles and books made him a good income.

are an exception'. Haire was famous for his sayings which, in a witty non-threatening way, promoted sexual reform and made people think. Others did the same; AE Housman described chastity as 'the most peculiar of all sexual aberrations'; Dr William J Robinson, the editor of the *American Journal of Sexology*, said there was no greater 'sin' than sexual abstinence, and a novelist linked the Bible's story of 'original sin' with ignorance and fear of sexuality:

> Holy Mother we believe
> Without sin thou didst conceive:
> Holy Mother, so believing,
> Let us sin without conceiving.[24]

Haire wanted sin-free use of contraception and joyful sexually liberated life, but in 1997 Sheila Jeffreys was not amused by what she called 'the new "science" of sexology' which she blamed for undermining feminism. Lesley Hall (1998, 136) called this 'condescension' and gave examples of sexologists' commitment to women's rights to show that Jeffreys and others were wrong to assume that women of the past 'were blank wax imprinted with the ideas of male sexologists'.

Sterilisation was another important rallying point for reformers and this needs to be put in context: Haire declared in the 15 July 1922 issue of the *British Medical Journal* that he had 'sterilised four males and four females without any ill effects', but by the 1930s the mood had swung against sterilisation and Haire masked vasectomies as 'rejuvenations' and stressed their healthy, reactivating aspects. In August 1930 Haire told CP Blacker that he had responded to JBS Haldane's letter in *The Times' Weekend Review* and had been careful not to say he performed sterilisations – it might be considered advertising – but mentioned 'observing cases both before and after the operation'.

Haire told Havelock Ellis in September that he was bewildered by the Eugenics Society's clamour for legislation to allow voluntary sterilisation when it was not forbidden by British law. He thought they were mainly influenced by Lord Riddell, the *News of the World*

---

24 Alexandre Boutique began his 1894 novel *Les Malthusiennes* with this verse, quoted by McLaren (1990, 194–95).

publisher, who believed that, in a test case, sterilisation would probably be regarded as a form of 'mayhem'. Haire performed sterilisations when they seemed justified but was not prepared to be involved in a test case which might result in an unfavourable judgement, even the loss of his right to practise.[25] He emphasised the need for an international body which could intervene in such a case so that the whole world's press would bring the matter to the public's attention. He meant the WLSR. Havelock Ellis asked Haire to give his objections to Major Archibald Church and report back: Church was a Labour member of parliament who with Eugenics Society backing planned to present a sterilisation bill. As requested, Haire told the politician in a 'casual conversation' that Ellis feared that legal red tape would 'sterilise sterilisation.' Reporting back, Haire told Ellis that Church was 'a very intelligent person' who said that the Eugenics Society was thinking of 'getting some well-known surgeon, who was so well established and so rich or so old' that he could volunteer as guinea pig in their sterilisation test case. Haire was ready to help privately and responded to Havelock Ellis' 17 May 1932 request for a doctor in Sydney to do a sterilisation by suggesting that Dr Bruce Mayes (from the Royal Hospital for Women) or Dr Keith Kirkland 'would consider the matter sympathetically'. Although Mayes 'was really a gynaecologist', he had spent a good deal of his time with him in London studying contraception.[26]

Havelock Ellis resigned from his position of Fellow of the Eugenics Society over their stance on sterilisation in January 1931 but Haire noted this had not 'dampened their ardour' and Major Church still promised to introduce the bill in the House. When Church presented the bill on 21 July 1931 it was defeated by 167 to 89 in the House of

---

25 Because many hospitals had links with the Catholic Church or with others opposed to sterilisation, it was usually necessary to perform sterilisations in a nursing home or at the patient's own residence: Haire (1936, 162).

26 Professor Bruce Toomba Mayes was born in Toowoomba, west of Brisbane and occupied the first full-time Chair of Obstetrics at the University of Sydney, and became know as the 'man who took the womb out of Toowoomba'. Sydney Medical School's tribute does not mention that he studied with Haire: sydney.edu.au/medicine/museum/mwmuseum/index.php/Mayes,_Bruce_Toomba]

ESCALATING TROUBLES

Commons but the Eugenics Society continued their campaign.[27] Haire resigned from the Society in the Spring of 1934 because he disagreed with their position on voluntary sterilisation when, despite his advice in 1931, they continued to support a sterilisation bill.[28] It was defeated because it lacked the support of the three key factions: the scientific community, the left (particularly the geneticist JBS Haldane who had helped to scupper it)[29] and the Catholic Church.

Blacker made it clear in *The Lancet* on 10 June 1933 that he and the Eugenics Society were repulsed by the Nazi sterilisation program[30] and Britain's Departmental Commission on Sterilisation (headed by Laurence Brock) took the view that doctors who performed this operation might risk prosecution on the grounds of mutilation (Brock Report 1934). Surprisingly, Haire had decided in May 1934 to include a very contentious book in 'The international library of sexology and psychology' series, *The case for sterilisation,* because there was much interest in the subject and it would probably sell well if some of the 'more frightful' Americanisms were removed. Haire's decision was even more frightful because the book was written by Leon F Whitney, the Secretary of the American Eugenics Society, who with fellow members Charles Davenport, Harry H Laughlin and Maria Kopp, helped to legitimate the Nazi extermination policies.[31] One of Hitler's staff asked

---

27 See Macnicol (1989, 159) for the reference to Church's statement that his ultimate aim, 'a Bill for the compulsory sterilization of the unfit', significantly wrecked any chance of the Commons accepting the motion.

28 Bradshaw (1992, 192), quoting *ESA* – SA/EUG/C.139. On 2 May 2007 archivists at the Wellcome Library found no letter of resignation from Haire but said there had been a reference to it on the original C.139 file cover, which had not been kept when the files were copied.

29 Haldane did this at the 1934 Norman Lockyer Lecture: Jones (1993, 219).

30 Blacker said the Nazis' anti-Semitic policies were 'ridiculous' and because, unlike America's eugenists (some were strongly pro-Nazi), Britain's Eugenics Society attracted a number of Jews. See also Kevles (1995, 172).

31 See Kuhl (1994) and Penchaszadeh (1996, 115–17). Whitney, Davenport and Kopp approved of Nazi policies but not anti-Semitic components, while American Eugenics Society extremists Madison Grant, Lothrop Stoddard and Clarence G Campbell strongly supported all Nazi policies.

for a copy of the book 'in the name of the Fuhrer', Whitney 'complied immediately' and Hitler sent him a letter of thanks (Kuhl 1994, 85). Whitney approved of Hitler's plans for wholesale sterilisation but 'the wilder flights' of Whitney's enthusiasm were 'curbed by the editor' according to David Eder who reviewed the book in 1935. Eder had delivered a paper on sterilisation at the WLSR's 1929 congress in which he advocated 'investigation rather than imprisonment, freedom not restriction'.

Also surprisingly, in March 1934, three months after the Brock Committee's recommendations were accepted, Blacker referred a patient to Haire for sterilisation.[32] They had an angry interchange of letters: in the first Haire asked Blacker to agree that the procedure was warranted but Blacker refused on 5 March because 'if the recommendations of the Brock Committee passed into law it would be very difficult for a medical man to furnish him with the required certificate.' Haire would not operate without it, saying 'I do not feel inclined to take on the task of pulling your chestnuts out of the fire for you' and asked why Blacker had sent him the patient. Blacker replied that if Haire did rejuvenations he did not see why Haire could not sterilise the patient even though Blacker would not agree that it was warranted. In his final letter Blacker disingenuously claimed that Haire had misrepresented the Eugenics Society's views and said, 'We think that the legal position is uncertain. This is very different from definitely stating that it is illegal'.

It is strange that Blacker asked for Haire's help, in view of his comment to Julian Huxley in 1928: 'I should like to have a talk to you about Norman Haire sometime. He is a problem. Between ourselves, I think he is to be avoided. I play the same game with him as with Stopes, i.e. I am most amiable on all occasions and review their books favourably but have nothing to do with them'. Blacker was far from

---

32 Haire wrote to Havelock Ellis on 11 January 1935 'Some time ago Blacker sent me a case, but would not give a certificate. I am willing to see any of them you would like me to see. If they can afford a consultation fee, of course they ought to pay it, as I am entirely dependent on my earnings for my livelihood. On the other hand I never refuse to see a patient for nothing if they really cannot afford my fee. Only I do not see any good reason why patients should economise by not paying me a fee, and then spend the money on some unnecessary luxury'.

amiable in a medical gazette in 1924 when he damned Stopes' work by saying: 'Her books are read extensively and secretly in girls' schools and by boys in the same spirit that indecent literature is generally enjoyed ... They can, in fact, in one sense, be considered as practical handbooks of prostitution!' (quoted by Rose 1992, 114, 254, fn 28). Haire thought Blacker was his friend and apologised to him in September 1930 about a *faux pas* he made at Sanger's conference:

> Although I am intellectually aggressive and enjoy nothing better than a good scrap, I am really very tender-hearted and would not willingly hurt anybody's feelings. I cannot tell you how ashamed and distressed I am that a frivolous and quite unnecessary allusion of mine should have caused you pain – particularly as you have always been so nice to me. What I said I said quite thoughtlessly, just as one might tell a joke against Jews or Scotchmen, without stopping to think that there might be a Jew or Scotchman in the room who would be hurt.

Haire's sightseeing in Zurich was spoiled by his remorse and he woke early 'with a heavy conscience' and asked Blacker to accept his assurance that he had been thoughtless not malicious. I wonder what Haire said: Did he call him 'Pip', the name his friends used; was it a national slur (Blacker's ancestors were Peruvian aristocrats); or a reference to his Catholic background; was it anti-war (Blacker had served in World War I in the Coldstream Guards and was decorated for gallantry); or anti-psychiatry (Blacker was a psychiatrist); or did he make fun of Blacker's habit of running five miles before breakfast? (Kevles 1995, 170–71).

Rejuvenation was another rallying point for reformers but one advocate wrote to *The Saturday Review* on 26 December 1931 because he feared it might benefit the 'wealthy old reprobate, rather than the great poet.' Ironically, in 1934 William Butler Yeats, the Nobel prize-winning poet, became Haire's highest profile rejuvenation patient. As a boy Yeats had been sexually anxious and asked friends to call him 'WB' not 'little Willie' and remembered little of his childhood 'except its pain'. He was awkward and delicate with bad eyesight; a poor scholar with 'a keen sense of his physical inadequacies' made worse by his father's bullying until, at the age of 15, his sexual feelings began 'like the bursting

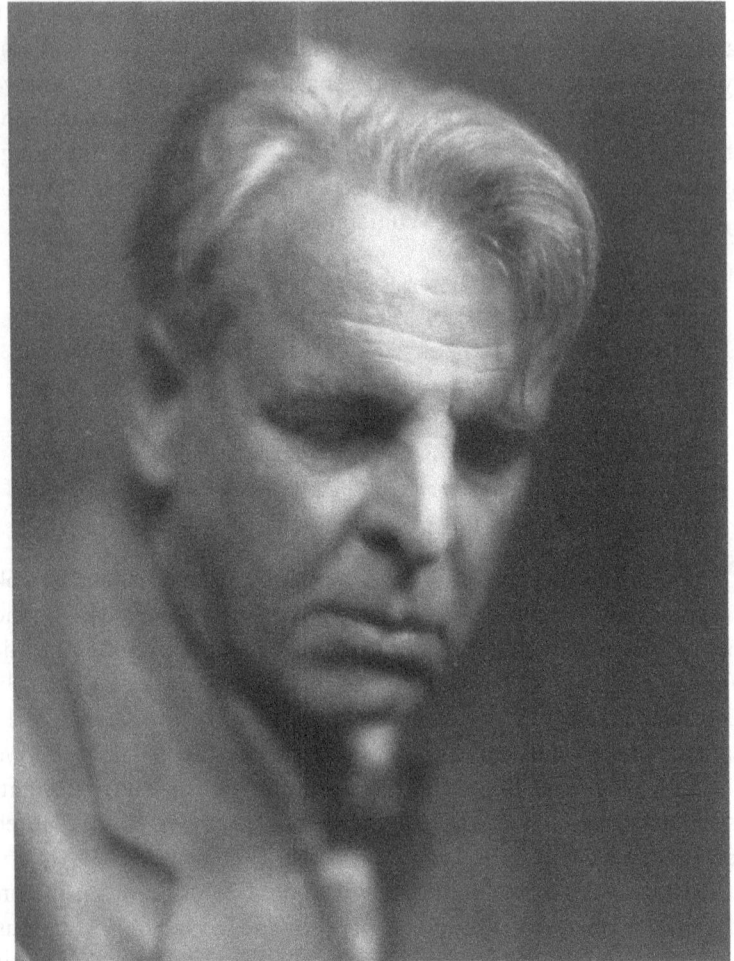

Figure 9.1. WB Yeats before the 'rejuvenation' operation.

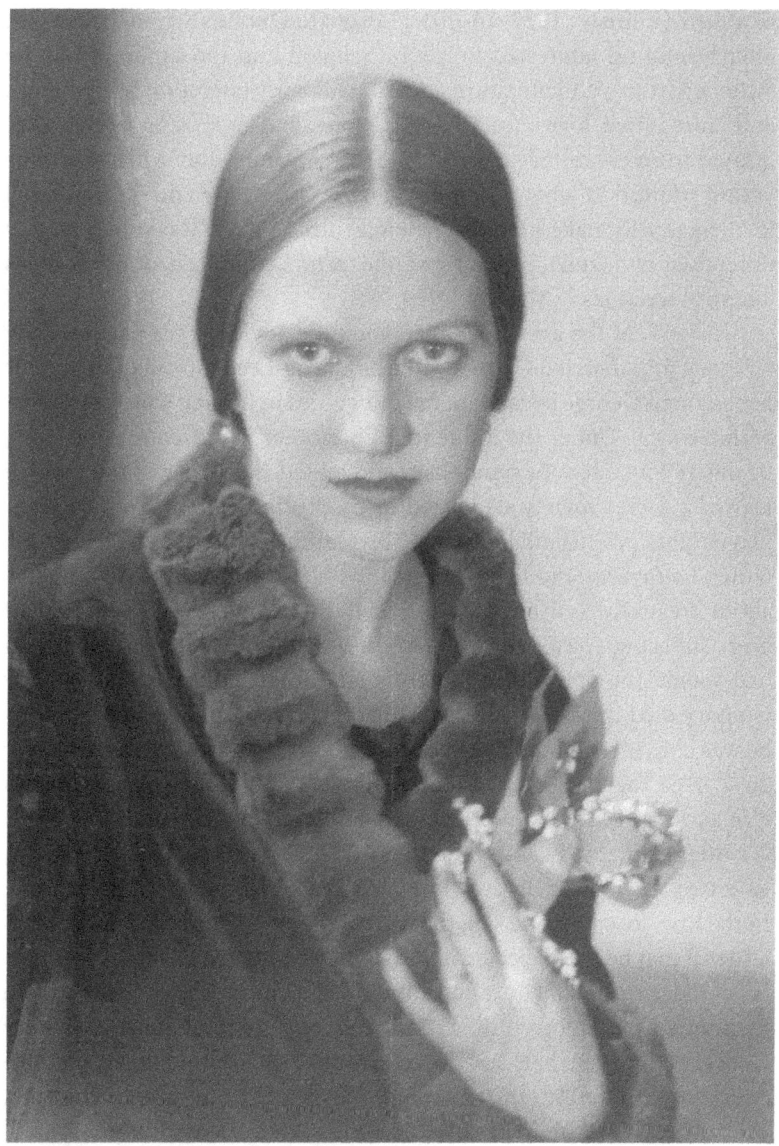

Figure 9.2. Ethel Mannin. Photograph by EO Hoppé, 1925. Reproduced with permission of Getty Images 53371233 (rights managed), Time Life Pictures.

of a shell' (Ellmann 1979, 24–25). He went to Dublin's School of Art but, after becoming interested in mystic religion and the supernatural, he switched from art to literature, focusing his early poems on Irish themes and unrequited love. Yeats expert Professor Roy Foster (1997, 182) quoted from cancelled passages in Yeats' *Memoirs* about his miserable young adulthood when, 'tormented by sexual desire and disappointed love', he would make himself ill by masturbating. He was thin, possibly tubercular and, at 43, began to wonder if he had inherited his mother's 'nervous weakness' (Maddox 1999, 199).

In 1917, at the age of 52, Yeats took the advice of his patron, Lady Gregory, and married Georgie (Bertha) Hyde-Lees, a woman in her 20s he renamed George because of the difficulties in finding words to rhyme with Georgie. Under the influence of her other world 'communicators', he derived a system of symbolism and joined the Order of the Golden Dawn, a secret society dedicated to cabalistic magic. He was a poet, playwright, politician, journalist, revolutionary, occultist, late-in-life father, *bon viveur* and lover, but in 1934 he was preoccupied with fears about creativity and impotence. For the previous seven years he had been suffering from lung congestion and raised blood pressure and had spent long convalescences in Spain, France and Italy. After Lady Gregory died in May 1932 he wrote no poetry for almost a year and, as he was convinced of the links between poetry and potency (Saddlemyer 2002, 476), the idea of being remade and sexually recharged appealed to him and made him intensely excited and hopeful (Ellmann 1979, 276).

Stephen Lock, who in the 1980s edited the *British Medical Journal*, gave two versions of the way in which Yeats heard about rejuvenation. In the first, Joseph Hone said that early in 1934 Yeats had complained to a friend that he was dejected and had no wish to live a long time unless he could continually recreate himself. To cheer him up, the friend mentioned the Steinach operation, and Yeats read about it in Trinity College Library: when his doctor would not comment, he had the operation in London. In the second version, Jon Stallworthy said that Yeats heard about the operation from his artist friend Sturge Moore.[33]

---

33   Locke (1983, 1965), quoting Horne (1943) and Stallworthy (1963).

However, Moore could not have been the informant because Yeats sent his artist friend the details on 10 July 1934 after he'd had the operation:

> The book I told you of is *The conquest of old age* by Peter Schmidt, translated by Edward Cedar Paul [Eden and Cedar Paul] published by Routledge. The surgeon I went to is Norman Haire 127 Harley Street. He is expensive and I think Dulac could tell you of someone else probably as good who would charge much less. You will find Norman Hair [sic] in *Who's Who*.

Yeats' spelling was quirky but he was not anti-Semitic – Foster told me in 2001 that while some of Yeats' friends were anti-Semitic, 'Gogarty and Pound virulently so,' he had never found any such evidence in Yeats who was 'Anything but!' Yeats was merely stating a fact: Haire charged high fees to the rich to offset the free treatment he gave the poor. Yeats and Haire had much in common: they had unhappy childhoods and were anxious about their sexuality and as adults they became tall, overweight, smokers who were sometimes impotent.[34] They were celebrities and members of the Eugenics Society,[35] they had beautiful voices, spoke inspiringly and liked racy stories, theatre and parties.

Haire operated on the elderly poet on 6 April 1934, then put his work to the test by asking Ethel Mannin to meet his patient. In the second volume of his Yeats biography, Foster described her as a Marxist with a young child from a former marriage and 'a free spirit determined on sexual radicalism' who 'collected' and had affairs with 'interesting' people such as Bertrand Russell. She was the first lover to feature in Yeats' 'second puberty' and, 37 years later, she described their meeting:

> The occasion was an invitation to dinner at the Harley Street house; I was to put on my most alluring evening dress and all my sex-appeal, for the famous poet to test out his rejuvenated reaction to an attractive young

---

34 The operation was primarily to reverse this: Yeats may have had mild diabetes which by the 1870s was known to cause impotence and Haire's obesity, diabetes and heart problems probably made him impotent too.

35 Haire was a member from 1921 to 1934 and Yeats joined in 1936. See also Maddox (1999, 198, 263–64, 283–84, 304–05, 318–19, 334–35).

woman, he said, blandly. I was flattered, I suppose; certainly I counted it an honour to meet Yeats, and I went along. It was an unconvivial, somewhat strained occasion, for Haire was not interested in poetry, and Yeats liked to drink very much more than he liked to eat, and we left early and spent the rest of the night drinking Burgundy, after which Yeats was always at his raciest and most eloquent (Mannin 1971, 67).

At the time of the rejuvenation, Mannin was 34, Yeats was 68 and his wife was 42, the same age as Haire. Unfortunately, after keeping the letters for three decades, Mannin burnt them. Her daughter, Jean Faulks, told me in 2001 that she was very sure about this letter-burning in the 1960s and remembered 'quite vividly' seeing her mother 'put a bundle of Yeats' letters on her kitchen boiler' and saying: 'All of these letters I am burning are about Yeats' rejuvenation operation which I find quite disgusting and revolting. After I am dead, someone will probably throw up their hands in horror at what I have done but I just cannot keep these letters and risk them being published later on'. Ironically, given Mannin's shocking deed 'on the boiler', in 1938 Yeats wrote a eugenic diatribe he called *On the boiler*, which called for the Irish government to send 'doctor and clinic' to 'limit the families of the unintelligent classes' (code for Haire and sterilisations), much to the horror of progressive members of the Eugenics Society such as Julian Huxley and Naomi Mitchison (Bradshaw 1992, 189–215).

In 2005 Patrick O'Connor told me about more letter destruction by his father (Paddy O'Connor) who was secretary of Britain's Abortion Law Reform Society in the 1930s where he met Haire. Patrick's mother was also a member and they became close friends with Haire but Mannin, in a letter to Paddy, referred to 'the horrible Haire.' In the 1960s, a few years before he died, O'Connor senior destroyed all his correspondence, commenting 'Who would be interested in it?'

In 1934 Yeats foolishly told his friends 'I had it done' and everyone knew what 'it' was and a friend worried that he had gone 'sex mad.'[36] On hearing the news, Dr Oliver Gogarty (whose 'incontinence of speech' was notorious) said scathingly that 'the poor old fool' was now 'trapped

---

36 The 'it' quote is Maddox (1999, 265) quoting Hone (1942, 437); the 'sex mad' quote is Lock (1983, 1968) quoting JB Lyons.

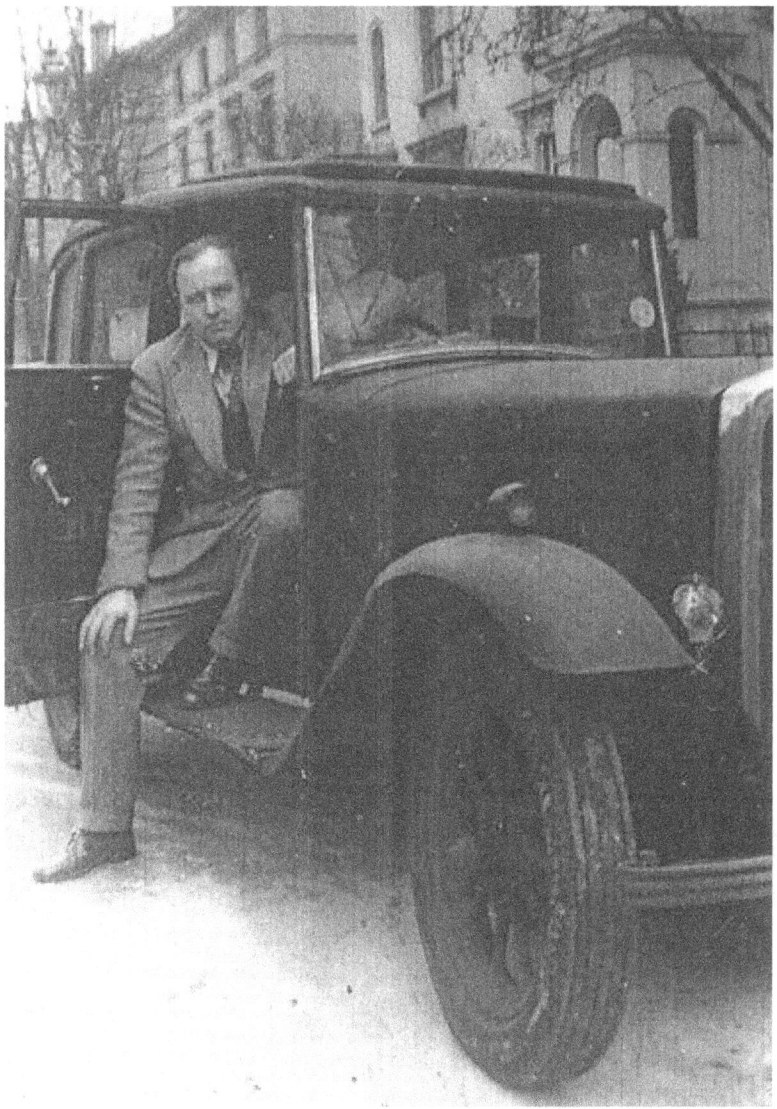

Figure 9.3. Haire's friend Armans Stiles 'Paddy' O'Connor posing with his car. Reproduced with permission of his son Patrick O'Connor.

and enmeshed in sex'. Gogarty had not dreamt Yeats 'would become so obsessed' by it when he parodied his poem into

> I heard the old, old men say,
> Everything's phallic. (quoted by Foster 2003, 499)[37]

Gogarty complained that Yeats had not consulted him before he 'submitted to that humbug Steinach'. After Yeats' death he criticised the old man for having too much interest in sex but he had also ridiculed him as a young man for having too little interest:

> What a pity it is that Miss Horniman
> When she wants to secure or suborn a man
> Should choose Willie Yeats
> Who still masturbates
> And at any rate isn't a horny man. (quoted by Foster 1997, 330)

Gogarty was alluding to the lopsided romance in 1917 between Annie Horniman, the heiress who supported the Abbey Theatre, and Yeats who was mainly interested in her wealth. Irish author Frank O'Connor joked that the operation was like putting a Cadillac engine into a Ford car and Dublin's newspapers ridiculed Yeats as 'the gland old man.'[38] This was a common mistake as many people associated the word 'rejuvenation' with Voronoff's monkey-gland transplants. In May 1934 Yeats wrote that it was too soon to know if he had benefited by the operation but felt that his blood pressure was down[39] and was not irritable and that was new. In June he was 'still marvellously strong, with a sense of a future' (Wade 1954, 823) and while in London he visited Haire for daily injections, commenting to Mannin on 30 December: 'perhaps the injections do not matter but they were arranged before we met'. He informed his wife in January 1935 that 'Norman Haire has done

---

37 The reference is to Yeats' 1903 poem 'The old men admiring themselves in the water'. Yeats referred to hearing elderly men say 'Everything alters'.

38 O'Connor's Cadillac quote was in Ellmann (1986, 40) and the gland old man quote was in Lock (1983, 1966) quoting Macliamoir and Boland.

39 Steinach claimed the operation would rectify irritability, depression, high blood pressure and diminished sexual powers.

me much good, I expect increased working powers etc. I am happy.' In April he told Mannin, 'I feel very well, full of energy and life but I am soon made breathless if I am not careful . . . I was worse before the operation' (Wade 1954, 836).

Yeats authorised Haire to speak about the operation, and twelve years later Haire discussed it with Richard Ellmann, Yeats' biographer. Yeats had been unable to write anything new for about three years and thought he must have the operation because 'versemaking and lovemaking were always connected in his mind'. Yeats thought the operation was a success and believed that his new poems were among his best work and his widow emphasised that the effect on his mind was incalculable. Ellmann said, 'on the physical level it cannot have had much effect', for Norman Haire said what a woman friend of Yeats' confirmed, 'that the operation had no effect upon his sexual competence. He could not have erections, Haire told me'. In her insightful biography Brenda Maddox criticised these views and said that one of the best bits of evidence that he achieved his sexual ambition is the letter he wrote to Ethel Mannin on 30 December, thanking her for their reassuring encounter which had left him with a 'feeling that he had been blessed'. Maddox noted that Ellmann 'tended to be protective of the family member who was his main source of information'. Maddox also questioned Ellmann's interpretation of the evidence because Yeats' wife 'may not have been the best judge' of Yeats' abilities in bed.

It would have been bad for business if Haire *had* said that Yeats 'could not have erections' after his rejuvenation and he probably said that Yeats was impotent *before* the operation. Ellmann was quoting Mannin who had a motive for changing the meaning by removing the last seven words from Haire's comment which might have been 'Yeats could not have erections *until he came to me for treatment*'. Mannin and Yeats had volatile temperaments and she had evanescent friendships, frequently changing her views. Mannin is probably the 'woman friend' who was Ellmann's and Haire's informant in the late 1940s. By this time she had married Reginald Reynolds, the love of her life (Huxter 1992) and, as Yeats was dead, she probably preferred to say her relationship with the poet was based on conversation, not copulation.

In 1930 Mannin had been overawed by Haire's 'brilliance' but in 1939 she found close friendship with Haire increasingly difficult and in 1948 he thought she was 'muddle-headed'. Her friendship with Yeats was also strained by 1936: she was angered by his political timidity and, after he had started a relationship with Lady Dorothy Wellesley, he called Mannin an 'extreme revolutionist' (Maddox 1999, 309).[40] The rejuvenation operation, by making Yeats sterile, would have removed fears about unintended fatherhood and this was 'a useful side-effect that cannot have escaped Yeats' notice'. This would have been irrelevant if his affairs were platonic. Maddox noted that he 'had at least four serious sexual liaisons after the Steinach operation', but whether he achieved full intercourse in any of them remains a matter of speculation. He clearly wanted to, telling Olivia Shakespear: 'I shall be a sinful man to the end, and think upon my death-bed of all the nights I wasted in my youth.'[41] Maddox could find little 'poetic or biographical' evidence that he ever ceased to regret his 'onanistic youth. What he dreaded was not death but impotence'. Yeats wrote to Mannin, with whom he had shared 'the bed's friendship,' that 'the knowledge that I am not unfit for love has brought me sanity and peace.' Six months after his operation Yeats told Virginia Woolf 'I finally recovered my potency'[42] and, during a serious illness, he wrote to Mannin in June 1935:

> I am forbidden all exercise, & all work that is a strain – congestion of the lung has left me with an enlarged heart. Furthermore the doctor has enjoined 'for the present' complete 'celebacy'. I said 'If I were a mathematician I could take to drink'. He said 'Yes they do drink but I will give you a bromide' . . . I do not accept his diagnosis, he is young, theoretical & over incisive.[43] However any captain in a storm. I shall

---

40 Yeats' remarks about Mannin being 'an extreme revolutionist' applied even more aptly to Maude Gonne, the object of his 50-year passion.

41 Yeats' 3 January 1932 letter quoted in Wade (1954).

42 Maddox (1999) quotations: 'Bed's friendship', 267, quoting Gould (1988, 215); 'Useful side-effect', 267; 'Told Virginia Woolf', 309, quoting Nicholson (1966, 188); 'Sanity and peace', Jeffares (1998, 338), quoting Yeats (30 December 1934).

43 When Yeats links 'incisive' with a physician, he is almost certainly playing on the word 'incision' and his recent surgery (LaSalle 2001).

probably obey him until I have seen Norman Haire. 'For the present' meaning until I get back to normal health, & I believe I can do that quicker than my doctor thinks possible. I am of a healthy long lived race, & our minds improve with age.

The celibacy reference has been excised from Allan Wade's *The letters of WB Yeats*. Significantly, Yeats did not promise to be abstinent and on 19 December 1935 he wrote to Mannin from Spain to let her know he was now 'well enough for work & pleasure', adding that 'Haire examined me ... and approved my state'. Yeats returned to Ireland and decided he 'must escape the telephone, committees & the like; & attempt before it is too late a masterpiece'. Yeats often stressed the link between lust and verse and made this explicit in 1938 in *The spur*:

> You think it horrible that lust and rage
> Should dance attendance upon my old age;
> They were not such a plague when I was young;
> What else have I to spur me into song?

Ellmann (1979, 275) commented: 'Lust and rage are here not the lasciviousness and irascibility of an old man's brain grown febrile, as some critics have said, but pure passions, spontaneous and complete as peasant life'. These strong emotions were vital to Yeats and he expressed the fervent hope in *Prayer for old age*:

> That I may seem, though I die old,
> A foolish, passionate man. (quoted in Finneran 1989, 282–83)[44]

The last two lines of his final poem *Politics* make it clear that passion was the driving force of his life:

> But O that I were young again
> And held her in my arms. (quoted in Finneran 1989, 348)[45]

---

44 Reprinted with the permission of Scribner, a division of Simon & Schuster, Inc, from *The collected words of WB Yeats, Volume I: The poems*, revised by WB Yeats, edited by Richard J Finneran. Copyright 1934 by The Macmillan Company, renewed 1962 by Bertha Georgie Yeats. All rights reserved.

45 Reprinted with the permission of Scribner, a division of Simon & Schuster, Inc,

On 4 January 1939, a month before his death, he told Lady Elizabeth Pelman he was happy and filled with an energy he had despaired of regaining. WH Auden gave this eloquent assessment in his poem *In memory of WB Yeats*: 'You were silly like us; your gift survived it all.' Yeats' fascination with the occult might explain his ready acceptance of the rejuvenation 'miracle.' However, as Maddox astutely judged, 'Of all the bizarre procedures Yeats used over the years to stimulate his muse, the Steinach operation was the least dubious'. Quite justifiably, she felt 'he was probably as much rejuvenated by the surgeon as by the surgery'.

Viriginia Pruitt (1971, 290), a professor of English literature, discussed the 50 poems by the rejuvenated Yeats and began her study by quoting the envious complaint made by the 'fitfully inspired' poet who featured in Anthony Burgess' trilogy *Enderby*:

> The only people who can write verse after the age of thirty are the people who do [newspaper] competitions... You can add to that, of course, the monkey-gland boys, of whom Yeats was one, but that's not playing the game, by God. The greatest senile poet of the age, by God, by grace of this bloody man Steinach.

Steinach's procedure was a vasectomy not a monkey-gland implant but Pruitt was also muddled when she asked if Yeats had been the 'victim of a fraud' or if his writing was surgically assisted – the 'splendid poetry of his later years' was merely 'a cheat, the product of a chemical "high", more of a "late", monstrous bloom of an impersonal technology than a remarkable personal achievement'. Yeats' managed his achievements despite his brief hormonal highs, not because of them, just as James Joyce, Brendan Behan, Dylan Thomas and Scott Fitzgerald made theirs despite their addictions to alcohol, drugs or other substances. Yeats' decision to be Steinached is not surprising; having explored the risky world of the supernatural and the occult, science offered a safer option and, given his fondness for Burgundy and other mind-altering drugs,

---

from *The collected words of WB Yeats, Volume I: The poems*, revised by WB Yeats, edited by Richard J Finneran. Copyright 1940 by Georgie Yeats, renewed by Bertha Georgie Yeats, Michael Butler Yeats and Ann Yeats. All rights reserved.

such as mescal and hashish,[46] his interest in a body-altering operation is understandable. Finally, Yeats was not the victim of a fraud (defined as intentional perversion of the truth) because Steinach and the rejuvenating surgeons believed it worked. Critical opinion is divided about the merits of his *Last poems and plays* (Henn 1965, 318) but Pruitt (1982, 99) found his lyrical verse 'far better than the poetry of his youth, passionate and moving as the poetry of his middle age'.

In her 1977 study, Pruitt drew on Ellmann's analysis of Yeats' concept of 'The mask'[47] to give a metaphysical explanation for the 'miracle' of Yeats' poetic resurgence – he had 'spent his youth being old', held back by timidity and illness and, by delaying marriage and children until he was in his 50s, he 'did not come into possession of his youth until he was middle-aged'. Yeats' delayed development explains his yearning for an old-age outburst of poetic creativity but Pruitt did not consider how Yeats managed the 'astonishing triumph' of transforming his dreams into action and dismissed it as 'an extraordinary case of the finest poetry being produced by false science' (Coote 1997, 537). As Steinach's theory was then accepted, Haire and Yeats would have expected a cure – a case of placebo *à deux* – and Haire's sound advice provided Yeats the justification to banish unwanted diversions and follow his instincts: 'I am writing better and more than I have done for years', he informed Olivia Shakespear in August 1936; 'I have proclaimed myself an invalid and got rid of bores, business and exercise'. Yeats believed the physiological basis for his 'lust' and creativity was restored by the operation and 'his prodigious creative vitality may have been sustained by that conviction' (Pruitt & Pruitt 1983, 122).

Yeats could have been experiencing placebo effects – medical treatment which performs no physiological function but may benefit the patient psychologically. The word, from the Latin 'I shall be

---

46 Yeats was introduced to these drugs by Havelock Ellis in the 1890s. See Maddox (1999, 17, 75–76) and Foster (1997, 109, 178, 182–83, 196, 204).

47 Ellmann (1948) described the 67-year-old Yeats' struggle in 1933 to come to grips with reality – after a life spent 'turning away', he felt he must 'reveal what he had concealed'. 'Usually in the past he had attributed his writing to his mask, but now he suggests that the mask is his uncreative ordinary self which has so often accommodated itself to the demands of convention'.

acceptable or pleasing', suggests an interaction between deceptive doctors and credulous patients. Henry K Beecher, in a 1955 study in the *Journal of the American Medical Association,* claimed that about one out of three patients find relief from placebos alone and Margaret Talbot explored various explanations for it in *The New York Times* on 9 January 2000; people who get relief after seeing a doctor or swallowing a pill are conditioned to repeat this. A second is that placebo pain relievers stimulate the brain's own analgesics (endorphins), and a third finding is that taking a placebo that is administered in an atmosphere of hope will relieve stress-related conditions like asthma and hypertension. Talbot quoted Walter Brown: 'What we're really talking about with the placebo effect is the reduction of distress, the reassurance from being in a healing situation that you're finally in somebody's hands'. Hard data supports the notion that an alliance between a doctor and patient is therapeutic and that a compassionate and optimistic physician can be a 'walking placebo' and that words can be physically comforting.

Haire was the archetypal 'walking placebo' according to Stella Cornelius who, throughout her life was 'a shining beacon of peace and unity'.[48] In 1998 she told me about visiting Haire in 1943 when she was a newly married 23-year-old and her husband was a seriously ill European refugee. They found him 'an awe-inspiring professional who was extremely understanding and sympathetic, a charismatic figure who cared passionately about his point of view and was very persuasive in trying to get his views across – he wasn't objective at all.' Doctors in the 1940s had said her husband would die in two years but he lived for another 35, she believed, as a result of Haire's advice: 'It was the dark ages as far as talk about contraception and sex education was concerned but he helped with non-directive information. He was the only doctor I'd ever met who talked about what we now call lifestyle. He talked about diet and was a mine of information about food, both shopping for it and eating it. He recommended salads three times a day, to be eaten first and then progress to other foods if you still felt hungry. Haire was concerned about nutritional needs not weight'.

---

48 Malcolm Brown, 'A shining beacon for peace and unity' (Obituary for Stella Cornelius), *Sydney Morning Herald,* 8 January 2011.

Even without the operation Yeats would have benefitted from Haire's advice to smoke less, eat wisely and lose weight. He also had to cut down alcohol, sedative bromides and hashish, all of which impair sexual performance. Haire would have reassured Yeats, and 'advice can cure'; good diets can restore physical health just as counselling can restore mental health. Haire (WLSR 1929, 561–63) stressed that while 'everybody' recognised indigestion and sleeplessness can ruin happiness, it was less understood that grave damage to health and happiness 'may result from slight disorders, such as a diminution of potency in the male' and that most sufferers hesitate to discuss this with their family doctor or their close friends. He said that, if they visited a competent doctor, the mere fact of 'getting it off their chest' was already the first step towards cure and that in many conditions no other treatment is needed. He knew of no more gratifying experience than to see a patient, who had come in to see him in complete misery over some imaginary or over-estimated sexual disturbance, and then see him walk out an hour later, restored to happiness after a simple discussion of his condition.

Haire attended a meeting to discuss impotence which was arranged by Alfred Adler's Medical Society of Individual Psychology and, in the 27 June 1931 issue of the *British Medical Journal*, he acknowledged the part psychology played in it and the measures people took to compensate for physical defects. He always paid 'special attention' to impotence because it was 'so common' and it caused 'so much unhappiness', mostly because of the associated stigma. In 2007 Angus McLaren neatly encapsulated this by saying that 'Western culture has simultaneously regarded impotence as life's greatest tragedy and life's greatest joke'.

In his marriage manual, Theodoor van de Velde listed its physical causes including diabetes, kidney disease, TB, gonorrhoea, obesity and 'chronic excess in the use of alcohol, nicotine, morphine and cocaine' as well as several 'vocational or industrial toxins' but said that in impotence 'the most important factor is neurosis'. Havelock Ellis emphasised that, while people took no notice of a man's nervous dyspepsia, if a man's lack of virile 'potency' has nervous causes 'it is almost a crime.' When it was suggested that Scotland's bearded sage Thomas Carlyle 'suffered from some trouble of sexual potency', his admirers rushed forward to defend Carlyle from this 'disgraceful' charge; they were more shocked than if it had been alleged that he was a syphilitic. Haire noted the paradox that while most people condemn frequent sexual intercourse as immoral and degrading, they 'regard a man who is incapable of it with a special sort of contempt' who, as a result, develops a strong sense of inferiority. It reduces their joy, upsets their psychological condition and may also cause unhappiness in their wife or mistress by denying them satisfaction. He felt that anything to help this condition deserved the attention of the medical profession and that Steinach's methods would increase sexual potency in a large majority of cases and bring great benefits. These were the early years of psychiatry and, even if qualified assistance had been available, it was unlikely that Yeats would have admitted to being impotent and sought help. Steinach gave Yeats a face-saving rescue and enabled him to achieve his 'second-puberty' as a result of patient–doctor trust, trips to London to see an expert, careful examination and attentive discussions, belief in the operation, treatment in a hospital and then convalescence in the company of alluring women. The surgery sparked Yeats' imagination but Haire's part should not be overlooked: many of the benefits should be attributed to this doctor–patient interaction in which a sympathetic doctor's advice was heeded by a compliant and respectful patient. Nine months after the operation Yeats sent his wife a Christmas message from London's Saville Club: 'I go daily to Norman Haire for injections [approximately seven words very heavily deleted] now is the time to get my body back to the normal. I am full of themes for poems'. The name of the injections has been censored, possibly by Yeats, but in this letter to his wife he would have been more likely to have erased the name of an aphrodisiac than that of an innocuous tonic of vitamins or minerals.

Mirko Grmek, a history of medicine professor at the University of Zagreb, wrote that in the case of elderly men 'these could increase libido, even potency in some cases, and revive mental functions'. Sometimes moderate doses had a favourable influence on the aged organism, but these effects are very irregular and short-lasting. This was not a rejuvenation, 'but a sort of eroticisation'. A careless application of hormones may in fact be dangerous. Although the French-trained rejuvenator Charles-Edouard Brown-Séquard felt 'thirty years younger' after having tried rejuvenating effects on himself, he died five years later (Grmek 1958, 102).

Yeats died five years after his rejuvenation but he and Brown-Séquard were old men: 73 in Yeats' case and 77 in Brown-Séquard's. In 1921 Haire gave 'a course of injections of testicular extract (Testogan) and Yohimbine' to a 64-year-old man who had been 'quite impotent for eighteen months'. These substances are still available: Yohimbine is a preparation of plant origin used as an aphrodisiac which has serious side effects;[49] Testogan is a hormonal solution which vets use to stimulate old stallions and bulls and it is also one of the illicit steroids used by some body-builders and athletes. If Yeats was injected with such drugs, any benefits would have been miraculous. Gillian Shenfield, Professor of Clinical Pharmacology at Sydney's Royal North Shore Hospital and a Haire relation, made these comments:

> Yohimbin has some evidence of effect for impotence but is not generally thought to work. It puts the blood pressure up but is a short-lasting drug so that both positive and negative effects would be short-lived unless the injections were repeated daily . . . Testogan is not in any of the human pharmacology texts I have consulted but . . . I suppose if vets use it, the preparation may have some activity. However, testosterone does not help human impotence unless the man is testosterone deficient. In that case, in appropriate cases there should be no unwanted side effects. If he is not deficient to start with, there could be side effects. In theory, blood pressure might increase but I've been unable to find any reports of this occurring. (Shenfield 2002).

In 2002 Ralf Dose sent me details of the drug's composition and marketing: Bernard Schapiro had developed an impotence remedy at Hirschfeld's Berlin Institute in the 1920s; it was Testifortan (pills and

---

49 Yohimbin is not approved for sale in Australia by the Therapeutic Goods Administration (the regulatory agency for medical drugs and devices) and is a restricted import. *Choice* (December 2010–January 2011) listed risks as 'high blood pressure, rapid heart rate; while high doses can cause low blood problems and heart problems'. Bulgaria and Costa Rica offer it for sale online.

injections, for the medical profession) and Titus Pearls (pills, sold to the public). The combination had been judged by professionals to be powerful, and it sold well. Testifortan only ceased production in 1989 and consisted mainly of organ extractions combined with Yohimbin. Haire, being in frequent contact with the Hirschfeld Institute may have had his own supply of Testifortan. Thus, Testifortan may well have been the injection given to Yeats. Titus Pearls were imported to England first by Hirschfeld (which was a financial disaster). Titus Pearls was exported to Australia in the 1930s and advertised there.[50] In 1986 Charlotte Wolff discussed the lucrative sales of Titus Perlen (Titus Pearls) in the 1920s and the controversy about its advertising and efficacy in the 1930s.

Steinach's beliefs about rejuvenation were wrong and Haire acknowledged this in the 1951 edition of the *Encyclopaedia of sexual practice*: 'Time and experience have shown that the Voronoff and Steinach methods there described were of little practical value.' When Stephen Lock mused about the kind of treatment Yeats might have received in the 1980s, he probably would have been told to stop smoking and 'almost certainly, he would not have escaped being given beta blockers' – to reduce angina attacks and lower blood pressure – which can cause severely unpleasant side effects in a healthy person. In addition, drugs for Yeats' blood pressure would have made his impotence and depression worse while denying him the medically sanctioned catalyst to create splendid poetry. Lock felt that we should be thankful that Yeats had 'escaped modern medicine', which is often better at treating the body than the spirit. Yeats himself commented on this: 'I have a slip-shod Spanish doctor who says "I am not a mechanical doctor, I work by faith". He said to me the other day "I am a bad doctor but I have done you more good than the good doctors did" . . . Heaven knows if he meant to say that, but the last part is true'. The Spanish doctor helped but Haire did much more to transform the poet's depression, impotence and inertia into a final dramatic blossoming. Yeats' dramatic 'second puberty' probably resulted from a combination of the placebo effect,

---

50 Information about Hirschfeld's Institute and this drug can be found online at www.hirschfeld.in-berlin.de/institut/en/theorie/theo_19.html [Accessed 10 December 2007].

Haire's sound advice, and the impact of those unknown injections. Haire deserves credit for his services to poetry.

Unfortunately, serious illness restricted Haire's ability to work, and just as his debts were mounting he was forced to make a dramatic decision.

10

MOUNTING GLOOM ON MOST FRONTS

In these years Haire completed a contraception textbook and bought a country estate but good fortune was outstripped by bad: he developed diabetes, the WLSR collapsed, his birth control clinic closed, he had money difficulties and the war started. Despite his sustained struggle to keep the Cromer Welfare and Sunlight Centre operating, it was forced to close 'on account of lack of funds after the depreciation of the pound sterling' (Haire 1936, 28). The North Kensington Welfare Clinic fared better and in March 1935[1] celebrated a decade as 'a pioneer medical service' for working mothers. Although it also operated 'almost entirely by voluntary contribution', the Kensington clinic enjoyed a network of prestigious supporters with close links to government health agencies.

Hirschfeld, having fled from Germany, was living in exile in Nice when he died after a stroke on 14 May 1935. Additional details emerged in 2010 after the death of his great-nephew Ernst Maass, whose son Robert donated a cache of Hirschfeld memorabilia to the Magnus-Hirschfeld-Gesellschaft archives in Berlin. These contained two letters from Haire to Maass and the draft of a sympathy telegram he sent from the Hotel Palais D'Orsay in Paris. Haire sent it to honour the man 'whose heroic life' was 'devoted to rescuing the sphere of sex from the influence of prejudice and unreason' and whose work had 'enlarged the bounds of science and abolished much unnecessary suffering and thus made an

---

1 The 2 March 1935 letter to *The Times* was signed by Dame Janet Campbell (a British Ministry of Health expert), William Davison (1st Baron Broughshane, a Conservative MP), Countess Angela Limerick (a co-founder of the Red Cross), Dr Charles Millard (an early advocate of vaccination, birth control and euthanasia), Sir JAL Duncan (a Scottish Conservative MP) and Lord Hanworth (Ernest Murray Pollock, 1st Viscount Hanworth, a judge and a Conservative MP). They did not mention London's two founding birth control clinics which Stopes, and the Malthusians under Haire, had established in 1921.

essential contribution to the cause of human progress.' Haire's first letter to 'Dear Mr Maass' was dated 18 May 1935:

> Thanks for your letter of 15th May. I was very sorry indeed to hear of Dr Hirschfeld's death – friends have already written to give me the news both from Paris and Holland. One can only be glad that the end came so suddenly and without pain. I have written to some of his friends to tell them the sad news. Can you tell me what is happing to the Institute? And has Dr Hirschfeld made any provision for Karl Giese in his will? I expect you know that Dr Hirschfeld, Frau Bækgaard, and myself were paying for Karl Giese to study medicine in Austria. I should be obliged for any further news you could give me. What is happening to Tao Li, and what is his address?

Haire was referring to Ellen Bækgaard, a dentist from Copenhagen and a WLSR committee member, who had motherly affection for Karl Giese, Hirschfeld's handsome young secretary and his long-time lover and heir. In 1931 Hirschfeld began an affair with a young medical student called Li Shiu Tong who came from a wealthy Chinese family. Haire knew him as Tao Li, the name Hirschfeld used which means 'beloved disciple'. Hirschfeld willed all his personal possessions to Tao Li and both disciples lived in an uneasy *ménage-à-trois* at Hirschfeld's Institute. Haire had made arrangements for the working-class Giese to begin a new life in London as a medical student and in preparation Giese was studying for his matriculation in Vienna; Hirschfeld hoped that Tao Li would also study in Britain. The contributions to help Giese study began in 1934 with Hirschfeld giving £40 and Haire and Bækgaard each providing £50. Haire wrote to Maass on 29 May 1935 to ask for 'the exact details in your late uncle's will with regard to Karl Giese' and reminded him about this three-way arrangement to pay for Giese's medical studies. Haire 'gathered' that Hirschfeld left money for the continuation of his work by the two young disciples and, if that was so, he suggested that the first charge on the money should be for Karl's training so that he would be fit to continue Hirschfeld's work. Haire asked Maass to send him and Mrs Bækgaard a copy of the will (or the part relating to the payment of tuition fees) so they could know 'exactly how matters stand'.

Haire paid tribute to his mentor in *Marriage hygiene* (1935, 120–22) and acknowledged his indebtedness to him for providing advice, teaching and experience, which he always gave willingly, just as he had for earnest students who sought help. Haire did not always follow Hirschfeld's advice but he always considered his opinions very carefully. Haire did not observe the protocol of only speaking well of the dead and made these ill-considered comments: 'Like the rest of us, he had his imperfections. He was not always tactful; he did not stop to think how his actions might be interpreted by persons of ill-will; he could be very selfish and exigeant in small matters; his appearance was, I think, unprepossessing. But these were small faults. They are faults one can forgive and forget'. The comments about 'imperfections' were ironic because Haire's actions were often misconstrued and his own lack of tact was criticised, particularly by people who never spoke about sex.

Ralf Dose sent me these letters and the telegram and explained that Haire and Bækgaard had stopped their contributions because they assumed that Giese would receive money from the Hirschfeld estate. However, this never happened nor did the disciples study in Britain. Giese settled in Brno where he mourned for Hirschfeld, his 'gentle fanatic': he was denied an exit permit and committed suicide after Hitler's army occupied Czechoslovakia in 1938. Tao Li continued his medical studies at the University of Zurich but remained a perennial student and never graduated. Details of his disturbed life emerged after his death in Vancouver in 1993 at the age of 86 (Dutton 2003; Haeberle 2004, 2–4). German authorities contacted him in 1958 to discuss any claims he might have to be reimbursed for property confiscated or destroyed by the Nazis but Tao Li refused to have anything to do with the proceedings and demanded that his address be kept secret. He wandered the world and each time he moved he took the Hirschfeld archive with him. He relocated to America in 1941, then studied in Zurich again from 1945 to 1960 and finally moved to Canada in 1975. He annotated some of Hirschfeld's papers but never published anything and made no provision for the collection's safe keeping after his death.

By chance a man looked inside the discarded suitcases on a rubbish tip, felt they were of value, took them with him when he moved to another city and then posted a note on the internet: eventually, in February 2003 Ralf Dose flew to Canada to collect the materials which are now safely housed in the Hirschfeld archives in Berlin. These discoveries of Haire's 1935 letters and the Hirschfeld papers in Canada have helped to fill some gaps in the two men's histories. Haire had privately provided financial help to Giese and attempted to help him settle in Britain, just as he had quietly paid Ernest Jerdan's medical fees and acted as his mentor. Haire was a generous man but he must have really struggled to help Giese because he was still weak from rheumatic fever and his debts were mounting.

As Jewish refugees poured out of Europe, Haire did what he could as a volunteer in the emergency association which the London Jewish Medical Society had established in April 1933. He had to ignore his own work and was soon 'seeing refugees all day' and attempting to find work for German doctors and dentists. Medical historian Professor Charles Singer wrote to Haire explaining that he could not possibly agree to support another refugee doctor because had been spending more than his income on refugees and had guaranteed seven others. Haire replied on 15 February 1939 and agreed that many were 'difficult and *anspruchsvoll* [hard to please]' which made him 'a little hard-hearted in self defence.' They knew what had happened to their colleague David Eder, the president of the association which, by March 1934 was dealing with around 200 medical refugees: Eder had successfully lobbied the BMA on their behalf but it was detailed, delicate work which had an enormous physical and emotional impact on him and he died in April 1936 (Cooper, 2003: 210–214).

Haire never managed to convince Havelock Ellis of their desperate plight. Shortly before the old man died, Haire tried again in his 20 June 1939 letter: 'I have been very busy with medical refugees. It is very depressing to see all our old friends and acquaintances, who took part in international congresses, in distress, and to hear every week that some more of them have committed suicide.' He mentioned the deaths of Karl Giese and Dr Felix Abraham from Hirschfeld's Berlin

Institute, and said that two survivors had come down to his cottage: Willem Stekel, a pioneering Austrian psychologist and psychoanalyst who was practising in London – until his suicide the following June – and 'poor old' Helene Stöcker, a German feminist, pacifist and sexual reformer. Haire and others who were supporting the refugees found it had become increasingly hard to find additional resources to help the new refugees and despaired of finding a solution to their problems (HC – 3.17).

The death of one of Haire's relatives several years earlier was having unexpected ramifications. In 1934 Haire had read a book called *The case is altered*, based on the November 1929 murder of his second cousin, Sybil da Costa (also known as Sybil Starr): the author was William Plomer, a young South African, who became a celebrity in London after Leonard and Virginia Woolf published this lurid novel and Haire wanted to meet him. Sybil had been Plomer's 'handsome and lively' landlady who, with the help of a female friend, ran a boarding-house to support her six-year-old daughter and her de facto husband James Achew (also known as James Starr), a 'furtive, dark-eyed American with Red Indian blood'. She stayed with him despite his 'insane jealousy' and, when his violence intensified after Plomer moved in (Alexander 1989, 161–62), she telephoned Haire in great distress to say that her lover was accusing her of unfaithfulness with some of the boarders and tradesmen, and was threatening to murder her although there was no ground for his suspicions. Haire advised her to go to the local police station and she rang again to say that the police could do nothing because he had not yet attacked her (*Woman*, 7 July 1947).

Plomer (1958, 39) had learned from Haire that his cousin Sybil was also one of his patients, she often borrowed money from him, her partner suffered from general paralysis of the insane (the final stage of syphilis) and 'was useless, useless to her' and that she had thrown her life away by sticking to him. Plomer was fascinated by violent crime and relished the details of her murder.[2] Initially Plomer declined Haire's

---

2 Plomer (1932, 280–93) spent a chapter detailing the way her partner cut her throat as she lay in bed and her struggle up the stairs with the child to her friend's door where she gasped ' "Natalie – I knew – this would – happen" ' And with that

invitation to meet but accepted it in January 1935 after hearing that he was a 'notoriously indiscreet' sexologist. When the novelist quizzed him, Haire unwisely spoke about a patient who got sexual satisfaction by having a partner defecate on his face. Haire asked: 'But don't you find it rather difficult to find anybody who is willing to join you in that?' "Oh, very difficult", was the answer. "And when I *do* find anybody, of course, they're *never* my type!"[3] Plomer called Haire 'Doctor Pood' (1958, 26–41) but, as the tale was anonymous it was not 'indiscreet' and, since Plomer agreed to meet him in the hope of being titillated, he should be called 'Mister Prude'. Haire's risqué banter was unlikely to have upset his homosexual visitor who claimed 'literature has its battery hens: I was a wilder fowl'.

Haire wanted to buy a place in the country and in 1933 Dora Russell began to send him lists of cottages for sale on the South Downs but he finally bought a much grander place in Hertfordshire – Nettleden Lodge. In October 1935 he offered to drive Margaret Sanger to see his 'old Tudor place', about an hour's drive north west from London, which he had bought 'with 46 acres' and had restored and modernised, telling her 'it really is lovely'. It still is lovely; although the woodlands surrounding it have been sold, it remains a haven for birds and animals and retains its tranquillity. When I visited Nettleden Lodge the owner said that because it is so low-lying, it is much colder than surrounding areas. Despite being much shorter than Haire, I had to duck my head underneath the wooden beams to enter the upstairs rooms and felt that his preparedness to accept these weather and height challenges showed just how much he must have loved this retreat. He provided a map to help visitors find him but asked unexpected visitors to telephone first to make sure their visit would be convenient.

---

she fell dead across the living body of her child.'

3 Plomer also became the literary editor of Ian Fleming's James Bond books and Moffat (2010, 249–50) explained how this happened. In 1943 when Plomer and his friend Fleming worked in Naval Intelligence, Plomer was arrested for soliciting a soldier and Fleming's intervention saved him from ruin. After the war Plomer resumed his job as a reader for Jonathan Cape and returned the favour by recommending they should publish Fleming's novel.

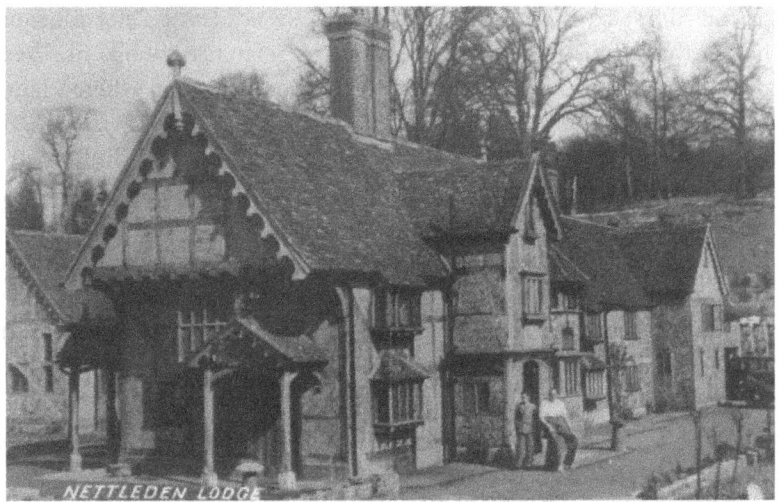

Figure 10.1. Post card of Nettleden Lodge, 1937 with Haire sitting and his uniformed chauffeur standing.

When Berta Ruck visited Nettleden Lodge, Haire collected her in London in his chauffeured Rolls. She had fictionalised him[4] in *The unkissed bride* (1929) and Ethel Mannin sniggered that it was 'ludicrous' for Haire to feature in a book with such a title. In her character vignette Ruck gushed about the 'ultra-Oriental' style of his house; 'black-and-gold lacquer predominated; dragons snarled over satin draperies' and 'fat white porcelain idols' contemplated their navels (Ruck 1929, 11). The surgery's door led to big, expensive, newly furnished rooms, 'in which he stood in a square of morning sunlight flung through the open window onto the room, the black carpet, the oriental trappings, the placid Buddha and the man's fair head'. She called him 'Dr Saxon Locke' which cleverly refers to locks of hair and Britain's Norman and Saxon invaders: Norman was not blue-eyed, fair or Saxon so it was an in-joke

---

4 Ironically, Virginia Woolf gave her a small role (as 'Bertha Ruck' on a tombstone) in her novel *Jacob's room*. Berta's husband sued her and on 27 December 1928 an apologetic Woolf wrote to say she was extremely pleased to discover that Ruck 'had survived the burial.'

to call him 'Saxon' and, as English literature academic Peter Morton noted, the double pun of the pseudonym's reference sounds like 'sex unlocked' – his goal – and refers to the Lock Hospital where Haire treated VD patients.

Dr Locke was about 33 with 'clear blue eyes', big, fair, and broad-shouldered, wearing a white linen jacket. In 1928 Ruck had kept a travel journal for the book and in it she wrote, 'To say he looked clean is inadequate . . . yet that was the first word that came to your mind as you looked at this man'. She described Locke/Haire as big, with breezy speech, 'childishly white and regular teeth' and clever grey eyes behind tortoiseshell-rimmed glasses; a friendly *enfant terrible* who tells the truth at all costs and delights in shocking everybody; 'after a while, people grew acclimatised and ended by liking the good-heartedness beneath the wilful unconventionality'. The plot depended on Locke's far-fetched social experiment into which he 'flung himself' just as Haire did in articles on future marriage or polygamy which had scandalised 'many a breakfast-table'.

Ruck included a vignette of the real man in her autobiography (1935, 164–65). When Haire sent his car to take her down to his country place he warned her 'that rude or not' he always slept on car journeys after lunch. Although he joked about bad manners, his lethargy was really a symptom of his poorly managed diabetes. She was struck by his love of Asian things – the ashtrays and cigarette boxes were Oriental, and so was the bowl of Japanese fish. Even his dogs were chows and they came in the car but sat in front with the chauffeur so they would not 'disturb their master's slumber'. Gwen Otter, a Chelsea party-giver, had warned her that Haire was a gynaecologist; and that some people were '*terribly* upset with him' because he gave 'too much importance to people's sex-life'. She admired this emphasis 'because most doctors gave it too little importance' but she was horrified by her first impressions of him and thought 'what an *awful* man!' Then she, like so many others, began to like him because of his 'generosity, his kindness with unfortunate people, his interesting, determined and original mind'. She forgave his hatred for things she cherished or revered; 'in spite of furnishing his house with Buddhas' he was an idol-breaker while she was 'a Utopian'.

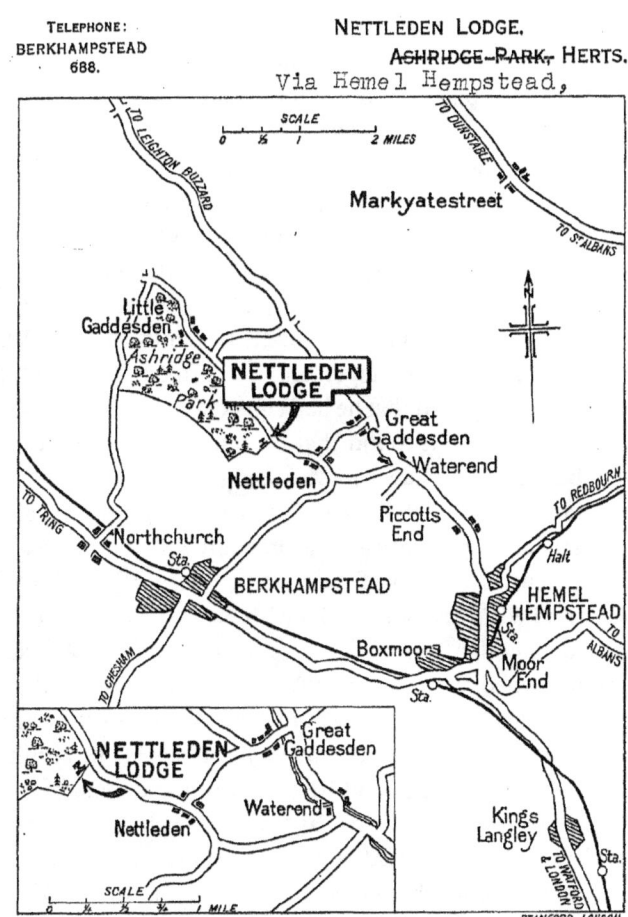

Figure 10.2. Haire sent visitors this map of Nettleden Lodge, Herts via Hemel Hempstead.

They could spend peaceful afternoons together, as they had when she visited Nettleden Lodge which he was having made into a private country estate. He planned to live there and enjoy all the amenities of rural and urban life – perhaps even build a swimming pool – and drive each day to his London consulting-rooms.

He admitted that owning 'a piece of land did tend to lure you, a once revolutionary, back to the side of conservatism'. Then he made a cryptic observation: 'They say success corrupts men' but corruption came 'much more bitterly from the lack of success' and added: 'I do not accept any statement because it is made. I examine it.' As a rationalist, his views were based on logic and this ruled out blind political acceptance. He explained that he had considered himself 'rather vaguely as slightly left wing' but found that his left wing friends accused him of being 'bourgeois'. His decision to change or hide his political views is understandable after the Nazis began their pogroms against Jews, homosexuals and communists; he probably felt that he had enough handicaps – just as Sammy Davis Junior, when asked about his golf handicap, replied, 'I'm a one-eyed Jewish Negro. Will that do?'

Nettleden Lodge was once the gatehouse of the Ashridge Park Estate (now owned by the National Trust) which nestles in the Chiltern Hills, and in this refuge Haire could sunbake naked if he wished. In the foreword to a book on nudism (Welby 1945, 11) he admitted that, although from early childhood he had swum and sunbaked naked at designated Sydney ocean baths, 'at times and places reserved for the male sex,' he was embarrassed on his first visit to a nudist camp. George Bernard Shaw facetiously opposed nudity, saying in *The Times* on 14 September 1929 that, after the exhibitionism and immorality of the Victorian age, 'women had now taken a large step towards nudity and sex appeal had vanished. Bring back clothes and it would be increased'. In March 1935 *The Times* reported the Pope's view that nudity was a 'tendency to paganism in life which many were leading with a pagan devotion to pleasure and amusement', but progressives praised the health benefits of light, air and sun bathing (Zweiniger-Bargielowski 2006). Jean Simpson[5] in her history of Nettleden quoted a woman

---

5 Jean Simpson (1998). In 2008 she told me that Haire extended the house and

who, as a child, remembered adults saying that when they walked on footpaths in the valley near Dr Haire's lodge in 1940, they had seen 'patients all lying out on the lawn completely naked!' The Lodge became a children's home for wartime evacuees but Canon Howard Senar, who wrote a book about the region in 1983, believed it was a nursing home (unlikely) or a resort (like nearby Champneys, Britain's first nature cure resort). There are other possibilities: villagers might have spread rumours about nudity in this hidden place at the bottom of a valley or they may have seen Haire and other members of Sex Education Society sunning themselves.

In October 1935 illness struck again and Haire explained to his editor at the publishers George Routledge & Sons that he was now living at Nettleden Lodge. As a result, Haire would have missed Dr Arthur Hill's paper on the control of septic abortion which Kelvin Churches mentioned in his 1976 lecture on 120 years of abortion in Melbourne. Churches said the 32-year-old 'Bung' Hill, a dapper young Australian and former medical superintendent of Melbourne's Royal Women's Hospital, 'strode up and down the stage with the confidence of an experienced actor' in his address to the Royal Society of Medicine in London on 29 November 1935. This could have been a description of Haire as both men were charismatic supporters of abortion law reform, provided artificial inseminations, inserted Gräfenberg rings and cared passionately about women's health and had great theatrical presence.

They were just two of the 'whole colony' of expatriates 'living in England or longing for England.' Percy 'Inky' Stephensen, a writer, editor and publisher, fumed 'What's the matter with them all?' but he would have worried less if, 'in exchange', Britain had sent 'Thomas Burke, Shaw, Wells, Chesterton, Belloc, Hardy and Galsworthy'. Inky considered Australia's sense of cultural inferiority had spawned 'our

---

linked the barn to the house. In 1936 he built a driveway to the road above the house; in autumn 1941 he leased it to the Soldiers, Sailors, Airmen and Families Association (SSAFA) for use as a children's home. It housed 40 children aged from 18 months to 14 years, a matron and ten staff. A man who lived there in 1943 recalled nectarines, peaches, vegetables, a pony and cart, and a dormitory in the ballroom. In 1945 the SSAFA reported that most children, terrified by air raids, recovered completely after a short stay.

émigrés' in Harley Street, in London's West End theatres or in the halls of Oxford, 'aspiring to set the Thames on fire'. While Haire once had these aspirations, he was now sick and had financial worries. In response to the Russell's request for donations to support their school, he commiserated and listed his own difficulties relating to the spiralling restoration costs which had left him with a huge overdraft. Although he had earned a very good income, he had spent his savings 'and more'. Even worse, diabetes had struck 'just at the wrong moment' and he was likely to earn considerably less 'when it would be most disastrous'. He apologised to Dora Russell in December 1935 for being unable to send money but offered to help in other ways.

Haire wanted his portrait painted and commissioned P Tennyson Cole, an artist 'of a sound old-fashioned type' who specialised in celebrities including the King. Haire also persuaded Havelock Ellis to have 'four or five sittings' with Cole who made two portraits of Ellis, one of which Haire planned to hang in his big room (a barn refurbished as a ballroom) as soon as Nettleden Lodge renovations (including a hare in bas-relief over the dining room fireplace) were complete. In January 1936 Haire invited Ellis to his country 'cottage' to view the portraits and watch the movie he took several years earlier of Lafitte-Cyon walking with him in their garden at Haslemere. Haire reissued the invitation in April 1937 for them to come 'any weekend during the summer' but warned him that the first full-face portrait looked like 'a benevolent old gentleman who might be anybody's grandpa' and so he had commissioned a second, side-on painting but this one made him 'look queer' – what Max Nordau or Cesare Lombroso would have called 'degenerate', but it did 'get the Satyr. Unfortunately, it doesn't get anything else'.[6]

Havelock Ellis said there was much truth in what Haire said about both of these portraits although the painter was anxious to do his best and thought him 'a fine subject'. He agreed about the Satyr likeness and his close friend Olive Schreiner used to say he was like the Satyr

---

6 Haire had been disappointed when he met Havelock Ellis in 1919 to discover that, while Ellis' upper face was 'noble', his beard masked a mouth and chin which struck him as being 'weak and sensual'.

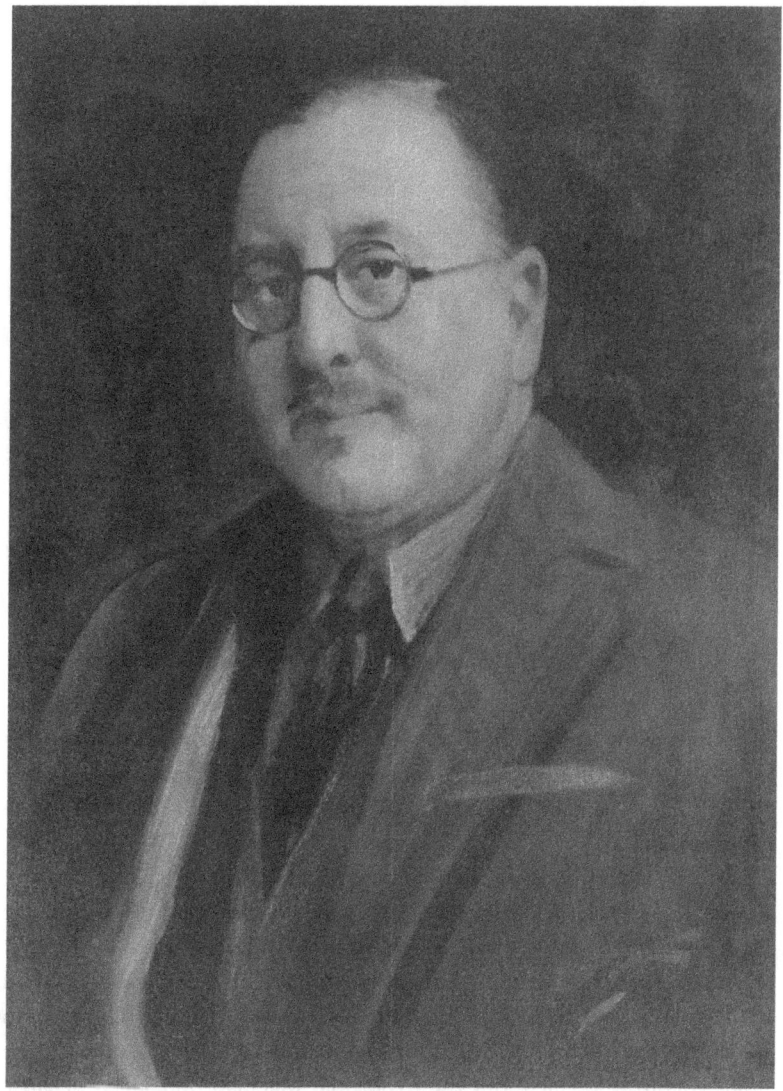

Figure 10..3. Norman Haire in his 40s, from a painting by P Tennyson Cole.

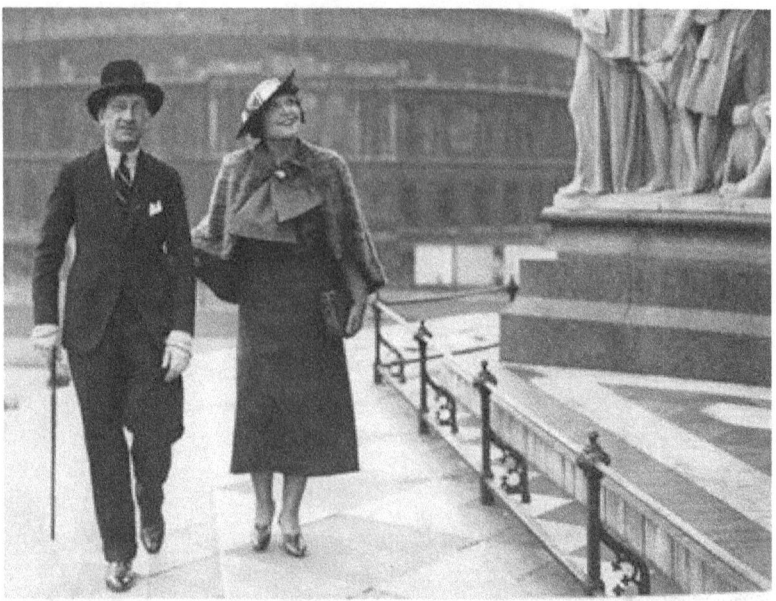

Figure 10.4. Conchita Supervia and her accompanist Ivor Newton when they laid flowers at the Albert Memorial on the statue of Rossini. Reproduced with permission of Patrick O'Connor.

in a Rubens picture in the National Gallery. Edward Carpenter in his autobiography said he looked like the Greek god Pan, but a fellow student at St Thomas Hospital once remarked to him: 'You remind me of Jesus Christ.'

When Haire was commissioned by a Sunday newspaper to write an obituary for Havelock Ellis he disregarded convention by writing: 'He used jokingly to allude to his resemblance to pictures of Jesus Christ. It was not only in appearance that the resemblance existed. Few men had greater right than Havelock Ellis to echo Christ's words: "Come unto me all ye that labour and are heavy laden, and I will give you rest."' The 'joke' was in poor taste but the hyperbole was also misplaced because the philosopher often saw people's sexual problems as material for his prolix, esoteric masterpieces. In contrast, Haire frequently went out of his way to provide 'rest' to the sexually anxious by responding to their questions, giving lectures and writing lucidly. Haire's obituary was rejected by the newspaper because they found it blasphemous; Haire told Lafitte-Cyon that the paper paid him and substituted a 'respectable' one.

Haire, who was revising *Hymen*, sent a note to the editor and his wife in October 1936, asking them to visit, and the couple hoped to do so very soon. Haire had 'mellowed and developed' the book and, as these undated notes show, he was also aware of the threats posed by deteriorating world events. He thought it seemed likely that there would be attempts to prevent people marrying or mating if their poor physical or mental health meant they were likely to produce 'defective offspring'. He said this should be achieved by education, rather than compulsion, for once the state is given legislative power there is always the likelihood, 'as we have seen in Germany', that such powers might be used for political ends. The revised edition was never published.[7] Haire's progress reports ceased and the editor asked the reason for his silence. Haire sent an apology; he was on a very strict diet which made him very depressed, he found it hard to work, his correspondence kept piling up and he felt hungry all the time. The editor sent his sympathy in early December and hoped he would get used to it as he got thinner.

Haire's problems intensified after one of his patients died in childbirth on 30 March 1936. She was Conchita Supervia, a talented opera singer.

Frank Forster referred to this tragedy in his 5 July 1978 letter to Dora Russell. He also mentioned receiving a 'fascinating letter' from Sir Edward Ford, a bibliophile and former Dean of Medicine at Sydney University, and promised to show the letter to the university's Rare Books Librarian.[8] Supervia's death certificate gave the cause of death as

---

7 Bongiorno (2012, 170) was chilled by the proposals Haire made in *Hymen* for the treatment of 'defective babies' and 'sexually abnormal people' and asked rhetorically if 'One wonders whether Haire saw the irony when he found himself assisting Jewish sexologists forced to flee Hitler's Germany.' Bongiorno quoted secondary sources in other references to Haire and he did not mention the 25-page draft of a 1936 revised version of *Hymen* which reflected Haire's changed opinions.

8 Searchers could not locate it in Ford's papers at the Royal Australian College

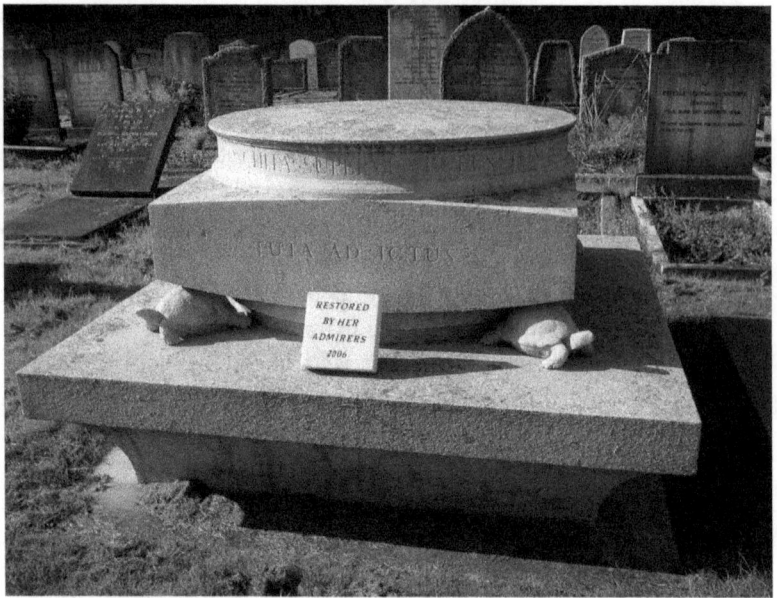

Figure 10.5. Conchita Supervia's grave in Willesden Liberal Jewish Cemetery, London.

'(a) Pulmonary Embolism and (b) full time childbirth'. The certificate listed Haire as her doctor and gave her age as 35, although she was 41.[9] Dr Irvine Loudon (1992) is an expert in the field and, in response to my question in 2006, he described her death as 'an unavoidable accident' – in the 1930s it was the fourth most common cause of death in childbirth, the other three being (in this order) puerperal sepsis, puerperal haemorrhage and toxaemia of pregnancy. He said, statistically, pulmonary embolisms in childbirth were always more common in women over than under 30 – but this was only a very slight difference.

Although Haire was blameless it must have been shattering. Many papers published eulogies and on 31 March the *Manchester Guardian*

---

of Physicians and the National Library of Australia, or in Forster's papers in the Royal Australian College of Obstetricians and Gynaecologists.

9 Barcelona's birth register gave 9 December 1895 as her date of birth (as Concepcion Supervia Pascual). Patrick O'Connor sent me these details.

paid tribute to Mme Conchita Supervia, the famous Spanish singer who had died in a London nursing home. She was the wife of Ben Rubenstein, an English timber broker and fruit farmer. Mme Supervia was expecting a child, and on Sunday went into the nursing home 'very happy and very well' but the baby was stillborn. A clot of blood developed, and despite the efforts of doctors, Mme Supervia died. 'NC' [probably the music critic Neville Cardus] wrote that opera had suffered a sad loss and described her sparkling presence, her sense of allusive and animated gesture, and said she had a voice that 'expressed with nice nuance a personality which was at bottom an actress's'. She was buried with her stillborn child in her arms, the directors and chorus of the Royal Opera House sent flowers, and mourners included Spain's Ambassador. Her coffin was draped with the red, purple and yellow new Republican flag of Spain and topped with orchids from the garden of her home in Rustington, Sussex.

Sir Edwin Lutyens, a distinguished British architect, designed her tomb which rests on four tortoises (her mascot) carved by Sir William Reid Dick, then the most famous sculptor in England.

In 1966 her accompanist Ivor Newton described how her husband's florist shop near Wigmore Hall 'would light up and become all smiles' whenever she called in. The couple had invited him to see the baby's nursery and, 24 hours before her death, she was 'lively, confident and very happy and invited him to "come soon and see my little Easter egg." ' Georgio, her 17-year-old son from her first marriage, made this sad but wise comment: 'Mama has been spared a lot. She couldn't have borne to grow old. There's a lot to be thankful for. She would have hated to lose her looks and her voice. She couldn't have borne life in obscurity'.

Haire was stricken, telling Havelock Ellis on 3 April that he was 'rather depressed at the moment' – the previous Monday he 'lost a confinement patient, Conchita Supervia', from a post-partum pulmonary embolism, his third such death in over 15 years – 'and on the same day, David Eder died'. Havelock Ellis responded immediately and was sorry to hear that Haire was going through a period of depression. He was saddened by the death of Eder who had also been a good friend of his and had been a very kind friend to Lafitte-Cyon when she had been his patient. He sent belated thanks for the invitation to Nettleden Lodge, which Margaret Sanger had described after her visit, but he was unlikely to come because the demands on his decreasing energy seemed to increase and he had financial and literary worries. He explained that he had not written the foreword because he received many such requests every week and had decided the only way out of the difficulty was to refuse them all. He ended his letter with some good news: the College of Physicians proposed to make him an Honorary Fellow and he enclosed a flyer for the *Studies in the psychology of sex* which was about to be reissued by Random House in America in a compact, much cheaper form.

Haire began his 9 April reply: 'Yes, many of us will miss Eder's kindness. For me, as for many others, he was an ideal father-substitute'. He told Havelock Ellis he knew about the publication of the *Studies* – John Lane had arranged for their publication in England and he supposed (wrongly) that they would appear in 'The international library of sexology and psychology', which he edited. He again tried to entice Havelock Ellis to visit his cottage to see the film of himself and some other films of sexological interest: he would send a car for him and he could come either for the day or stay overnight because there were plenty of guest rooms. Haire was sorry about his literary problems and hoped his financial worries were over: 'If not, and I could be of any assistance, I should regard it as an honour and a privilege'. Fortunately for Haire, who said the previous December that he was too poor to give such help to the Russell's school, Havelock Ellis did not ask for help.

Haire's troubles continued; in April 1936 he apologised to his editor at Routledge about his slowness with the book's revision; he had been sick and he had lost his secretary who had been with him for seven years. He meant Ruby Lockie who had worked for Haire and the WLSR. She, like Haire, had brave, rational views and these showed in a letter in *The Eugenics Review*.[10] When a local paper said a nurse's action, in saving a baby's life against a hundred to one odds, showed 'courage and self-sacrifice' Lockie asked, 'What can one do to divert altruism into wiser channels and to biologically more desirable ends?' Unfortunately for

---

10   Ruby Lockie (1936, 161) gave an address in Denham, Buckinghamshire so she may have resigned from her job with Haire because of travel difficulties.

Haire, her successor 'was a terrible dud' who got everything muddled.

Haire hoped to be able get on with *The future of marriage* soon and would let his publisher know as soon as he had finished it. It remained unfinished perhaps because he was completing a long-delayed book for Allen & Unwin: *Birth-control methods (contraception, sterilization, abortion)*. It was published in May, two months after the deaths of Conchita Supervia and David Eder and, just as he had kept on editing the WLSR proceedings after Jerdan's death in 1930, Haire did not let emotion interfere with his work. He posted one copy of the manuscript to Havelock Ellis and another to Sir Eardley Holland, a gifted writer and a distinguished pioneer of obstetrics and gynaecology and asked if they might write a foreword. Haire later said both men sent 'kind letters' but neither man agreed to do so.

Havelock Ellis' rejection was so painful that Haire wrote 'Private file' on two letters relating to it. Haire's writing was known for its lucidity but his 3 January 1936 letter to Havelock Ellis was the incoherent outpouring of a severely depressed man: he first asked Ellis to comment on the page proofs and then wrote: 'The second, which I hardly dare to make, for I stand still in great awe of you, I don't know quite why, is that you will honour me by writing a short foreword if you think the book sufficiently worthy.' Havelock Ellis was renowned for his *Studies in the psychology of sex* and, in a preface to his article about sterilisation in *The Manchester Evening News* (20 March 1936) he was described as a courageous pioneer, 'among the noblest of Englishmen.' However, he did not respond nobly in this case. Ellis suffered agonies of shyness himself and was ill-at-ease if more than two or three people were present and could never make a public speech. His decision to ignore Haire's call for help indicates either cruelty or a lack of perception. Haire always responded to requests from Havelock Ellis and would have interpreted the refusal to provide a foreword as a personal rejection and an indication that his mentor thought the book was unworthy – two severe blows to a man who was on edge and lacked confidence.

Ten days later Haire wrote to Havelock Ellis and tried to save face over the rejection: he had been hoping that Ellis 'would feel there was a special reason for writing an introduction in this case' but could 'quite understand' that he could 'accord' to all the requests he received. He meant to say 'could *not* accord' but this slip shows he was still agitated. Haire wrote again on 3 April to thank him for sending his sterilisation article, saying that he had read it with great interest because they seemed to be alone in their view that sterilisation should be seen as a medical rather than a legal matter. Haire had discussed this 'at considerable length' in his book and 'in truth' had hoped, 'on account of this alone', Havelock Ellis would have written the preface to emphasise this. Aldous Huxley had now written a foreword but had not referred to sterilisation at all. The now-calm Haire sensed that anger about the proposed legislation had galvanised Havelock Ellis to take a rare public stance in his dissenting newspaper article and he was chiding his mentor for ignoring the opportunity to use the foreword to further his views.

When Aldous Huxley agreed to write the foreword Haire expressed his gratitude and explained his motives for writing the book. He had never earned enough from writing to make it worthwhile when he could be attending to patients and earning far more. He was not writing it to make money but because he thought he had 'more experience of birth control than probably anybody else in the world, certainly than anybody else in Europe'; and also because he believed he could write 'more lucidly and convincingly than most doctors'. He wanted it to sell well because it should help remove some of the misery that burdens most human beings. To help make it within reach of all, he was pressing the publishers to produce it at the lowest possible price. Haire thanked Huxley for reviewing *The encylopaedia of sexual knowledge* so favourably and Huxley agreed to introduce the new book despite his fears about possible misuse of birth control. The publisher shortened and softened it, leaving an introduction in which Huxley said that efficient contraception was a technological achievement of the 20th century and the spread of knowledge about it was one of the most significant social changes of recent years. Puritans likened sex to a 'dangerous addiction' but 'to those who believe that charity is more important than chastity, and that the obsession with chastity represents a perversion of morality, the puritans' objection to birth control will seem merely irrelevant'. He concluded by saying that Dr Norman Haire's 'compact and sensible little book sums up all the best information on the subject'.

Richard Aldington congratulated Haire for writing 'without prudishness, in language intelligible to everyone, without sentimentality or cynicism, of these intimate physical things on which so much of human sanity and happiness depend'. He praised Haire for showing 'faith in life', for while he showed 'how not to have children that are unwanted', he also showed 'how to have those which are wanted'. Haire thanked Havelock Ellis in May for his kind comments about his book, one of several letters he had received including 'one especially nice one from HG Wells'. He said the book was going well and would be reprinted: this was a preface to another diffident request which was also refused by his mentor. Haire asked Havelock Ellis again in October but this time he said it was at the request of the publishers who wanted 'a really important favourable opinion' to quote in the advertisements for the book's second printing. Finally Havelock Ellis broke his rule to reject all such requests and responded with qualified praise which began: 'The author of this book is widely known as a sometimes daring pioneer' and then he noted two features: it was based on wide experience and the techniques were explained in a 'characteristically lucid and forthright manner.' The book included 'two brief but significant chapters' on sterilisation and abortion and 'It would not be easy to find a more practically useful book on this subject'. This suggests that Havelock Ellis was still somewhat resentful and his ambiguous last sentence could be taken to mean that, while he felt it was suitable for lay readers, discerning readers would be able to find better books on the subject.

Haire thanked Havelock Ellis on 27 October for his letters and the paragraph on his birth control book which he had received after returning from Lugano where it had been too hot to sit in the sun for long. He had crossed the Channel in a roaring gale and was not pleased by the clouded skies of England and, even though a visit to Nettleden Lodge at that time would have been bleak, Haire was still looking forward to Havelock Ellis' visit to view the P Tennyson Cole portrait of him.

However, the overseas distribution problems remained and Haire was irked when American customs confiscated the review copy he sent to Dr Abraham Stone, the editor of *Journal of Contraception* (Rose

1936). Haire told his publishers that the book was 'freely available in Australia' but initially this was not true; Australian authorities only decided it was 'not to be regarded as a prohibited import' in February 1937. In London the publishers enthusiastically endorsed it, saying there were too many books on birth control written by people without adequate background training and experience and 'few books were really good, lucid or practical', implying that, in contrast, Haire's book provided all of these missing essentials. Haire complained bitterly in 1933 when Allen & Unwin called him an 'eminent gynaecologist' but he was silent when they now advertised him as 'the medical pioneer of birth control in this country'. People had waited a long time for such a book but the wait was worthwhile because Haire skilfully combined his intensive and extensive experience and knowledge gained by long years of study and clinical testing. While the book was primarily intended for medical practitioners and students, it was equally useful for 'Mr and Mrs Everyman'.

Haire's book contained the same daring he had displayed in *Hymen*, such as this earthy plea for genital cleanliness: some people said secretions were natural and did not need to be removed and this would be valid if women were naked and their genitals were exposed to sunlight and fresh air or if men shared dogs' liking for 'stale urinary and vaginal odours'. But civilised women are swathed in underclothes which allows 'natural discharges to cling about the parts and decompose, giving rise to stale fishy odours which are repugnant to most cleanly civilised men, however ardent their sexual desire may be'. The book evaluated all forms of contraception and Norman Himes praised him and RL Dickinson for warning women not to use strong chemical douches such as Lysol or coal tar disinfectants. Stopes also meant these harmful products when she said, 'never put anything in your vagina you would not put in your mouth'.[11] This was memorable but excluded the use of safe spermicides, and one girl, on hearing Stopes' aphorism years later, asked her teacher if it included tampons because she wouldn't put *them* in her mouth.

---

11 Stopes said this to 'bemused, mainly male readers of *The Lancet* in 1938' quoted by Gary Dexter at www.spectator.co.uk/books/14297/surprising-literary-ventures-41/ [Accessed 12 October 2012].

Haire told Himes in May 1936 that the deteriorating conditions in Germany threatened the future of the WLSR's quarterly review *SEXUS* and said he would try to review two of Himes' books in *The Socialist Review*. After sending Himes 'hearty congratulations' for his great pioneering work, *Medical history of contraception*, Haire complained that the American customs had seized every copy of the 1934 edition of *The encyclopaedia of sexual knowledge* and that his chapter on contraception had been omitted from the American edition because of the 'obscenity laws of your funny country. Not, of course, that your country is funnier than this – it is simply funny in a different way'. Himes suggested some witty ways to fool the censors; he should take a chance and send the book to him. He would fight the case if the customs men held it up, although there was 'more than an even chance' that it would get through. Haire should mark on the package: 'Book. Value less than one dollar'. If he did this, customs men might not examine it, because they do not assess duty on objects (at least books) which cost so little. He also suggested 'another stunt' to get other copies into the USA – send them to Spain and mail them from there, marked 'book'. It would be assumed that they are in Spanish and there is no duty on foreign language books and this would probably work for other countries such as Sweden and Denmark. He suggested Haire should try the same tactics with his encyclopedia.

Himes told Haire that Morris Ernst, a New York lawyer who co-founded the American Civil Liberties Union, was taking action over the holding up of shipments of the journal *Marriage Hygiene*. They had tried to get a court test but the government would not bring action and was probably waiting to see the result of the appeal of the Japanese pessaries case. The outcome was a victory for American birth control, and Hannah Stone discussed this in 1937. After the US Customs seized a package of 120 contraceptives from Japan in 1933, Margaret Sanger protested and the law was contested by Morris Ernst. As a result Judge Moscowitz decided that 'the US Tariff Act could not reasonably be construed so as to prevent the importation by physicians of articles for the prevention of conception when intended for lawful use'. Haire promised to post Himes a copy of the first edition of *Birth-control methods* which had been published in May 1936 and said a second edition was coming out in June. Allen & Unwin had spent fruitless months trying to broker a deal with major American publishers. Haire wrote to Norman Himes and listed birth control books by American authors which had been published – Dickinson (1924), Cooper (1928), Konikow (1931) and Stone and Stone (1935) – saying that he didn't see why his book was refused and asked him to suggest a publisher. Himes agreed but said soothingly that American publishers were 'squeamish and it takes persuasion'. Himes suggested two more publishers but the answer was the same: no American publisher was prepared to break the law.

In June 1936 Haire asked Allen & Unwin to send review copies to American medical journals and in November he suggested they might contact Morris Ernst. Haire tried again and asked if they would put the book in the hands of Miss Joseph, a literary agent who had been recommended by George Sylvester Viereck. This suggestion showed a stunning lack of judgement: during his America tour Haire had warned Hirschfeld in February 1934 that 'Viereck is acting as Hitler's main agent in America'; it is odd that Haire would listen to suggestions made by a man who *Time* called in May 1931 'a venom-bloated toad of treason' and who *The New York Times* denounced in May 1934 for organising a New York rally attended by 20,000 'Nazi friends.'

Allen & Unwin were prepared to follow Haire's wishes but reminded him that any copy they posted Miss Joseph would be held up by customs. Haire replied that if they replaced the dust jacket with an innocuous-looking one ('not about sex') he was sure his book would reach its destination. He added 'George Sylvester Viereck seemed to think that Miss Joseph would have no difficulty in finding a publisher, and he is a man who is pretty smart on the business side of publishing.' In December 1936 Haire was happy to leave the decision to Allen & Unwin but urged them to do something soon and the publishers astutely decided to re-assign the American rights to Haire because they would prefer to do something which was not customary than leave him feeling dissatisfied. Haire was ill, Viereck was dropped by his Jewish literary agent and his publisher, then unmasked (*The Chicago Daily Tribune* 28 May 1940) and jailed (*The New York Times* 14 March 1942). Haire's dream of an American edition of his book crumbled and so did his 'The international library of sexology and psychology' series after John Lane's The Bodley Head press was placed in receivership in December 1936. It was bought in 1937 by an Allen & Unwin, Jonathan Cape and JM Dent consortium.

However, his book did well in Britain when Haire asked the publishers in May 1936 to send the book to London's medical booksellers and ask them to display copies in their windows; he suggested doing the same for 'rubber goods shops' (which sold sex aids and condoms) because 'more people purchase birth control books from shops of this sort than from all the other booksellers combined.' A major distributor of condoms offered to include thousands of advertising flyers for the book with their weekly consignments, and also sell the book, if the name 'Durex' was mentioned. Sensibly the publisher added a footnote: 'Very good condoms are made by the London Rubber Company, 221 Old Street, E C 1 and sold under the trade mark Durex'.

In May 1936 the publishers advertised in medical and birth control magazines and in weeklies such as *New Statesman* and *Time & Tide* but the booksellers WH Smith & Son refused to stock or display any books on birth control although they would supply copies of Haire's book if customers requested it. Although the Australian Customs agreed not to ban the book,[12] it was difficult to buy a copy because distributors Gordon and Gotch would not stock or supply such books (Willett 1997). The popularity of *Birth-control methods* caused problems for two London department stores; when curious customers at Selfridges damaged the display copy, the publishers gave the store 'a free copy which can stand on the counter simply for the purpose of being thumbed' and copies for sale were kept under the counter, and the same strategy was used by Harrods. Allen & Unwin spent a huge amount on advertising[13] and

---

12   Australian Customs sought to determine whether Haire's book (which 'deals fully with the subject of birth control in language plainer than is usual in books of this nature') should be banned under the *Blasphemous, Indecent and Obscene Publications section of the Customs Act*. The Collector of Customs was advised on 12 February 1937 that the book would not be regarded as a prohibited import (NAA – D596/2, Item 1936/9416).

13   Advertisements were placed in: *Health and Strength, New Health, Health and*

they agreed to spend another £50 if Haire would do the same. Haire was also working on a much bigger birth control book, to equal the length of Marie Stopes' 1923 book *Contraception* and he hoped to have it ready for publication by Allen & Unwin in a few months. The details of the forthcoming work were announced opposite his book's title page: 'Methods and technique of prevention of conception: a textbook for medical practitioners and students', by Norman Haire, CH M, MB and Sidonie Fürst, MD. Oxford University Press' cancellation of the contract for this book was discussed in chapter 4.

It would cover the history of birth control, male and female reproductive anatomy, physiology of reproduction including 'hormonic methods', male sterilisation (by female sex hormones), male and female 'hyperhormonic' sterilisation (by 'extra-genital hormones' and 'immunisation by semen'), the birth control movement and the organisation of a clinic. Haire would write the clinical chapters and his co-author, who gave a paper on the 'Problem of the unmarried woman' at the 1930 WLSR congress, would write about the history of the movement and the physiology and chemistry of birth control. However, after seeing her first chapters, he told her about his concerns and told the publishers that the writing was 'very poor and unsuitable.' He had spent about £20 on translating and typing and it was 'so bad', he doubted whether she would or could re-write it in a suitable form. Haire had to forgo his dream of outdoing Stopes with his textbook and Sidonie Fürst had to flee from the Nazis; she became one of the German Jewish doctors who, with Margaret Sanger's assistance, came to America.

There are few details of his work in 1937 but two stories stand out. One was told years later by Constantine FitzGibbon, described in *The Times* 25 March 1983 obituary as 'an alcoholic novelist and much-married historian.' In his autobiography FitzGibbon (1967) recalled his visit to a Paris abortionist who refused to abort his pregnant partner. The doctor said it was too late and too dangerous and advised them to

---

Efficiency, Parents, Manchester Guardian, Bristol Observer, Edinburgh Evening News, Literary Guide, Freethinker, Vogue, Britannia, Daily Worker, Daily Herald, Sunday Referee, Left Review and the medical papers Haire suggested. Three papers refused: *The Birmingham Post, The Nottingham Guardian* and *The Daily Express.*

continue the pregnancy under the care of Norman Haire. FitzGibbon had heard of Haire who 'was not only a very famous gynaecologist' but also wrote 'liberal-progressive' books and 'advocated birth-control and, in certain circumstances, abortion'. FitzGibbon hoped that he would solve 'our gigantic problem, and perhaps even do so for very little money, since the extreme luxury of his offices made it plain that he himself had more than enough'. But he soon discovered that Haire 'did not intend to allow his left-wing principles to affect his right-wing bank balance' when he mentioned the fee, up to and inclusive of the baby's birth. When FitzGibbon 'spoke of an abortion, hypocrisy was snapped down as a knight in armour might snap shut his visor. Did I not know it was illegal in England? It was, he led me to believe, unethical of me to have even mentioned such a word in the pile-carpeted splendours of his millionaire's consulting rooms'. They agreed that Haire should look after his partner and Haire scribbled a prescription for some medicine she was to take, recommended that she do the exercises listed in one of his books on prenatal care, and said she was to come back in a month's time. Their premature baby died and FitzGibbon was angry because Haire appeared at nine in the morning shaved and smelling of cologne, he was rich and charged high fees but, most of all, because he was *not* an abortionist.

Haire mentioned another story as an amusing instance of people's failure to recognise homosexual messages: just before the war a British publisher produced a list of public urinals in central London 'for the guidance of gentlemen suffering from a frequent desire to urinate.' A large number of his homosexual patients used the book to discover public toilets and pick up casual sexual partners ('cottaging'). Haire claimed not to know the author's identity and said he could not 'imagine an American publisher being so naïve.'[14] Routledge published the book in 1937, the author was 'Paul Pry' and the title was *For your convenience: a learned dialogue instructive to all Londoners and London visitors, overheard in the Thélème Club and taken down verbatim*. Historian Matt Houlbrook analysed it in *Queer London* (2005), calling it 'remarkable' and 'perhaps the first queer city guide' of public urinals, indicating the ones

---

14 Haire in Albert Ellis (1952, 7).

that were safe from police 'earshot' and 'observation' and accompanied by a hand-drawn map (flanked by a pair of sweepers with erect brooms) with urinals highlighted as little green cottages. Houlbrook said that Tom Driberg had reviewed the book for the *New Statesman* in 1937 and that this communist, openly gay, life peer, journalist and spy – who Winston Churchill said was 'the sort of person who gives sodomy a bad name' – had apparently identified Pry as Thomas Burke, a once-famous writer who had interviewed Haire.

The critic Richard Aldington lived for many years in self-imposed exile in Paris and in 1933, when he made a rare visit to London, Haire asked The Bodley Head press whether they might like Aldington to write a book on sex and censorship in art, or one on censorship in literature but nothing came of this. Aldington was a close friend of Lawrence Durrell who, in an August 1958 letter to his friend, referred to Haire's language, saying the only cut the publishers had 'insisted on' in *Mountolive* (the third part of *The Alexandria quartet*) 'was the word "fellatio" which I shouldn't have thought anyone knew, save the late Havelock E and Haire'. In 1981 the editors of Durrell's book added a footnote: 'Havelock Ellis and Norman Haire were pioneering writers on sex' (quoted by MacNiven & Moore 1981, 50–51).

Haire was famous for 'saying what you mean' and some people considered this was rude and broke the protocol for polite conversation. He carefully avoided slang and used medical terms or the 'more polite synonyms' for urination, defaecation, copulation and the genital organs and disliked people who used foreign language phrases to hide meaning or fool the censors. Haire translated euphemisms when he found them and, when Hirschfeld wrote *inter fæces et urinas nascimur* in his 1935 book, Haire added a footnote: 'We are born between urine and fæces.' He considered the use of Anglo-Saxon terms as 'mere expletives' showed poor vocabulary and he swore 'almost not at all', perhaps saying '*bloody* or *damn* once or twice a year'; to him swearing was distasteful because he was 'brought up in a suburban and bourgeois atmosphere where it was regarded as a heinous offence'. However, few noticed this restraint, only his blunt words which they found shocking. This was counterproductive because people were less likely to take him seriously and they may have considered that his crusades for birth control and sexual reform were just one of the acts he performed so well.

Haire relished his raffish reputation and gave 'Sexology, London' as his cable address. In 1963 the fashion designer James Laver commented on Haire's risqué conversations back when they were Gwen Otter's guests at the elaborate 1920s 'Sunday luncheons' in her Chelsea apartment. The guests at her salon were usually artistic luminaries, such as Katherine Mansfield, Ethel Mannin, Aleister Crowley and 'the well-known gynaecologist' Norman Haire, 'a great mountain of a man' whose attitude to sex was simple: 'he thought there ought to be a great deal more of it'. Laver said Haire's 'ordinary method of greeting any young man was to clap him on the shoulder and say: "Well, my boy: sex all right?" And he loved to startle dinner parties by remarking with enormous conviction: "Incest? Very good thing!"' Mannin (1971, 67) took him seriously when he asked if she had tried bestiality, and asked why she had not tried it adding, 'They say you can train a peke to do anything!' He meant a Pekingese dog and if she had thought about it for a moment she would have known that he was joking.

Mannin described a Rationalist Press Association meeting in the 1930s when Haire said 'out loud in public such words as masturbation, homosexuality, orgasm' which left them all 'a little breathless'. She had dinner at his house before the meeting and heard some of what he intended to say and thought it would be 'fun if he could' but doubted he would dare. She said, in the Bright Young Things talk of *Vile bodies*, at first his address was 'too, too, shy making' and she sensed waves of shock, but by question time everyone had become remarkably frank. Mannin said afterwards that he seemed to have had a 'loosening' effect on the audience. He was pleased because most people 'were so dreadfully mentally constipated' and they had all thoroughly enjoyed themselves (Mannin 1930, 189–90).

Sydney's salacious *Daily Mirror* focused on Haire's ribaldry in its 7 May 1987 article 'NSW sex reformer shocked Londoners with naughty jokes.' Ethel Mannin was now dead so the author had either attended the meeting or recycled her story with some variations. According to this 1987 report, the first meeting of the WLSR was held in 1921 in

London and its principal speaker was Dr Norman Haire, 'a large roly-poly Australian who was well-known for his outspoken views on sex'. He had told outrageous stories at the pre-meeting dinner that evening but no one expected him to repeat them before a large, mixed audience. At first he was greeted with a stony silence, but, once the ice was broken, it was a different story. The glares, the nervous giggles turned to whole-hearted laughter. By the end of the evening, complete strangers were chatting away to each other about their sex lives. Haire knew that talking 'reasonably' on the subject wouldn't get him far and that people needed a good jolt to start them thinking. So he prepared a surprise and, as the talk began, Haire walked to a blackboard and unrolled a large chart. 'Now look closely', Haire said. 'What we have here is the male sex organ of the West African Negro. Enormous, isn't it?' Anticipating the outburst of horror, he said, 'I see some of you ladies are getting restive. But I assure you there is no hurry. The boat for Africa doesn't leave until Friday'.

There are problems with this story: the WLSR was not established until 1928 so Haire was probably addressing the British Society for the Study of Sex Psychology, and an urban myth website Snopes.com has many versions of this 'Last boat to Africa' legend whose roots trace back to Cambridge University and the anthropologist AC Haddon (1855–1940) who, while lecturing on the Torres Strait Islanders, said that in some islands the women proposed marriage. On hearing this, some female students tried to slip out of the classroom. He called after them, 'No hurry, there won't be a boat for some weeks.'[15] Accoding to Snopes.com, folklore classes at Michigan State University collected 17 versions between 1947 and 1956.

The best known Australian version relates to 'Pansy' (Roy) Wright. According to his biographer Peter McPhee (1999), as a newly appointed professor of physiology at Melbourne University, Wright used this tale from 'an old store of medical ribaldry' in 1939. McPhee quoted Beatrice Faust's view that Wright might have used it to deter female students

---

15 Exposed [Online] Available: www.snopes.com/college/embarrass/shortage. asp, compiled by Barbara and David P Mikkelson whose sources range from the scholarly (Brunvand 1960, 1962) to salacious *Playboy*.

from attending medical school by creating an atmosphere in which they would feel ill at ease. It has also been attributed to Sydney University's Charles Birch and the University of Western Australia's Harry Waring.

The lead up to World War II was an anxious period and Haire's optimism had vanished by the time he wrote the introduction for René Guyon's second book in 1939. The first was published in 1932 when the old taboos were dying and liberal minded people were discussing the dangers and misery of sexual ignorance. Even 'religionists' were acknowledging the need for sex education, laws were being liberalised and many countries had set up birth control centres, but 'only six years later, our high hopes have been rudely dashed' by German barbarities. In the 1939 introduction, Haire criticised the switch to pro-natalist policies in totalitarian Russia and Germany and stressed the impact this had on democracies, which were also restricting sexual liberty and imposing censorship but he was naïve to think that Guyon-style 'sexual emancipation' was 'bound to triumph'. However, Guyon's views *have* been influential with more moderate versions of them appearing in the works of Alfred Kinsey, William Masters and Virginia Johnson (Etzioni & Baris 2005, 226). Guyon also influenced Haire, and a review of the 'provocative' 1933 book appeared in *The Journal of Sex Education* (February 1949, 166–67) and Haire published eleven parts of Guyon's *Sex offences in the future penal law*.[16]

Norman Himes had visited Nettleden Lodge in 1937, following directions Haire had thoughtfully sent him with a map and instructions if he was coming by train or car. Himes shot two rolls of film during his visit and sent the negatives to his host. From the tone of Haire's 11 March 1938 letter to Himes it appeared that everything was going extremely well; he could not say when he might return to America

---

16   Extracts of Guyon's work were published in *JSE*, 2(2), October–November 1949, 54–59; 2(3), January 1950, 101–07; 2(4), February–March 1950, 151–57; 2(5), April–May 1950, 194–99; 2(6), June–July 1950, 243–49; 3(1) August–September 1950, 9–16; 3(3) December 1950 January 1951, 123–27; 3(5) April–May 1951, 225–28; 3(6), June–July 1951, 271–74; 4(1), August–September 1951, 32–34; 4(2), October–November 1951, 80–82; 4(3), December 1951–January 1952, 149–52; 4(4), February–March 1952, 149–52; 4(5), April–May 1952, 194–200 and 5(1), September–October 1952, 16–19.

because 'the more successful a doctor becomes, the less easy it is for him to leave his practice for any length of time'. Haire returned the negatives and thanked Himes, explaining that he had made prints but did not enlarge them because shortly after his visit a press photographer had taken some very professional pictures, one of which is shown in figure 10.1. However, all was *not* well, as shown in his 29 January 1938 letter to the Secretary of the BMA offering to help in a national emergency. He gave details of his birth, qualifications, work and previous war service and added:

> As I suffer from (1) diabetes and (2) a somewhat damaged heart following an attack of rheumatic fever in 1932, my resistance to strain and fatigue is limited, and the conditions under which I could do useful work, without a breakdown, are correspondingly restricted. There are, however, many jobs in which I could be useful. I might, for instance, usefully replace some younger or healthier colleague in a hospital post, and, having a considerable experience of anaesthetics in the earlier part of my career, I am still quite a competent anaesthetist. I would be willing to do any job which would not involve a breakdown in my health and thus render me a hindrance instead of a help.

The BMA did not respond, so on 4 September 1939, the day after war was declared, he wrote to the Minister of Health's Medical Department offering his services as an obstetrician or anaesthetist in one of the new small obstetric hospitals in Hemel Hempstead. He also explored the possibility of leaving the country; he usually avoided British winters and, if he could depart for health reasons, it was best done quickly. Overseas travel was denied to British subjects during the war although invalidity was one of the few eligible categories for an exit permit.[17] Haire's doctor Harold Avery supplied a 'medical certificate stating that he had been treating him for a breakdown and that he considered that he should

---

17 The rule governing the granting of wartime exit permits applied to British subjects aged from 16 to 60, who were not allowed to travel abroad unless they were invalids or mothers accompanying young children or wives travelling in company with, or to join, their husbands stationed permanently overseas (Sir J Anderson, UK Hansard, 22 August 1940).

undertake a sea voyage'. Haire's application, now in Security Service files of the National Archives of Australia, was 'strongly supported' by Sir Warren Fisher, Robert Boothby and Haire's solicitor Mr Oswald Cox. Fisher was the Permanent Secretary of the Treasury from 1919 to 1939 and became Britain's first Head of the Civil Service, and Boothby who was a friend, a WLSR lecturer and a distinguished politician who in 1940 became Parliamentary Private Secretary to the Minister of Food and devised the National Milk Scheme.

There is an intriguing coda in two letters sent to Sir Hugh Walpole on 27 and 28 May 1940. Haire explained in the first note to 'My dear Hugh' that he had only just received his exit permit and was 'still not quite sure' whether he would be travelling on a Blue Star ship to Australia or America. If he went to America (where he could not work) he would send Walpole a cheque for $1000 to reimburse him for the money he had lent but if he went to Australia (where he could work) he would not need the money. He asked Walpole to let him know if he owed him 'anything for the cost of cabling etc' and ended with these words: 'The debt of gratitude which I owe you for your immediate readiness to help me I cannot of course repay, but I assure you that I do appreciate it, & shall be for ever grateful. Yours ever, Norman Haire.'

The government had commandeered all merchant shipping and Haire travelled as ship's surgeon on a refrigerated cargo vessel bound for Australia. The second letter, from Haire's solicitor, informed Walpole that 'Doctor Norman Haire left hurriedly for Australia this morning, and just before he left, he asked me to write and let you know. At the same time he asked me to convey to you his sincere thanks for the help you were going to give him, had he gone to the United States of America'. Sadly, Hugh Walpole, whose health like Haire's was undermined by diabetes, over-exerted himself doing voluntary war work and died of a heart attack on 1 June 1941. Haire's companion and contraceptive supplier, Willem van de Hagt, the administrator of the Rotterdam zoo, survived the city's destruction by German bombs on 14 May 1940.

Haire's enemies wrongly claimed he left in 'cowardly haste' but only combatants and the intrepid would make a sea voyage during the war and the speed of his exit was determined by wartime regulations: he had to wait for months before the permit was granted and then had a 24-hour rush to board his allotted ship. Haire was seriously ill, but it was insulin, not the sea voyage, that helped to restore his health, and his Australian homecoming was to provide many other surprises.

11

HAIRE'S HOMECOMING

Haire responded to the hostile rumours that he had fled in terror by sending his solicitor the facts: people who disagreed with him but could not find valid arguments to oppose his views had 'consistently sought to discredit [him] by whispering campaigns of baseless slander', for instance by saying that he had 'left England for fear of bombs'. Actually he had been very ill since 1935 and was forced to work in Harley Street for four half days a week, resting the remainder of the time at his country house and going away to a warmer climate during the winter because his health responded to a more suitable climate. The rumours lacked credibility because it took courage to make such a trip when 200 ships had been sunk in the first year of the war and, in contrast, when British suffragette and birth control advocate Edith How-Martyn died, her obituary notice in *The Eugenics Review* (April 1954, 15–16) mentioned with no comment that she had received her 'long-awaited permit' and travelled to Australia for health reasons in 1940 after the outbreak of the War.

Ethel Mannin probably started the 'loose lips' campaign to sink Haire's reputation, although she herself spent many months in the neutral Republic of Ireland. In 1971 she resumed her spiteful campaign, claiming that in 1940 Haire had 'fled back to Australia, where he was to die in 1952'. He had 'often declared that Germany was his spiritual home' and planned to settle there when he retired but he went to Australia instead 'when it was expected that Germany would invade England during World War II'. She said that those who saw him off said he was 'shaking like a leaf and hysterically declaring that he had "so much to lose", which as a Jew he had' like many others also 'on the Nazi black list' (Mannin 1971, 65).

British authorities did not inform Haire that his travel permit had been approved until the day before the *MV Melbourne Star* left

Birkenhead so he had only 24 hours to pack his luggage, close his house and take the long trip north to the Merseyside port. Because of his hasty departure and the port's remote location, it is unlikely that anyone 'saw him off', witnessed him 'shaking like a leaf' or heard him say anything. Mannin's suggestion that he should go to Germany in 1940 was ludicrous and Haire did not die in Australia. However, Frank Forster seemed oblivious to these facts and recycled Mannin's story that Haire had 'pleaded health reasons, but there were others who thought he was "ratting out"'. Betty Roland (1990, 50) was not malicious but mistaken when she said Haire left after 'a well-aimed bomb' had 'demolished his house in Harley Street' – he left on 28 May 1940, the Blitz started on 7 September and his house was not bombed.

When Haire finally received permission to go, the shipping details were given to British security agents who forwarded the information to their Australian counterparts. The National Archives of Australia has about 40 of these 1940s surveillance memos about Haire. Officials in Australia House sent the first one, marked 'secret', from London on 27 May 1940 to Australia's Prime Minister's Department and sent copies to three other departments, informing them that 'Dr Haire (formerly Zajac) [with 'Zions' inserted on the line above] would be sailing from Britain to Sydney on the SS *Strathallan*' and information they had received from the Director of Britain's Passport and Permit Office 'suggests that Haire is a secret member of the Communist Party[1] and in addition he is President of the Sex Education Society which has close connection with extreme political elements. It was understood that Dr Haire was a Captain in the Australian Medical Corps 1915–1919 and that he remained in England at the termination of the Great War' (NAA. A367/1, C69409).

Australia's security service, which was then called the Investigation Branch of the Attorney General's Department, could not find Haire's military papers or his birth certificate and on 16 July suggested that

---

1 I asked archivists at the People's History Museum/University of Central Lancashire, which holds the Communist Part Party of Great Britain archives, if Norman Haire had been a member and they replied on 25 February 2010: 'There is no record of him joining the Communist Party at this end'.

the Department of the Interior might be able to prevent him landing in Australia because he was 'in ill health and the Australian birth cannot be verified'. The memo was incorrect about the boat in which he travelled and it made another mistake by saying that he had *remained* in England in 1919 because this was the date when he *arrived*. Although in June 1940 the Menzies government, under the *National Security Act*, declared the Communist Party was an illegal organisation, these security officials seemed more worried about Haire's presidency of the Sex Education Society than his politics. Haire's executors burnt the Society's records so there is no list of its 600 members and no way of knowing if they had 'close connection with extreme political elements' but perhaps their wish to uplift humanity was thought to be extreme.

Shortly after Winston Churchill delivered his 'We shall fight on the beaches' speech and Britain was entering the most dangerous phase of the entire war, British and Australian authorities took the extraordinary decision to divert extensive resources to monitor Haire's movements. On 19 July, a confidential cable alerted all Australian states to be on the lookout for Dr Haire who was expected to land in Sydney at the end of July. Security investigators were waiting in Sydney to meet the *Strathallan* at 10.15 pm on 1 August but when it berthed their search of the passenger list and baggage revealed 'no trace of him being on board at any stage of the vessel's voyage.' They did not find him on this former liner which was now a troop-ship because he travelled on the *Melbourne Star*. Army officials in Perth notified their counterparts in Brisbane on 27 July that Haire had disembarked in Fremantle and would continue his journey to Brisbane by an interstate vessel. Brisbane sent the notification by air to the director of the Investigation Branch in Canberra on 31 July but it was too late to call off the Sydney search. The Perth authorities gave this evaluation of his trip from London to Freemantle:

> He had informed the Military Passport Officer that he was on holiday, taken to get away from the turmoil of war, but was evasive as to his purpose of choosing Australia for his trip. Asked if there was conscription of doctors in Australia.

Master of *Melbourne Star* stated no suspicious circumstances were attendant on Haire throughout the voyage . . . said he was keenly interested in the war situation – listened keenly to the news broadcast – appeared depressed at any news unfavourable to Britain. He states he has no grounds for actual suspicion, but has the impression that Haire had to leave England in a hurry. Admits that Haire mixed well with officers, crew and passengers . . . The Chief Steward sent a cable at Durban for transmission on behalf of Haire. The following is a copy:

> (DLT[2]) Haire 127 Harley St., London. Remember files and ask Stephen do same books at college specially entrance lounge and trunk full upstairs tell all arrive Brisbane end July reply Durban if necessary – Norman Haire 19.6.40.

Manners – Ship's Carpenter and a West Australian, states that Haire mixed with the crew a great deal, and spent a lot of time with him (Manners). Haire could speak German, French and a little Italian. Did not on any occasion discuss politics. Appeared to be quite a good fellow and pro-British. Stated that while at Wyndham Dr Haire operated on a lady ashore and 'saved her life' . . . The main topic of Haire's conversation was sex.

A Blue Star Line brochure described the 'luxurious and spacious' accommodation on the *Melbourne Star*'s trip on the 'direct route from Britain via South Africa to Australia.' It was a cargo boat but also offered passengers 'a delightful, restful experience' with 'dainty, commodious, well-planned and decorated' accommodation, 'excellent' cuisine and games, exercise, music and other entertainment. On its 1940 trip Haire was the ship's surgeon, along with ten paying passengers: Donald Woodrow (banking), his wife and their two children; Lillian Pearce (home duties); and Neil Hutchinson (jockey), who had all embarked at Birkenhead. They were joined in Durban, South Africa, by Percy Allsop (banking) and his wife; Marjorie Gordon (actress) and Lucelle Jansen (artist), an 'alien' from Belgium (NAA. K269, 26 July 1940). The Allsops

---

2 'DLT' is an abbreviation for Daily Letter Rate: telegrams were charged one third of the full rate and were delivered on the second morning after the day of filing. It applied to most destinations outside Europe. Perhaps Haire's June 1940 telegram really was a code message.

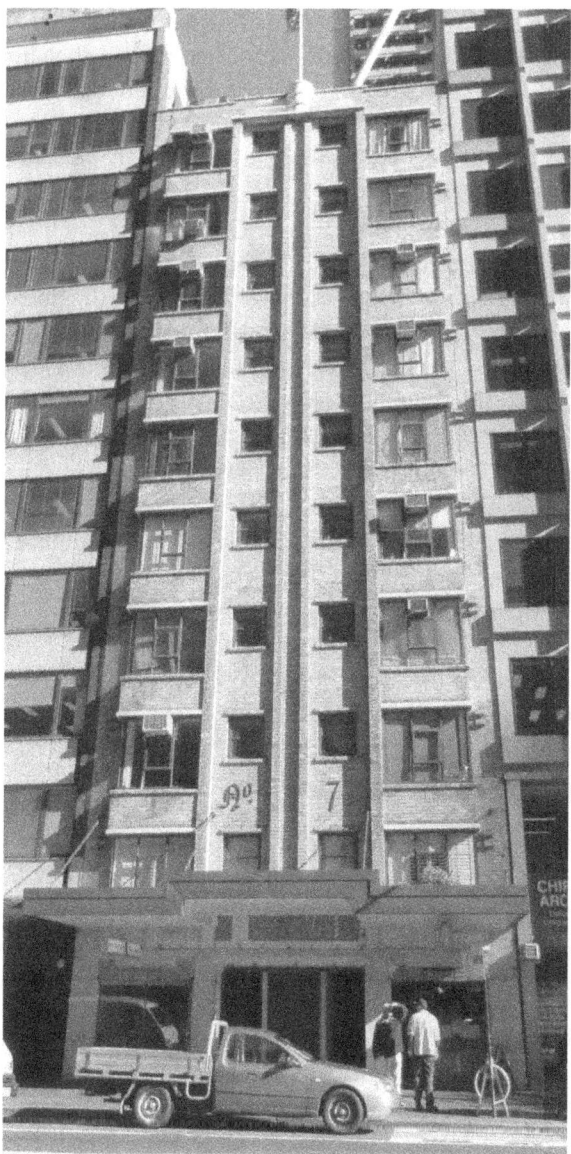

Figure 11.1. 7 Elizabeth Street, where Haire had an Art Deco apartment in 1940.

may have had links with the Burton brewing dynasty and the actress, whose real surname was Kettlewell, got her start in the chorus of the D'Oyly Carte Opera Company. Their names sound like a cast list of the performers in a farce but Haire's conviviality and his recitations around the grand piano would have provided light relief for passengers and crew on their three-month voyage through hostile waters.

In Australia, Investigating Officer Detective Creswell said that the ship's crew believed his 'inquiries of a general nature' were directed at Haire because of his 'decidedly foreign and Jewish appearance' and possibly as a result of the 'inquiries which may have been made at Durban'. Haire had worked as a locum while the ship was in Wyndham and said he was in no hurry to go to the eastern states. After landing in Fremantle, Haire bought a newspaper which reported that Japan might attack Australia; they did bomb Broome and Darwin and within three years the *Strathallan* and *Melbourne Star* were sunk by torpedoes.

Perth's security service reported to their Canberra office on 31 July that Haire was 'residing at the Hotel Esplanade in Perth' until 3 August and would then proceed to Brisbane by train and spend two days in Melbourne. When Haire passed through Adelaide on 7 August, with a ticket from Perth to Brisbane, the security officers in Adelaide said that he did not contact anyone in Adelaide and the train guard told them that Haire was simply on a health trip. The reports were badly written and unintentionally funny, as this example shows:

> The guard approached Dr Haire at the request of police officers who were exercising supervision over him whilst he was changing from the Perth to the Brisbane express, with a view to learning any further details respecting him. The Military authorities have reported his departure from Melbourne to Southern Command, Military Headquarters.

The clandestine police supervision and the subterfuge of making the train guard ask the questions was farcical and the security services kept press articles in their search for news about him but the press were guessing too: *The Argus* reported on 22 August he would spend 'a holiday of some months in Queensland', the *Sydney Morning Herald* announced his Sydney arrival on 25 September and on 5 October *Smith's Weekly* described Haire as 'War's most picturesque gift to Australia to date.'

Detective Creswell claimed Haire looked 'Jewish' and 'decidedly foreign', while *Smith's Weekly* found him 'tall, forceful, rather rakish looking, and originally dressed' and described him as a gynaecologist who was a 'brilliant research worker and thinker' in sociology and sexology. He had returned to his native land and had a flat at no. 7 Elizabeth Street (figure 11.1) and practised in Macquarie Street. Now that he was no longer discussing intellectual issues with Bertrand Russell, AS Neill and Hugh Walpole, Norman Haire might form a similar circle of advanced thinkers in Sydney. He was related to the Jacobsens (intimates of Princess Catherine Radziwill) and the Zions and, after his success in London, 'there should be ample room' for him to practise in Sydney. The article praised Haire although he could not give them an interview because he was 'settling down to practice' in Sydney and had to comply with medical ethics.

Haire's sister Estelle was married to Jack Jacobsen but few would brag about Princess Radziwill, a Russian-born adventuress who had tried to snare the elderly Cecil Rhodes and had been jailed for fraud. However, Haire's 7 Elizabeth Street accommodation *was* special, in a nine-storey Art Deco block of 'luxury flats for moderate incomes' designed in 1940 by Emil Sodersten with interiors by Marion Hall Best who launched her career there with beautifully designed curtains, rugs and furniture. These 'bachelor flats in the heart of Sydney' had phone connections to the manager's office and the Normandy Café where tenants were served by waiters in evening dress. After the restaurant closed, the bohemian tradition continued in the 1950s when Lorenzini's wine bar provided free olives and an outlet for intellectuals and students in a stodgy city.

Haire had returned to Australia expecting to become an invalid or die but his health improved with the help of insulin to control his diabetes. He defied the bad advice his medical specialist had given him not to use insulin and began to inject himself with it, half an hour before each meal, and 'the effect was magical'. He was transformed and soon could 'work hard all the morning', rest after lunch and work again in the late afternoon and several hours each evening. He still had to restrict his diet by avoiding sugary foods and limiting floury and starchy foods but he was no longer hungry and his energy became almost normal again.

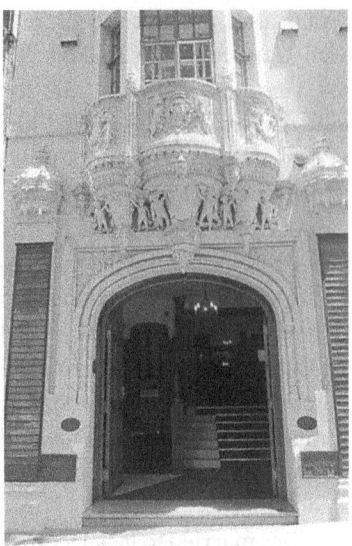

Figure 11.2. Hengrove Hall, 193 Macquarie Street, where Haire worked in the 1940s.

Haire set up his medical practice again in Hengrove Hall, a nine-storey block of professional rooms for doctors and dentists at 193 Macquarie Street. The 1929 building has a splendid view over the Botanical Gardens but it now looks like a crumbling stage set and the interior is a cluttered nest of single-room renters. Elizabeth Riddell (Haire's editor in the 1940s) said Haire's office on the fourth floor was 'dark and poky' and Jan Monson (who was his typist then) agreed in 2006, adding that it had not changed since she was there in the 1940s: Haire had a surgery, a waiting area and a workroom and she remembered him trekking from the surgery with test tubes of urine, down the public hall, past the lift and into the workroom.

His colleague Ernst Gräfenberg had escaped from Germany and asked for Haire's help when he reached New York. Haire was delighted by his escape but explained in June 1941 that he could not help him financially because he was poor and had 'had to begin all over again' in Australia and was not earning enough to cover his expenses: specialist fees were much smaller, his income from England had ceased and all his

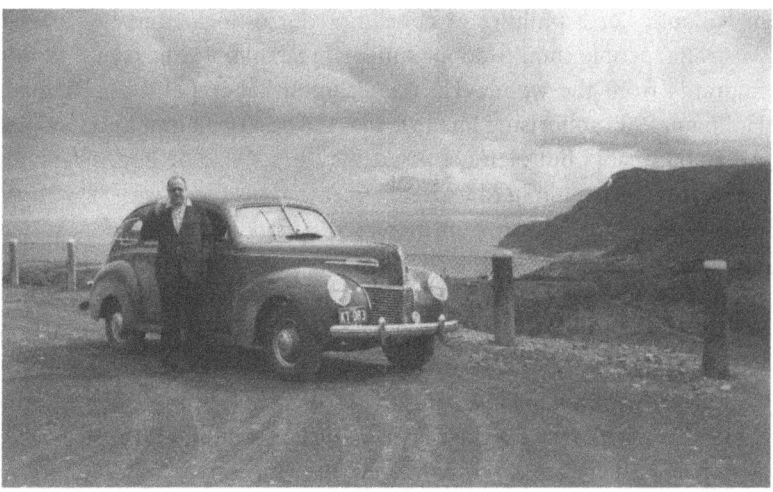

Figure 11.3. 1940s greeting from Norman to his brother Bert.

property there was non-productive, so he was 'poor again.' He suggested Harry Benjamin, who had a practice in New York, might be able to help him.

Haire sent a photograph in the 1940s to his brother Bert with a note 'Love to all and the Season's Greetings from Norman'. The car was American, not his trademark Rolls Royce and he was standing at the Bald Head Lookout at Stanwell Park on the NSW south coast.

In November 1940 Haire wrote to the *Medical Journal of Australia* offering to provide unsigned reviews of items in his field which covered contraception, population problems, sterility, sterilisation, sex education, marriage guidance, sexology and 'fiction, biography, autobiography, or *Belles Lettres* by medical writers'. The Australian War Memorial Archives has Haire's May 1941 article from *The General Practitioner* 'sent with the author's compliments' in which he discussed 'Australia's population problem.' While he thought Europe's birthrate should be reduced, he enthusiastically favoured an increase in Australia. He stressed the risks of abortion, advocated sterility treatment and good prenatal treatment and warned Australia to carefully encourage births 'of the right sort' – just as 'no sensible man' would encourage physically or mentally diseased migrants or 'offer inducements to idiots or imbeciles or epileptics or syphilitics or consumptives to flock from England to Australia', people should 'adopt similar precautions with regard to our migrants from the womb.' He was echoing Labor politician William Holman's 1905 aphorism, 'I believe that the best of all immigrants is the Australian baby', but Haire stressed they must also be eugenically fit. Edith How-Martyn told Margaret Sanger that his paper was 'very good' because, while it favoured an increased Australian population, it had 'trenchantly' pointed out the circumstances in which birth control was needed. Haire wanted How-Martyn to join forces with him because they might 'be able to do something' in spite of the growing preoccupation with the war.

Haire's papers include an unsigned tribute to him when he was 'only 49 years old' and described Dr Haire as an 'outstanding Australian' who would 'leave firm footprints in the uphill path of humanity's progress'; Australians were 'fortunate in having a man of Dr Haire's keenness and experience in their midst' who 'preaches and demands enlightenment'.

Dr D'Arcy Ryan, an anthropology lecturer, told me a less flattering story about Haire in a 1941 Sydney University Dramatic Society (SUDS) play in which Haire did *not* perform; he had a clear recollection of him when May Hollinworth was casting *Julius Caesar* for a SUDS production in the Great Hall at Sydney University – she had Haire down for Brutus which was not the part he wanted:

> In a dramatic but rather high-pitched voice, he proclaimed, 'But Maaaay!' (with a dying fall) 'I just can't FEEL Brutus! But ah! Cassius does speak to me!' May gave him one of her unfathomable looks and murmured, 'Methinks yon Cassius hath a lean and hungry look!' The subject was dropped and so, I think, was Haire.

Despite this, Haire was very 'in' with Hollinworth who directed SUDS from 1929 to 1943 and made it flourish. Margaret Whitlam was a university student from 1938 to 1942 and remembered him as 'a character; a pompous but amusing person who used to hold court at Sydney University Women's Union [Manning House] and it was really something to be asked to join the gathering at his table' and in 1999 she told me she was invited 'once'. Betty Shwabsky told me about another 1940s drama which she heard from Marion Dallison, a drama lecturer at Balmain Teachers' College: Haire once refused to act unless his 'boy friend' was also given a part, but the young man couldn't act and his attempts caused 'gales of laughter', though things had 'eventually worked out'.

In March 1941 Haire played a minor role as 'Dr Stefan Kurtz, another passenger' in Robert Ardrey's *Thunder Rock* at North Sydney's Independent Theatre, and returned in September with a major part as Cauchon, Bishop of Beauvais in Doris (later Dame Doris) Fitton's production of *Saint Joan*. Haire kept the programs listing his recital and theatrical performances but this one is missing, which suggests that the story Betty Roland (1990, 83) told about a cruel joke is true:

> Norman had both the figure and the presence with which to portray the arrogant prince of the church ... He had squandered a whole year's clothing coupons on yards and yards of scarlet silk, which he had made into a robe of suitable proportions. Unfortunately he had antagonised some of the cast by his overbearing manner and they avenged themselves by putting an empty petrol tin on the tail of the splendid garment while he was standing in the wings waiting to make his spectacular first entrance. The banging and clatter that accompanied him totally ruined what should have been an impressive moment and the audience showed its delight with laughter and loud applause. Poor Norman was deeply hurt and threatened to resign but Doris made the culprits beg his pardon, and honour was appeased.

Despite the actors' unprofessional behaviour, Haire played the part of a Hampstead nursing home owner in a new three-act play at the Independent Theatre in February 1942. It was *Lady in danger*, a comedy-thriller with spies, murder and a playwright heroine who was reprimanded by her journalist husband after he'd lost his job: 'I'll earn the salary in this family! You stick to play writing'. This was an in-joke made by Max Afford (1974, 181–82) who became one of the few Australians to earn money from their plays. Haire was so famous that he featured in a poem and as a character in a book, but in another in-joke Afford transformed this tall fastidious man into:

'Dr Gilbert Norton', a plump, pink-faced, genial little man in his mid-fifties who peers through rimless glasses. While he is neatly dressed there is somehow a suggestion of soiled linen underneath. His manner has a kind of professional heartiness that would be frowned on in Harley Street. He pauses and peers short-sightedly around the flat.

Haire moved house to number 10 Ithaca Flats at 4 Ithaca Road, Elizabeth Bay, and Paul Lowin, a homosexual who left money to establish one of Australia's largest prizes for music composition, was another troubled Odysseus who lived there in the 1940s. After fleeing from Vienna to escape the Nazis, Lowin became a mentor to Australian students and musicians at his musical 'at homes' (Skinner 1991, 2007). Haire also gave 'at homes' and Jock Marshall kept one of the invitations. Elizabeth Riddell probably introduced Haire to this 'different, sometimes difficult academic' who was a zoology professor and wrote for *The Telegraph*. Haire wanted 'a few intelligent people' to come for afternoon tea on 18 January 1942 and asked Marshall if he could come, adding, 'If not, a few are coming for a sherry from 5 to 7 on Wednesday January 31'. Marshall was 'very glad' to hear from him but had cellulitis of the jaw and, true to his 'one-arm warrior' reputation, had 'dashed off' a typed note while waiting for an ambulance. He was 'very sorry' to miss both because he would be in hospital but suggested 'a drink together sometime'.

Haire also attended 'at homes' in Mona van Wein's flat at the Wintergarden in Darlinghurst Road, Kings Cross, where she held open house on Tuesday evenings for new comers and regulars such as Betty Roland, Guido Baracchi (a wealthy communist) and Lotte Fink and her husband Friedel (Jewish doctors who had fled from Germany). They discussed art, books, politics and the theatre: wine and intellectual discussions were scarce in wartime Sydney.

Betty said he did not complain about his flat's limitations and cooked simple meals on a gas stove. She once shared a prawn omelette with him (in defiance of Jewish food taboos) and friends would 'invite him to a meal more in keeping with his past' when he would place a syringe and phial of insulin on a white linen cloth so he could gorge himself on foods which diabetics should not eat. He 'smoked like a

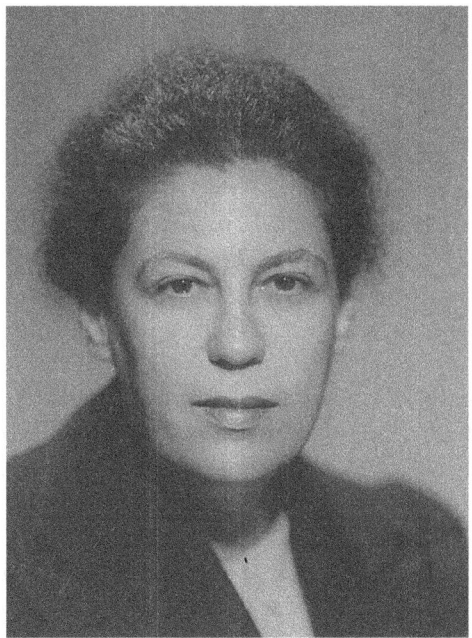

Figure 11.4. Dr Lotte Fink who, with Norman Haire, ran Australia's first sex education classes in 1942. Image reproduced with kind permission from Dr Fink's daughter, Dr Ruth Latukefu.

chimney' and his only ostentation was Vincent who lived with him and drove the Rolls Royce because 'Norman never trusted himself to drive' (Roland 1990, 82–83). After 35 years' practice as a sexologist he had concluded that relatives and friends were the last people to hear of or to suspect homosexual practices. Haire *was* homosexual but it was 'totally taboo', 'never acknowledged' and 'only the inner circle of his friends knew.' Ruth Latukefu (2003) said her mother said that Haire had a flat in Elizabeth Bay in 1940 and lived 'in a homosexual relationship' with his chauffeur, Victor (or Vincent) who also worked as a lift attendant at the David Jones department store.

In 2008 two women told me about their experiences of hearing Haire speak in the 1940s: Una Gault was a psychology student at the University of Sydney when she attended one of his psychology lectures and remembered his uniformed chauffeur in the front row wearing spats; Stefania Siedlecky belonged to a left wing doctors' group who invited him to address them. She said his method of delivering babies pleased her a lot because he sat with them and talked them through their labour if necessary; this was very different to most doctors who left everything to the nurses and rushed in to do the delivery when called. However, his method was expensive and Hesling (1960, 13) said Haire had laughed at complaints about his 100 guinea confinement fee and explained that the only time he had reduced his fee, a few weeks after the delivery the woman had come to show him the baby and she 'was wearing a *fur coat*'.

Haire was worried that the police might raid his flat and gave his lecturing anatomical diagrams to Lotte Fink whose daughter told me that they kept them safe, on top of her wardrobe (Latukefu 2006).

Security was intense during the war and on 2 October 1942 Haire sent a note to 'Chris' – Chris O'Sullivan, a journalist for *Smith's Weekly* who undertook a secret errand for a Russian agent in 1919 and is probably the only person to have organised a successful strike in the Kremlin[3] and perhaps the author who wrote the flattering article on Haire's return to Sydney. Haire told Chris that two military police officers had visited him after receiving an allegation that he was German and his real name was 'Von something or other'. 'Nothing more may come of it' but 'these days' under the National Security Regulations anybody could be arrested and interned for long periods without any reasonable cause and, 'if anything should happen', his secretary had a list of friends Chris should contact immediately. Haire knew he would do anything he could and suggested he could probably 'do something' through 'David in Melbourne' who would be [and here the handwritten addendum is indecipherable]. The note added, 'It is becoming a bit alarming'. His alarm was warranted because the Deputy Director of Security for NSW wrote to his counterpart in Canberra:

---

3   Ruth Latukefu is certain that Haire contacted O'Sullivan. His story was told on ABC radio's *Hindsight* documentary, Vintage Red. Since the CPA was a proscribed organisation from 15 June 1940 to mid-1943, if Haire was a member, he was unlikely to have divulged this to anyone outside the party.

Re Norman Haire: 1. It is not considered that a Restriction Order should be placed. 2. One of the main considerations is the difficulty of fitting Haire's actions into a breach of the Regulations; 3. Certain steps have, however, been taken which should ensure that no great harm to public morale will result from his future actions. [The authorities added a shorthand note to Haire's *Who's Who* entry: 'Any action was a matter for the State and any control would be best if it came from the State'] (NAA Series A. 367/1, Item C69409, 27 November 1942).

Australia's security services were suspicious of Haire's role in the Australian Association of Scientific Workers (AASW). Few people know about this association now which was established in Britain on 19 July 1939[4] and was widely supported by scientists and respected by government because it 'played an important role in Australia in a variety of projects';[5] the AASW Drug Committee pioneered the synthesis of essential drugs[6] and produced an anti-malarial drug which was 'as important as ammunition' in tropical warfare. Despite this, there were strenuous efforts to suppress the AASW and it was dissolved in 1949 (Moran 1986, 13–14, 19). The surveillance dossiers on the AASW[7] include a flyer for the 24 May 1944 celebration to mark its first five years; it was to be held in the University of Sydney's Great Hall, which shows its respectability. It had 12000 members in Britain and 'vigorous associations' in the US, South Africa and Australia where half of the AASW's 1200 members lived in Sydney and came from universities, industry and the public service.

Haire was the Convenor of the Sex and Society Sub-Committee for the AASW (NSW) and wrote in the 1943 annual report that it had

---

4 Turtle (1987, 28) quoting AASW (NSW), Annual report 30 June 1943. It aimed: 'To secure the wider application of science and scientific method for the welfare of society, to promote the interest of science and to maintain the status of the scientific worker'.

5 Johnston (1988, 312, fn 15) refers to a detailed history by Moran (1983).

6 See Fellows of the Australian Academy of Technological Sciences and Engineering, Melbourne (Eds), *Technology in Australia 1788–1988* (2000, 624).

7 Twenty records for the AASW at naa12.naa.gov.au/scripts/Search.asp [Accessed 20 February 2006].

been established in November 1942 and was mainly concerned with the problems of sex education in schools and was represented on several other organisations' committees dealing with this. The Sub-Committee was also preparing a pamphlet on venereal diseases and material for lectures on sex education. However, this pamphlet caused such a stir among members of the State Committee that it was not published. In 1944 Haire reported that his group held formal meetings from July to December of 1943 but not in the second six months when he was ill, although they met informally. They complained to the authorities about the contraceptive ban under National Emergency Regulations, pointing out that this would endanger women who were 'temporarily or permanently unfit to become pregnant' and claimed that partly as a result of their representations it was decided to allow doctors to prescribe contraception for such women. This exchange of letters followed the NSW Health Minister CA Kelly's claim in parliament, as reported in the *Sydney Morning Herald* on 11 December 1942: 'The lack of parental control was largely to blame for the spread of venereal disease'. This was a convenient excuse for doing nothing, which contrasted strongly with an October 1942 Australian Gallup Poll finding that '78% of the population favoured an outspoken press, radio and church campaign against VD' (Darian-Smith 1990, 190).

Haire's long unpublished rebuttal listed many factors causing the spread of VD but he said one of the most important was the difficulty in obtaining 'rubber prophylactics' (condoms) to prevent venereal disease or to prevent pregnancy. The government's wish to divert rubber and manpower from non-essential to essential purposes 'was understandable' but, in this case, 'emotional prejudices' prevented a consideration of all aspects of the problem. For many women, pregnancy and childbirth posed a threat to their health or life and, to prevent this, their doctor prescribed rubber contraceptives but these were almost unobtainable even with a prescription. If these women became pregnant, it might be necessary for her doctor (after consulting a colleague and corroborating the diagnosis) to perform an abortion. 'Every service man or woman, every munitions worker, every civil worker performing work of value to the community, who becomes infected with venereal disease, diminishes national efficiency' and every woman whose pregnancy jeopardises her life or health 'adds to the nation's burden'. He believed that if these considerations were brought to the notice of the Commonwealth and State Ministers (Health, Manpower, Supply and Customs) they would permit sufficient supplies to be manufactured or imported to deal with cases where this was needed for health reasons. 'In deference to a curious local custom' which forbade doctors signing their names on medical subjects in a newspaper, he had signed as 'Medical Sociologist'.

A year later the *Medical Journal of Australia* published an article in which Haire discussed recent pronouncements on venereal diseases and their prevention. Surprisingly he published it under his own name and, even more surprisingly, the *MJA* published his 23 October 1943 article although it was highly critical of their 9 October editorial on this topic. He criticised the National Health and Medical Research Council's suggestion that only health departments or official bodies should issue statements on sex education because they were 'always conservative' on controversial issues such as sex education and VD. He argued that if the BMA issued a publicly supportive statement it was likely to cause violent dissention within its ranks and members with religious convictions might resign *en bloc* in protest. For this reason, 'non-conservative statements' on controversial topics could only be expected from individual doctors or non-official groups who could freely express their opinions. He also criticised the editorial's recommendation that Leslie Weatherhead's 1931 book *The master of sex through psychology and religion* was 'one that medical practitioners can put into the hands of parents and intelligent adults'. While he said much in the book was admirable, he listed its multiple errors, including the idea that women were least likely to conceive in the middle of the menstrual period, a view that Haire said 'was directly opposed by modern medical opinion.' The author had 'no medical knowledge' and the problem with his book appeared to be that 'he was so anxious to consult medical advisers who were sound Christians that he took no trouble to be make certain they were reliable scientists'.

Haire's AASW group lectured on 'Venereal disease' and 'The population problem' to workers at the St Marys Explosives Factory in

Sydney's west. He said it (the lecture not the factory) had been 'sabotaged' by religious opponents so they had had to omit the usual advertising, but despite this both lectures were well attended and followed by lively discussion. They also held sex education lectures in six Sydney suburbs, the first in Chatswood Town Hall despite more 'sabotage' attempts to ban it because the 'room in which the lecture was to be held was not licensed for public lectures.' One of their members was a barrister and they took his advice to hold the lecture and take up a collection instead of charging at the door. They planned to do this at another series of sex education lectures for students and Haire hoped to be able to hold formal meetings more regularly (AASW 1944, folio 23).

Haire combined his work life with acting, writing and lobbying, and Sydney's family planning association, then called the Racial Hygiene Association, privately benefited from his knowledge but would not have him as a member because 'he wasn't very popular' (de Berg 1976). Their motherly mainstay was Lillie Goodisson who said in private 'he's a very naughty boy, but very helpful. I could say more but I won't'. Ethylwyn Dawson Wallace (the widow of Melbourne birth control advocate Dr Victor Wallace) told me this in 1998 and said that Mrs Goodisson was a warm and caring woman who knew when to keep quiet. This is not surprising in a conservative era when slang for sexual intercourse was 'having a naughty'. Australia was a backwater and Haire's advocacy of trial marriage and easy divorce was denounced in the *Canberra Times* on 14 December 1942 by the president of the Australian Council of Churches who saw it as 'spiritual sabotage' and 'a return to paganism' although 'the War was supposed to be a fight to preserve Christian civilisation'.

A few months earlier Haire had complained to his publisher Stanley Unwin that Sydney's four leading booksellers (Angus & Robertson, Dymocks, Swain's and Moore's Bookshop) did not have his book *Birth -control methods* or those in 'The international library of sexology and psychology' series. The publisher's agent had not ordered any and Angus & Robertson had borrowed copies from Haire to sell and replace later. Haire had been in Australia for two years and there was a 'considerable demand' for these books, from patients and as a result of his lectures and articles, but only Moore's Bookshop had them because they ordered stock directly from London. Haire suggested Unwin might urge their Australian agent to 'stir themselves' because in 1945 Angus & Robertson was publishing his little half crown volume, *Sex problems of today*, which would increase their demand, making it even more desirable that the Allen & Unwin books should be obtainable. Unwin reassured Haire that they would reprint 1500 copies of *Birth-control methods* as soon as they could get the paper; book production was painfully slow and their meagre paper ration prevented them from printing a larger run. In December the publisher told Haire that a new edition of the book was waiting on the Dutch docks for the appropriate import licence, that they were frequently 'harrying the unfortunate officials' and bound copies should be available the following February.

Haire's work on a VD pamphlet for the AASW was not wasted; in April 1943 he made a broadcast from radio 2KY's studio in Sydney's Trades Hall on 'The scientific approach to the problem of venereal disease in war-time' and the transcript is signed 'A Medical Sociologist per D Stewart'. Haire stressed that VD had not been prevented because the approach was not scientific, 'only moral and religious', but fortunately these moralists had not yet disapproved of attempts to cure it. 'D Stewart' was David 'Dave' Stewart, an adult education pioneer who established a branch of Britain's Workers' Educational Association (WEA) in Sydney in 1913 and was their general secretary for 41 years. His biographer was EM Higgins, a 'communist intellectual'[8] who in 1957 quoted an Anglican bishop who compared Stewart with Moses and said 'sanity, decency and goodwill' were his norm. Stewart and Haire had diabetes and their resulting mood swings might be linked to the row which caused an impasse over the rights of free speech versus the WEA's need to maintain itself as a non-partisan, non-sectarian, voluntary workers' educational movement (Clanchy 1990).

Higgins said that 'one of the most exhausting wars of attrition went on from 1942 to 1945 over classes on sex'. Dr Haire was wellknown

---

8 Higgins was a publicist and adult educationalist, the brother of the writer Nettie Palmer and nephew of Mr Justice Higgins, whose 1907 judgment established Australian workers' basic wages and conditions.

internationally as a pioneer in the study of sex problems and had offered to take a class for the WEA. A hundred and forty people enrolled but the Unitarian Church, which owned the hall where the class was held, complained about statements made in the lectures and would not allow a second course in the hall. The YWCA also refused to have Haire's classes 'under its roof' and the Railways Commissioner would not display a WEA advertisement which mentioned this course. Officers of the NSW Education Department warned Stewart that the Women's Christian Temperance Union were pressuring them to cut off the WEA's government grant if it sponsored Haire as a lecturer. Haire and several of his supporters on the WEA Council complained that Stewart was not resolute enough in helping to arrange further courses and protested about his insistence on changing the title of one course from 'Sex and society' to 'Sex and the individual'. Stewart was in an embarrassing situation: he did not want to submit to pressure from the objectors but he thought that Haire was needlessly offensive in his lectures and, while prepared to support his lectures on the physiology of sex, he denied his claim to be an authority on sociological questions.

Letters in the University of Sydney's archives from the Department of Tutorial Classes and extracts from the WEA newsletter, *The Australian Highway*, show the seriousness of the spat: it started when Stewart indicated on 1 January 1944 that Dr Haire had been wrong to claim the New Education Fellowship was the first to organise lectures on sex education in Sydney because 'the WEA organised a conference and public lectures on this subject as far back as 1917'. Haire asked for 'authentic details' about these early lectures and rudely commented in March 1944, 'Well, my article on sex education seems to have caused some severe reactions, especially in those who are allergic to sex'. The arguments went on for months and in June Haire commented: 'The WEA Conference was held in 1916 and dealt with "the teaching of sex hygiene". It was excellent as far as it went, but necessarily very incomplete'; the only other sex education classes listed in WEA annual reports were Marion Piddington's Eugenics Circle lectures in 1921 and 1922 and he dismissed these and the WEA's pioneering work as being 'by no means comparable with the NEF's. He then added if, after his 25 years' work on sexual education and sexual sociology, he was not an expert, he wanted to know who was and provided a list of his credentials. Sensibly, Stewart called a stop to the newsletter battle with a footnote: 'This article by Norman Haire closes this correspondence'.

Higgins explained what happened next in this complicated fight: Stewart recommended to the WEA's Central Council that Haire should be asked to get another sponsor for his course but the council disagreed and instructed Stewart to arrange a further class on 'Sex and society'. Stewart solved this impasse by hiring another lecturer and, in retaliation, 'Haire's class elected him as its delegate to the WEA Council'. When this was ruled unconstitutional because he received money as a tutor, he refunded his fees and offered to lecture free. After this, a move to get him co-opted to the council failed, he got himself elected to a newly formed 'cultural club'[9] and, as their delegate, attended every WEA meeting, 'sitting prominently and menacingly in the front row'. Council over-ruled Stewart's objections to having Haire as tutor for the course on 'Sex and society' but Stewart claimed that, by 'a curious oversight on the part of the printer', this class was twice omitted from a general advertisement. There was bickering in the council and executive, with Stewart fighting a losing battle. Council insisted that Haire should lecture on 'Sex and society' and represent the WEA on a deputation to the ABC asking for talks on venereal disease. 'Matters became so tense that minutes were challenged at every meeting and a minute secretary was proposed'.

No hint of this strife was evident to outsiders when the University of Sydney students' magazine *Honi Soit* advertised a series of lectures about venereal diseases. Norman Haire was to introduce the series on ten successive Tuesdays evenings at the Theosophists' Adyar Hall in Bligh Street, Sydney, beginning on 27 July. This course cost ten shillings

---

9   Australian Cultural Society, 86 Darlinghurst Road, Kings Cross. Patron: Rev G Stuart Watts; President: Jack Terry; Vice Presidents: Tony McGillick, Alice Holloway; Secretary: Betty McGillick. It aimed: 1. To encourage and develop culture in Australia; 2. To establish friendly cultural relations with the peoples of all allied countries, particularly with the peoples of the Soviet Union. In 1943 Haire gave ten lectures on sex education for them with a flyer noting that 'only persons over 18 years will be enrolled'.

and was being managed by the WEA. In the weeks before Dr Haire's series, the United Associations of Women would hold six lectures in the Masonic Odd Fellows' Hall with an admission of two shillings; the speakers were well known in Sydney and would include Dr Edna Nelson, the Director of the VD clinic at Rachel Forster Hospital; Rev CL Oliver, from St James Anglican Church; Dr Cooper Booth, the Director of Social Hygiene [VD], NSW Health Department; Haire's colleague, Dr Lotte Fink 'and the grand campaigner again – Dr Norman Haire'.

Haire made several correct but tactless observations about Australia in the 1940s in his book *Sex problems of today*: medical students' training in contraceptive technique was 'either totally absent, or quite inadequate'; there were only two birth control clinics, one of which (probably Piddington's) seemed to be a purely money-making concern; and the 'extortionate cost' of local or imported contraceptives (at ten times British prices) put them beyond the reach of many. Birth control was still seen in Australia as not quite respectable and contraceptives, like 'drinks are at a sly grog shop', sold at fantastically inflated prices. He was similarly direct if the *Canberra Times* on 22 April 1944 quoted him correctly at a lunch when he said, 'staff at homes for delinquent children were quite unqualified and without any skills and the homes were hotbeds of depravity – academies for the teaching of sexual activity'.

Despite the Haire versus WEA quarrel, he lectured at their 1944 forum in Newcastle which the *Newcastle Herald* described on 14 February. Haire had emphasised the importance of sex instruction in efforts to teach people about VD; he found sexual ignorance was astounding in all sections of society and recommended that parents and teachers should attend sex education lectures so they could teach children. He was also one of three speakers at the WEA's September 1944 Public Conference on Freedom in Education[10] with the *Sydney Morning Herald* reporting on 21 September that Higgins introduced Haire as 'a prominent rationalist', 'a noted sexologist, and President of the World League for Sex Reform' – the last description was doubly wrong because

---

10   *Canberra Times* on 25 September 1944. The two others speakers were from the University of Sydney: Dr AH McDonald, reader in ancient history, and John Anderson, the well-known professor of philosophy.

the WLSR had ceased in 1935 and Haire had been a co-president. The *Newcastle Sun* on 25 September quoted Higgins' praise for the speakers and called them 'outspoken critics of conventional complacency' who would steer the public to examine education as a whole. Higgins hoped that 'animated public controversy would continue over some of the views expressed.'

It did cause a reaction but Haire's censure of individuals, institutions and religions was foolhardy and confrontational if he was reported correctly in the *Newcastle Sun* on 23 September. In a marked contrast to his former careful stance about religious tolerance, he attacked 'the churches [as being] the main obstacle to freedom in education.' He told conference delegates 'If they had the chance, the churches would tyrannise over us just as much as any German or Italian dictatorship'. He argued that changes in education were opposed by the churches who 'had a vested interested in keeping people stupid and deluded in superstitious subjugation to the irrational dogmas of organised religion'. They particularly opposed anything to do with sex because they knew that sexual activity 'was the one activity in which the ordinary individual was sure to indulge at some time or other'. Haire supposed that he had been so savagely attacked, particularly by the Catholic Church, but also by the fundamentalist Anglicans and certain nonconformist groups, because he was 'the only person who had talked freely on this subject in public and who had not allowed himself to be bluffed into silence'. He complained that we taught the child to believe everything in the Bible, and told children lies about human reproduction. Sooner or later the child discovered we had lied to it and a mental conflict was set up. We taught the child almost nothing about its own body and the way to keep the body working efficiently and he said this 'rendered most people physically and mentally defective.' This belligerence may have been the result of Haire's declining health and the harassment he had experienced not just because of the WEA talks, but also in response to his articles in *Woman*, and the attacks he esperienced in parliament, described in the next two chapters. Others saw his benevolent side and even his 'populate or perish' critics would have been astonished to know that he helped infertile couples to have children; Haire was the

'Sydney Doctor' whose articles in *The Daily Telegraph* in November and December 1944 proposed establishing clinics 'in every city and large town in the Commonwealth so that every sterile couple may be within reach of investigation and treatment'.

In November 1944 Haire acted in a SUDS production of George Bernard Shaw's *The doctor's dilemma* at their club rooms in 700 George Street, Sydney. Haire was a method actor, insisting that he *was* Sir Ralph Bloomfield-Bonnington, and Hesling (1960, 12) said he was 'a very fine actor indeed; quite world standard'. Edith Cardus was the newly appointed SUDS producer when Haire starred as Sir Ralph, and the anonymous reviewer in the university's *Union Recorder* (1944) praised its high standard of theatrical achievement but noted that the cast was thrown out of balance by the almost incongruous difference in age (and size) between Haire and the other actors. The reviewer said, 'Norman Haire's acting as Bloomfield Bonnington, that blustering, pseudoscientific fool, is very close to brilliant' and 'his confident and able presence on the stage, as well as his expert delivery and experienced by-play, mark him as outstanding'. Haire slightly marred his performance by overacting occasionally which was 'entirely unnecessary, for B-B is sufficiently amusing as Shaw makes him, without requiring obvious exaggerations'. Haire sometimes displayed the same tendency offstage and the intensity of his fervour could be disconcerting but his passion, directness and honesty were also strengths which many people found endearing.

The *Sydney Morning Herald* noted discreetly on 25 April 1945 that Haire had withdrawn from his much-acclaimed role as Sir Ralph Bonnington-Bloomfield at the independent Theatre. The lawsuit against Haire on a concocted assault charge is the likely reason for his withdrawal and it is discussed in the next chapter, but the main focus is on his achievement as a columnist in *Woman* when, despite wartime censorship, he produced what Peter Coleman called 'probably the most free-thinking series of articles ever written for a mass circulation magazine'.

12

DR WYKEHAM TERRISS WRITES FOR *WOMAN*

In 1941 a Sydney newspaper proprietor made the brave but lucrative decision to start a sex advice column in the magazine *Woman*. Norman Haire was to write it under the pseudonym Dr Wykeham Terriss – a play on Wickam Terrace, Brisbane's equivalent of Harley Street or Macquarie Street. Elizabeth Riddell was the editor then and when I met her in May 1998, she was a lively 91 remembering Haire with affection, and said they were 'honest with each other and got along well'. She died a few months later and is now revered as a poet, author and journalist; she also deserves credit for recognising Haire's talent and standing by him.

Haire planned to call the series 'A Doctor looks at life' because a doctor did this each day when he met fresh people and learnt about their bodies and minds. He told Riddell this was the most fascinating aspect of his work and said his view of life was not the same as others' because the books, people's faces and newspaper editorials had 'different and deeper nuances' for him. He said for him and other doctors with a special inquiring temperament, medicine offered the greatest opportunities for intimate glimpses of human psychology. He would determine the page's content and might discuss a play, a book, or some current topic such as maternal mortality, the falling birthrate, or suicide. Next month, unless something of greater interest turned up, he would write about 'Illness as a weapon' (*Through a doctor's spectacles* HC – 2.09).

She thanked him on 21 March 1941 and said the magazine owners wanted to discuss prudery but 'had hesitated to do so without an authoritative voice'. They wanted him to discuss sex education and the dangers of venereal disease but first they needed to gain support from leading public health doctors, university department heads, professors and feminists. If it was forthcoming, they would start with this article and then consider other topics (HC – 2.17).

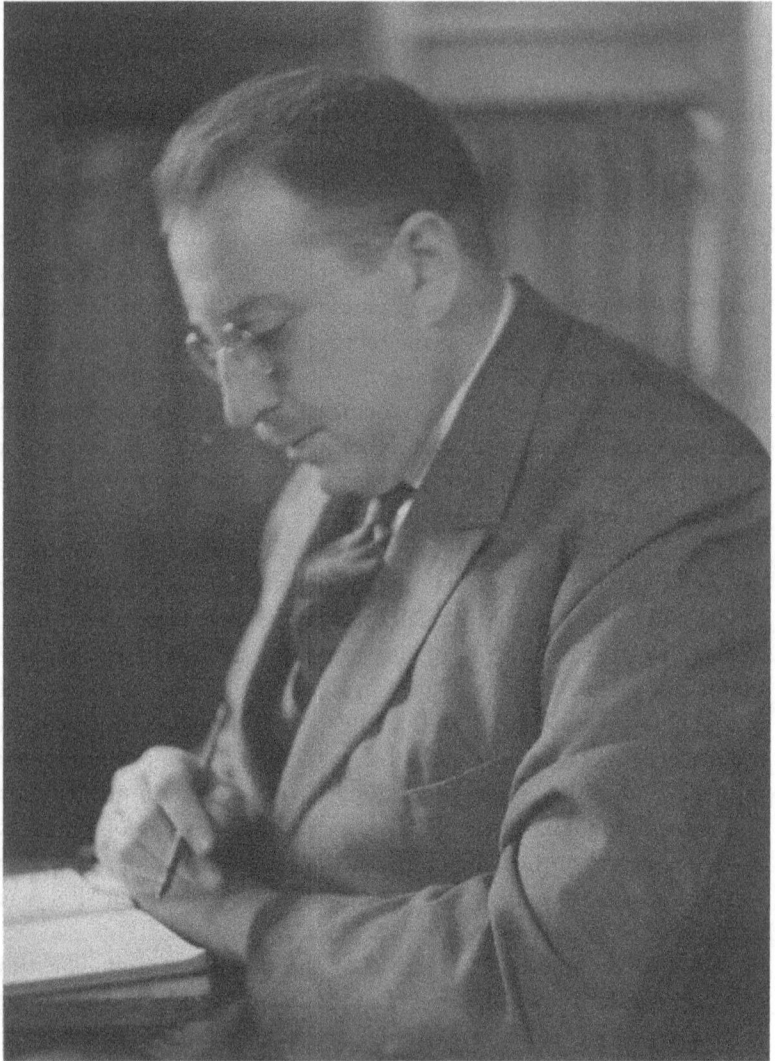

Figure 12.1. Publicity photograph of Haire, the doctor who looked at life.

Unfortunately, Haire's first article has not been retained[1] and even its date is unknown, but the readers' appreciative responses must have surprised the publishers because, when Riddell introduced the second article on 19 May, she provided an author profile, something a magazine would usually do when introducing the writer's first article. The 'hundreds of letters' praising the recent article 'What shall we do about this grave problem?' (VD) had prompted them to publish this 'stirring challenge to parents': 'What have you taught your children about the vital facts of life?' She described the author as a 'distinguished Harley-street specialist' who had recently returned to Australia and was using the pen name Wykeham Terriss. His work was well known in England, the United States, and Europe, where he had lectured to medical societies and universities; his writing had been translated into several foreign languages and his 'achievements occupy a full column in *Who's Who*'.

Haire also received fierce criticism and, while the first anonymous abusive letter distressed him, he gradually learnt not to worry and to ignore them. However, it was impossible to ignore the furious criticism that greeted his *Sex problems of today*, an inexpensive paperback for 'the intelligent reader without medical knowledge'. His aim was to provide a sex education book for workers, and this right to publish was a civil liberties issue that had already been won – in 1888 – in a landmark case when Justice WC Windeyer said in a Supreme Court of NSW judgement that Annie Besant's birth control literature was not obscene because: 'Information cannot be pure, chaste and legal in morocco [leather] at a guinea, but impure, obscene and indictable in a paper pamphlet at sixpence.' Windeyer also rejected the view that birth control was immoral, or that a book was obscene if it fell into the hands of the immature or the uneducated (Coleman 1962, 72–73).

---

1 The four Australian libraries listed as holding 1941 issues of *Woman* could not find this issue in 2003: Librarians at ACP Publishing Pty Ltd (formerly Australian Consolidated Press that published *Woman*) said the issue was missing and it could not be found in the State Library of NSW, the Northern Regional Library, Moree, or the Australian War Memorial. Haire wrote in *Sex talks* (1946, 105): 'About a year ago, in the first article I wrote for this publication, I pointed out the dangers of sexual ignorance, especially in wartime', and a footnote indicated it was 'not included in this volume'.

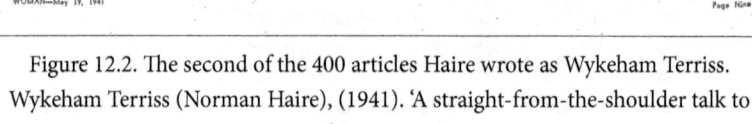

Figure 12.2. The second of the 400 articles Haire wrote as Wykeham Terriss. Wykeham Terriss (Norman Haire), (1941). 'A straight-from-the-shoulder talk to parents', *Woman*, 19 May.

It is extremely unlikely that his opponents knew about this famous judgement but it would not have stopped their abuse which culminated in this (unintentionally funny) telegram of complaint sent on 8 October 1942, a week after Haire was interrogated by security service officers:

ATHUR CALWELL
PARLIAMENT HOUSE CANBERRA
SEX PROBLEMS OF TODAY BY NORMAN HAIRE STOP ANGUS AND ROBERTSON PUBLISHERS STOP PRICE 2/6 STOP ROTTEN STOP CAN HOLLOWAY STOP IT STOP COPY FOLLOWING - - - BOHUN

This old-fashioned telegram, using STOP as a word to save having to pay extra for punctuation, was sent by Catholic Chemists' Guild member GR Bohun to Arthur Calwell, the Minister for Immigration, and it mentions Jack Holloway, the Minister for Health.

Riddell believed that the magazine hired Haire to boost circulation, although she was aware of the dangers – when the Catholic Church found out, they would forbid their congregation to buy the magazine. Once he invited her to morning tea in his Macquarie Street rooms and she had a vivid picture of another young man being there – she paused – 'I believe the expression is "he dropped his dacks"'. The stranger's action did not bother her, nor did phone calls from Haire's opponents and her response to warnings that the magazine had been proscribed from the pulpit was: 'That's good, it'll stir things up'. She said they paid him very little – 'he didn't want money, he wanted his voice to be heard'. She always felt that 'he worked for peanuts' and said he paid for the publication of *Sex talks,* one of three books compiled from his talks.[2]

While Frank Forster claimed the articles provided Haire a 'steady source of income', it was a really only a pittance, although they did allow his views to be heard. Haire claimed to have loyally turned down more lucrative offers from other papers but this was an exaggeration because, when he approached Macquarie Network and asked for a

---

2 *Sex problems of to-day* (1945) and *Sex talks* by Dr Wykeham Terriss (1946) used a pseudonym and *Everyday sex problems* (1948) was published under his own name.

similar platform on radio 2GB, they refused. Haire was paid £10.10.0 per article but said that he *lost* money – it reduced the time available for his medical practice which, in the second half of 1942, increased so much that he had had to rent a second suite and hire a second typist; his secretary sent out this form letter to readers who asked him for free advice:

> Mr Norman Haire instructs me to inform you he would have no time or energy left to earn his livelihood if he were to attempt to answer the many thousands of letters which he receives [often without a stamped reply envelope, about matters which could not be discussed satisfactorily by mail]. If you wish to consult Mr Haire, will you please telephone and fix a time. His fee is five guineas, payable at the time of consultation.

In February 1942 Haire wrote to correct 'a mis-statement' by a Sydney member of the medical association (then called the British Medical Association, NSW Branch) who said in a public meeting that the BMA did not allow its members to lecture to the public on VD and sex problems. Not surprisingly, they responded by saying that he should not use his name when addressing a public meeting. In his next letter Haire pointed out that the 'parent body of the BMA' imposed no such restrictions in Britain; that he had been a member for 20 years and had always lectured and written under his own name. The BMA (NSW Branch) then admonished him for allowing his name to appear in an advertisement for VD and sex education lectures. Haire argued that he had not breached medical ethics because he was dealing with issues such as genital cleanliness which was 'no more a medical matter than is washing the neck or ears.' This prompted a sterner reprimand from the BMA: he had contravened the Medical Ethic Committee's By-Laws, he should have sought its permission to give a lecture and it was for the Committee, not individuals, to decide whether a subject was 'medical or otherwise.'

Haire's neck washing analogy was typical of his direct approach and his comments were renowned for their succinctness. However, he should have tried not to alienate this key professional body and used more tact. For instance, after he received an 'almost unreadable letter', he unwisely told the woman who sent it that he had only one 'pair of eyes' which had to last till he died and that her writing had 'worn them out very much.' She complained and Riddell reminded him that *Woman* could not be associated with letters that were 'offensive' or 'insulting' to readers. Haire was very apologetic and said that it had taught him the difference between the written and spoken word – he dictated all his letters and it was meant to be 'jocular.' He told Riddell that the woman's writing had been 'really very difficult to read' – diabetes had probably damaged his eyes – and he promised to be more careful in future.

Later he had fewer restraints when he reviewed books in his own journal. He read about '15 or 16' a month and some were 'very good, some moderately good, and some very bad indeed'. He quoted an extract from one of the worst books he had ever read: 'Evolution produces fleas and lice to make the laziest of men to scratch their bodies.' The book was *Mystery of birth* by Josiah Olfield, a medical graduate who had also studied theology and spoke of 'pre-earth life' and 'post-earth life'. Haire quoted extracts of the muddled prose which was 'as clear as mud' to him and, on consulting *Who's Who*, found that 'while at Oxford he adopted the Fruitarian diet, and has since then strenuously advocated its adoption by the higher classes'. Haire wondered, 'Can it be the effect of the Fruitarian diet?' and called the book 'tosh, rot, rubbish and balderdash' (*JSE* August–September 1949, 46–47).

It was one thing to defy specific Catholic criticism but *Woman* could not afford to lose readers in a generalised attack on religion, so they refused to print an article Haire called 'Gloomy Sunday' and gave him the weak excuse that 'it would no longer be topical by the time it appeared in print.' Haire objected on 26 June 1942 but Riddell stayed firm and said their position about 'outspokenness' in his articles stayed the same. However, the main problem was the title which came from the 'suicide song' made famous by Billie Holiday in 1941.[3] *Woman* relented and the article appeared with a new title, 'Boredom a sexual danger'.

---

3 'Gloomy Sunday' was a Hungarian dirge composed by Rezso Seress in 1933 to a poem by Laszlo Javor in which the singer mourns the untimely death of a lover and contemplates suicide. Thomas Keneally (1982, 236) described it as 'a syrupy love ballad' which enjoyed notoriety in the 1930s and appealed to 'SS men at their leisure'. The song was banned by the BBC.

Even so, it was a brave decision because Haire was defying community norms by linking the increase in VD and pre-marital pregnancy with the closure of shops, libraries and places of entertainment on the 'day of rest' – he claimed even the trams stopped in the hours when church services were held and there was nothing to do apart from going to the beach or a park. He believed that much of the drunkenness and delinquency would disappear if Australia followed the example of Holland, a 'country of very pious churchgoers', where restaurants, cafes, theatres, cinemas and even shops were open on the Sabbath (*Woman*, 30 November 1942, 8).

His articles provided many teenagers with their *only* source of sex and health education and they frequently began with a chatty anecdote; for instance, he complained about big, boring meals on a boat trip to Europe as though it was a problem he was sharing with these stay-at-homes. The story was an entrée for his discussion about the importance of healthy diets with salads and fruit three times a day. Another time he warned readers not to fry food in fat and said that a notice should be placed in every kitchen: 'The frying pan is deadlier than the sword', and he advised readers to cook steaks quickly on a very hot griller to preserve their food value. Food had huge significance for him and he was touchingly honest; in response to a question about a weight-loss pill, he replied that no such thing existed although he wished it did 'for, alas, I, myself, am considerably overweight' and he acknowledged that the only cure was to 'eat less, eat sensibly and take more exercise'.

In November 1942 Riddell went to work for Ezra Norton's Truth & Sportsman Ltd, first in New York and then in London, on assignment for their newly launched Sydney newspaper, the *Daily Mirror*. Norton's dubious business dealings are discussed in the next chapter. However, he did help Riddell. As a New Zealand schoolgirl she had been 'flung into journalism' after Norton hired her to work for his Sydney newspaper.

Haire continued his friendly relationship with the new editor, Guy Natusch, a former parliamentary reporter from New Zealand. Support for his column came from rationalists and from Dr EH Burgmann, the Anglican Bishop of Goulburn, who wrote to *Woman* on 15 March 1943 to praise the 'good work' they had done by publishing the articles. He said 'all disease must be fought by knowledge' and venereal disease was no exception and had to be stamped out. He hoped they would not be diverted 'by those who are blind to the urgency of this great social problem'. He meant those people who cited Scripture and maintained that virginity before marriage and lifelong fidelity was the only way to eliminate this 'Social Evil' and also that the 'pure' would be saved but the 'sinners' who flaunted 'God's rule' would 'Reap the Wages of Sin' and deserved to die; an attitude which this limerick lampoons:

> There was a young lady so wild
> Who kept herself pure, undefiled,
> By thinking of Jesus,
> Venereal diseases,
> And the danger of having a child.

Unfortunately, the vital role condoms played in those 1940s anti-VD campaigns led to a perception problem – some couples would not use condoms as contraception because they associated their use with venereal disease protection and brothels.

The man who had sent Arthur Calwell the telegram, GR Bohun, 'a fanatical member of Catholic Action', attended Haire's 8 pm sex education lectures half an hour late (after shutting his suburban chemist shop) and then circulated his hostile, abridged reports to politicians. Other opponents included the League of Catholic Women and the Women's Christian Temperance Union, which fulminated against Haire in a newspaper called *The Propellor* in suburban Hurstville. Florence Kenna, the union's Superintendent of Moral Education, complained to the Prime Minister on 8 February 1944 that: 'Haire's renewal of propaganda for birth control and the use of contraceptives' in *Woman* the previous August was a blow to the good which had been achieved when the National Security regulations prohibited publicity for birth control. The union sent an urgent request 'that more rubber shall not be granted for the purpose above mentioned but only for essentials such as hot water bottles, eye droppers and rectal enema syringes'. In December 1942 *The Rationalist* had lampooned a similar tirade:

> Mrs Florence Kenna becomes hysterical at the thought that scientific knowledge should be given to the people; of Dr Haire's lectures, she says: 'Technical lectures, just full of filth. I investigated these lectures for 12 months. And what a job it was. Science he calls it. Bestiality, I say. If we are going to have these scientific talks of sex it's just reverting to the Dark Ages. I know what will result – anarchy, chaos, and a great cataclysm brought about by Providence. And about time too, with all this abominable stuff going around. We wrote to Mr Lazzarini, Home Security Minister, too ... There's no home security with men like Dr Haire around. I'm not resting with sending letters to Ministers about Dr Haire. I'm seeking fresh data about him.

In response to questions in parliament about Haire's sex education classes and whether it should be taught in state schools, the Minister for Education, Dr HV Evatt, said: 'the best place for children to obtain sex education was at their mother's knee'. However, Evatt gave a measured response in the *Canberra Times* on 19 May 1943 when he said that Haire had nothing to do with the Department of Education and 'this was still a free country in which he presumed Dr Haire or any other person could give lectures on any subject'. Few politicians were so liberal.

A Catholic Archbishop found the idea of 'sex instruction in schools abominable'[4] and Calwell made a revealing slip in a 20 September 1943 confidential letter to Holloway; he meant to say there were standards governing food purity and there should also be standards of public propriety but instead he called for 'standards of *priority* in public lectures'. He wanted Holloway to ask Evatt to strengthen the National Security Regulation and to include 'adequate provision in the Commonwealth Powers Bill, because this is a matter of far-reaching importance.'

The devoutly Catholic Calwell was incensed to find that the Darlinghurst Branch of the Australian Labor Party had sponsored Haire's King's Cross lecture and he concluded, as this was 'inimical to the Labor Party's interests', that they must have done so in ignorance of Haire's reputation. Calwell included extracts from Haire's 'deplorable'

---

4 Dr Bevotich, the Catholic Archbishop of Adelaide said this in response to a statement by the Secretary of the International Women's Committee (*Canberra Times*, 8 April 1943).

'Sex and the juvenile community'[5] article in his letter to Holloway and denounced the *laissez faire* attitude of responsible Ministers in the NSW Government, to Haire's 'notorious lectures'. Calwell offered to supply him with statements that Dr Cumpston, the Director-General of Health, had made *in camera* to the Broadcasting Committee.

Holloway forwarded Calwell's complaints to James Fraser, the Minister for Social Services and Health, on 27 September, with Bohun's 'anonymous report' about Haire's 'Morals in war time' lecture on 11 April 1943 which was free, 'open to both sexes' and presented on a Sunday night in King's Cross. The lecture's tone was 'vulgar' and included statements such as '99% of people are unchaste and the other 1% are liars'; Haire called a critic 'Fornication Flo'; criticised the federal government's decision to restrict the manufacture of 'French letters' and claimed he had received assurance from the 'Controller of Rubber' that there was enough rubber to 'fill every doctor's prescription.' Holloway added a cover note: 'I think he exploits the sex problem in a loose and dangerous way for the money he makes out of the practice. However, I could not stop him, because Dr Evatt says this is a state matter and one for the State Attorney-General to handle. You may feel like asking Dr Evatt what he thinks. Dr Cumpston knows this man and can tell you what he thinks of him' (NAA. A472/1, Item W1613, 1943).

On 16 June 1943 the *Canberra Times* reported that state health ministers had considered the National Health and Medical Research Council's recommendations for prevention and treatment of VD including social measures such as restricting the sale of alcohol to young girls. Health Minister Holloway presided over the conference and the *Canberra Times* reported on 10 April that he had previously defied the 'prudes and sadists' by saying 'it was the Government's job to help build a healthy community' and 'it seemed to be anything but in accord with Christian teaching to deny knowledge and enlightenment.'

Haire's effort to provide such enlightenment was anathema to Senator Fraser who told Dr Evatt on 18 October that he believed Haire's comments about condoms would undermine the wartime National

---

5 The lecture was published in *New Horizons in Education*, April 1943. A transcript is in NAA. A472/1, Item W1613, Dr Norman Haire, 1940-44.

Security (Venereal Diseases and Contraceptives) Regulations, which had been proclaimed in September 1942 – they remained in force until the end of 1946. Fraser sought a meeting with Evatt and Cumpston to find out ways to stop Haire 'delivering such lectures'. Although it had been decided on 27 November 1942 that a Restriction Order should *not* be placed on him, the Director of Security applied to the Deputy Director General of Security in Sydney on 30 October 1943 to place an order on Haire because he was 'lecturing on matter which may have a very deleterious effect on public morale' (NAA. A472/1, W1613).

The surveillance continued and Haire informed his solicitor about a 'whispering campaign' to silence him. He deplored the 'heresy hunt' for 'anybody advocating control of fertility' and in *Birth-control methods* (1945, 15) he lent support to Jessie Street who was pilloried for representing Australia at the May 1945 United Women's Conference in San Francisco. Haire also faced religious opposition from Father Peter Ryan and Father Leslie Rumble (who ran *Question box* on the Catholic radio station 2SM) and 'a few rabid Anglicans'.

In 1943, when he had joined the expert panel (as Wykeham Terriss) in the ABC program *The army wants to know*, these opponents made the ABC 'politely' drop him after five sessions. One of the panel members was John Passmore, an eminent philosopher who, in his 1997 memoirs, called this his 'strangest experience of all' and 'the biggest fraud'. Others on the panel were the war historian CEW (Charles) Bean, war correspondent Chester Wilmot (which posed special censorship problems), pianist Lindley Evans, composer Frank Hutchens, philosophy professor Alan Stout who also wrote about cinema, and law professor Julius Stone, with the popular broadcaster Wilfred Thomas as the chair. The ABC invented the names of the soldier-questioners *and* the answers: Passmore (1997, 199–200) did not know how the ABC 'got away with this'. He provided me with a postscript in 1999: while he was writing his memoir he went to the State Library of NSW to examine the broadcasts and found no reference to the ABC program. He said the story about Haire 'is very plausible. But whether it is true I do not know although if it was known to our group they would certainly have made a fuss about it, even if in war-time it was not always easy to create a fuss'. Perhaps regretting their 1943 timidity in removing Haire from their panel of experts, in 1944 the ABC defied their critics and asked him to lead an important debate on population which is considered in the next chapter.

Following this debate, politicians denounced him in parliament and behind the scenes their sabotage attempts segued into a dramatic court case on 22 March 1945. The *Sydney Morning Herald* reported on 4 April that Haire had been charged with assaulting a patient with her 'red handbag', the inference being that only a 'fast' woman would choose red in defiance of drab wartime fashion norms. Haire believed the charge was 'ridiculous' and told the maverick minister Stuart Watts[6] that, although he had a clear conscience and expected to win, it was very unpleasant and worrying.

Prestigious lawyers represented both parties: Shand KC appeared for the patient, Olga McKenzie and Dovey KC defended Haire. Wilfred Dovey had a 'fine presence', 'a rich voice' and a 'Shakespearian vocabulary'. He was a successful but 'irascible' lawyer whose career was marred by public criticism (Broun 1996) and he was Margaret Whitlam's father. In contrast, John Shand 'had a thin-piped voice' and an insinuating manner 'which could annoy and bring a witness into antagonism'; he was 'an expert on laws of libel and contempt', reputedly Sydney's most successful criminal barrister and later secured the acquittal of Shirley Beiger, a model who had shot her lover dead outside Sydney's Chequers Restaurant (Slee 2000).

Mrs McKenzie told the court that she did not keep her first appointment with Haire on 19 March and that on her next visit, while they discussed payment for her missed appointment, he 'grabbed her handbag and twisted her arm'. Haire said she became angry and assaulted him with her handbag which he grabbed thinking she was

---

6 Haire to Watts, 24 April 1943 (HC – 3.06). The Rev Watts was ostracised for claiming some members of the Anglican Church synod had 'a dark ages mentality'. The *Canberra Times* (4 November 1942, 3) quoted Haire's declaration at an Arts Club luncheon, 'It was a shame that public-minded citizens, like Rev Watts, should suffer in this way.'

going to hit him in the face and break his glasses. She said she had 'interviewed' Dr John Hunter, Secretary of the BMA, and then went to the police. On 20 April the *Sydney Morning Herald* pointed out that Mrs McKenzie was entitled to have the case heard in closed court 'but after consulting Mr Shand KC declined to exercise this right.' This gave *Truth* the opportunity it wanted. The managing director of this scandal sheet was Ezra Norton, who employed a bodyguard (Griffen-Foley 1999, 81) and had a 1920s reputation as a 'raucously ranting journalist' and 'blackmailer who survived prosecution after prosecution' (Lindsay 1960, 63).

Haire gave a list of his opponents to his lawyers but, amazingly, he did not believe the woman's charges were part of a 'premeditated plot' but said that, once his enemies and *Truth* found out, 'they decided to exploit it, and encouraged her to make the most of it'. Conspiracy seems *very* likely with Norton a willing conspirator: he despised homosexuals and loathed Freemasons (Knightley 1997, 41; Lawson 2000) and Haire belonged to Sydney's Masonic Club which doubled Norton's reasons for disliking him. Norton may have been paid by anti-Haire forces to ensure that a charge was laid and made even more money by selling the story.

Haire mentioned 'other forces in the background' who were trying to use the charge as an opportunity to discredit him but he was naïve not to suspect that Mrs McKenzie was the decoy in a well-planned plot. The 'assault' took place in private so there was only her word against his; she sought maximum publicity by having an open trial; although there was no serious injury – the detective who examined her arm noticed only 'a bruise above the wrist' – the case was heard with unprecedented speed; she was represented by a top-rank criminal lawyer who would not normally have accepted such a trivial case; she gave an address in a sleazy area near Central Station[7], and was a probably a paid *agent provocateur*.

Dovey asked if she issued the summons to expose Haire and asked how she could afford to be represented in court by King's Council if she could not pay Haire's fee because her 'husband was only a working

---

7   McKenzie's perhaps false address was Flat 5, 142 Liverpool Street, Sydney.

man'. She replied unconvincingly that her husband 'did not care if it cost every penny he ever earned so long as this man was reprimanded'. Dovey asked Haire if he was Wykeham Terriss –a strange and damaging question to ask his client. Haire replied, 'Yes – I am sorry that came out', and this interchange, which emphasised his unmasking as Wykeham Terriss, was the angle the *Truth*'s Brisbane edition on 29 April and their Sydney edition both stressed. Clearly Norton considered the case was sufficiently important to have two reporters covering it, one of them from interstate. Haire was fined £5 plus costs of £7.18.00 because the stipendiary magistrate was satisfied that Dr Haire had lost his temper and grabbed Mrs McKenzie by the arm: 'That is an assault' he said. This minimal fine was not the issue – it was the same cost Haire received for a consultation – but his opponents had achieved their objective which was to discredit Haire.

The day after the trial, Haire made an inglorious exit from the stage after a scathing review of a 1911 'pot boiler' that he had produced: George Bernard Shaw's play, *Fanny's first play*. It was 'taken from the mothballs' for the debut performance of the Student's Dramatic Society of the WEA and presented in 2KY's *Radiotorium*. Embarrassingly for Haire who had had a long association with the radio station, the Workers' Educational Association and May Hollinworth, she lampooned it (using her initials MJH) in the WEA's magazine *The Australian Highway* on 1 June. She hoped the next play would be 'chosen for its literary and entertainment value and not for the "message" it contains'. Ironically for Haire, the play was a spoof of propriety in which two of the young characters became joyfully liberated after going to jail for assault.

Woman remained supportive and he continued with the articles. He even wrote about abortion and said he had received 1000 abortion requests from Australian women between 1940 and 1946. When some of the readers accused him of being an abortionist, he wrote on 6 August 1945 that he had 'learned to ignore such scurrilous abuse' although he worried others might be bored by his frequent warnings. He was taking a particularly brave stance when Australian newspapers refused to print the word 'abortion' and substituted prudish euphemisms such 'an illegal operation' or 'bringing on the periods.' However, Gideon Haigh (2008, 11) was exaggerating to claim: 'For much of Australia's history it has been easier to obtain an abortion than to use the word in print'.

That December he praised the president of the New Education Fellowship (Beatrice Ensor[8]) 'the headmistress of a large public school', for her strong support of sex education broadcasts. But he was sarcastic about the Deputy Director of Public Health in NSW who was in favour of such teaching while saying it 'should not be done by the snivelling maniacs who like talking about sex'. Haire did not know that anybody had ever suggested that 'maniacs, snivelling or otherwise' should do this, although he thought it would be good if the various state Ministers for Education sent properly qualified educationists to Europe and America to study what was being done in sex education in '*civilised* countries'.

After the humiliating court case, Haire may have wanted to leave the country immediately but he needed permission and this took time. The first of seven letters applying for a passport is this undated, handwritten application that Haire sent to the Collector of Customs in Sydney:

> I am an Australian by birth but domiciled in England since 1919. In 1940, being ill, I returned to Australia on a health trip, but have been practising here since. I now desire to return to England, and shall be travelling as a ship's surgeon as soon as there is a vacant post. My English passport having expired, I am now applying herewith for a new passport. [He wrote on the bottom] Urgent – short notice will be given of ship's departure. (NAA. SP 42/2, C1946/10597)

His solicitors Lionel Dare & Dawes sent several requests but one dated 29 August 1945 seemed to meet approval. It included details of Haire's 1932 British passport, said 'his domicile was in England' and that the two houses he owned had been 'taken over by the authorities for war purposes' and asked what procedures Haire should follow to get his passport renewed. A week later Customs replied with details about the fees and photographs required; he would also need a certificate

---

8 Beatrice Ensor (1885–1974) was a theosophical educationist and a co-founder of the New Education Fellowship (later the World Education Fellowship). The NEF's *New Era in Education* is still published.

from the Deputy Chairman and Executive Officer of the NSW Medical Co-ordination Committee to confirm that it had no objection to his being allowed to leave Australia. When the Customs officials received this certificate and Dr Haire's application, they would send him further advice. It is ironic that while Haire's political opponents were trying to pass laws to stop his voice being heard in Australia, he was desperately trying to leave the country but the authorities would not let him go.

Haire's papers include the 'Ninth report of the Parliamentary Standing Committee on Broadcasting' relating to the question of broadcast talks on venereal disease and other sex matters, 11 March 1946. The chairman was the truculent SK Amour, a Roman Catholic and one of Labor's 'Donkey vote' senators; he and the committee, most of whom had close religious affiliations, feared radio provided a unique opportunity for home invasion. One witness deplored the 'morally subversive teaching' of groups without 'spiritual or moral uplift' and the risk of adolescents being influenced by a sex lecturer who admits he has no moral objection to abortion or masturbation, who has publicly displayed diagrams of his own method of contraception to an audience containing adolescents, who has given instruction of methods of sexually exciting the opposite sex and who has suggested companionate 'marriage' as a prelude to marriage. Haire highlighted the committee's next paragraph:

> Needless to say, we have refrained from hearing evidence from any spokesman of this group, in order to avoid the scandal inherent in the publicity which might have been given to its well known views, as disclosed in documentary records. We share the indignation of the witnesses who have been public-spirited enough to expose and denounce its activities. With patriotic and long-range vision, these witnesses foresee a calamitous repetition of history in the fate which would eventually overtake Australian if the degenerate tenets of these advocates of public instruction on sex matters were accepted and practised in this country.

They found 'overwhelming evidence that on social and national grounds alone, it would be unthinkable to provide facilities for the broadcasting of advice from this group'. 'Australia is a Christian country' and its ideals would be corrupted by any teaching which undermined these standards of morality, 'an activity all the more reprehensible when it is pursued for commercial gain'. Haire highlighted their hypocritical rationalisation: 'Lest this attitude might be misconstrued as a negation of democratic freedom, it is necessary to emphasise the universally accepted fact that there is a vast difference between liberty and licence'. This restrictive victory was announced in *The Argus* on 4 July 1946:

> Broadcasting stations have been requested to refrain immediately from broadcasting talks on venereal disease and sex matters. Announcing the Government's decision today, Senator Cameron, Postmaster-General, said it followed a recommendation from the Parliamentary Standing Committee on Broadcasting, which had taken evidence in all states, after various organisations had protested against the continuance of such talks.[9]

Four days later Haire received his passport and Guy Natusch, worried about the future of the *Woman* articles, sent him a note on 23 July saying that he understood Haire would leave for London the following Saturday and expected 'to be returning here about Christmas of this year.' Haire may have believed this or he may have invented a polite fiction.

He used one of his final articles in Australia on 5 August 1946 to write about the fundamental mistakes made by a very highly qualified 'doctor-novelist' (AJ Cronin) in his controversial bestseller *The citadel*. Cronin had portrayed one of the villains as a rich and 'fashionable Harley Street society doctor' who was 'nothing but a damned abortionist.' Haire responded with snide comments about 'novelists who are doctors' and said he believed the book did much harm by making people believe that rogue doctors represented the whole profession. These fears were misplaced; it was made into a film and the audience understood Cronin's exploration of medical ethics and his innovative ideas were said to have helped in the creation of Britain's National Health Service.

---

9 Restrictions were imposed and remained in force until the 1980s when talk-back radio blossomed and listeners' queries about sex were used to enlighten and entertain a wider audience (Bashford & Strange 2004, 98).

Haire left Australia on 24 August 1946 and never returned. He wrote more than 400 of these eagerly awaited weekly articles for *Woman* and he continued to send them from Britain. His 9 September column was written onboard ship and he thanked the proprietors and the editor for their 'courage' in giving him the opportunity to address readers for over five years. He was gratified by 'the thousands of appreciative letters' and had been ready for protests 'from those who think that ignorance is synonymous with innocence'. Approvals had greatly outnumbered the disapprovals and 'happily, the proprietors and the editor stood their ground' supporting his 'endeavour to bring enlightenment to the public' thus demonstrating 'beyond dispute that such enlightenment can be given in a clean and decent way'. With the exception of a few topics he was forbidden to discuss (masturbation and sexual 'perversion'), his discussions ranged from abortion, adolescence, birth, childcare, contraception, diet, divorce, infertility, impotence, marriage, menopause, menstruation, pregnancy, prostitution and sex education to VD.

Haire had correctly judged that his articles 'had a considerable effect in moulding Australian public opinion, in making people realise that it is not only desirable, but possible, to make sex knowledge available in simple and inoffensive form to the public'.

This chapter gave an overview of Haire's Dr Wykeham Terriss contributions to *Woman* which spanned a decade. The next one deals with his important contribution to a radio debate on population in 1944 which infuriated conservative politicians.

13

THE ABC POPULATION DEBATE

In the years Haire was writing for *Woman*, one date stood out because, in Dickens' words 'it was the best of times, it was the worst of times'. On 23 August 1944 he was the key speaker in a radio debate and the chair said there was no need to formally introduce him because he was 'well known to most of you as a public speaker and writer' (ABC 1944, 7). However, Haire's great triumph in being able to promote his views to the nation was clouded when political protesters made this debate on population the Australian Broadcasting Commission's 'largest controversy during the war years' (Thomas 1980, 110).

The ABC had only begun broadcasting in 1932, and radio was in its infancy: the ABC was hampered by wartime censorship and by Labor Prime Minister John Curtin's dislike of 'too much talking and too much serious music' so staff dutifully obliged with lightweight programs to 'cheer people up' (Bennett 1982). Considering this, the ABC executives were taking a big risk when they launched *The nation's forum of the air* as 'an experiment in democracy' to support tolerance, reason and justice and to 'establish radio as an active force in political education' (*ABC Weekly* 22 July 1944). The fortnightly debates were based on an American program in which experts spoke and responded to questions from a studio audience (Inglis 1983, 115). The commissioners had also examined Canadian radio debates and daringly adopted a North American model rather than the ABC's usual approach of imitating the BBC.

The format was proposed by the ABC's Director of Talks, BH Molesworth, who had worked in university extension courses and adult education and was considered 'something of a radical' because he had once lectured on Marxism in Broken Hill (Hodge 1995, 101). General Manager Charles Moses sent the managers a memo headed 'Controversial subjects' in March 1939 and suggested 'these should be allowed and not so rigidly censored' and that the results could be excellent if the other side had the right to reply. Molesworth agreed that such debates were 'amongst the most attractive material for talks' and said he thought the ABC's state offices were too timid and, as long as various opinions were expressed, there was no reason to prevent such debates. The scheme was approved by the ABC's executives and commissioners. In the words of ABC historian Ken Inglis (1983, 114), 'Molesworth loaded up the university men from the (ABC's) National Talks Advisory Committee and fired them in defence of his territory.' It was a great win because, although Moses welcomed controversial subjects, he shared Curtin's preference for light entertainment and often clashed with the ABC's intellectuals.

One of the brightest thinkers was William Macmahon Ball who had resigned in protest from his position as chief executive of Radio Australia when the government took over short-wave broadcasting in 1944. Four months later he returned to the ABC to run *The nation's forum of the air* and he chose the subject and the four speakers for the debate. John Hilvert said in his book on wartime censorship (1984, 156) that Macmahon Ball's job was difficult because his superior, the ABC's Director-General of Information EG Bonney, was suspicious of intellectuals and gave his first loyalty to the anti-intellectual Arthur Calwell[1] who became Minister for Information on 21 September 1943, a month after Curtin's landslide win. Macmahon Ball clashed with Bonney, a feared, skilled and ruthless administrator whose tactics were parodied in this jingle:

> My Bonney lies over the ocean
> My Bonney lies over the sea,
> And sometimes I get the notion,
> Bonney also lies to me.

As well as in-house tensions, the ABC was harassed by the Gibson Committee, an all-party Joint Parliamentary Standing Committee on

---

1 Vickery (2003, 131) felt that Bonney may have been reassured in his moves against Macmahon Ball because Calwell disliked academics and had said in his autobiography (1972, 262) that John Curtin never suffered from 'the disability of a university degree'.

Broadcasting, which Moses dubbed the 'Standover Committee' after Calwell became the chair. On 20 May 1944 Moses gave his approval for Macmahon Ball's selection for 'the debate on the birth rate': Dr Norman Haire was to be the 'leading speaker' in the second of the ABC's *The nation's forum of the air* programs in which 'frank, unfettered discussion of really important public issues' would be led by 'the best people in Australia', similar to the National Broadcasting Corporation of America's very successful *Town meeting of the air* series. Macmahon Ball wanted Haire to speak in favour of 'birth rationing' because he felt Haire could do it 'more successfully and effectively than anyone else available in Australia'. They hoped to get Dame Enid Lyons and Mr Colin Clark to put the counterview that 'a large and rapid population growth was urgent'.

Macmahon Ball approached Haire who agreed to speak but made it clear that he was 'ardent' about 'cautiously' increasing Australia's population. In the *The General Practitioner* Haire had argued that Europe should reduce its population while Australia needed to increase because the country could no longer rely on growth from immigration since Britain had finished its 'swarming period' (Still 1937, 286). Australians should 'encourage increase only among parents who are really fit to have children' and pay as much attention to breeding human beings as they did to breeding livestock. He believed that childless unhealthy parents who had refrained from 'polluting the race' were providing the same service to the community as healthy parents who had children. Haire asked if the debate would be broadcast live or pre-recorded and inquired about the date because he gave evening lectures for the WEA on Tuesdays in Sydney and Fridays in Newcastle.

Sensing his opportunity for a broader platform for publicity, he said he would be glad to participate in ABC debates about VD and sex education, adding that his details were in 'the British, International and Australian editions of *Who's Who*'. The ABC scheduled the debate to suit him and Macmahon Ball suggested a Wednesday evening in early August. Haire asked him not to stress his 'good qualities as a medical practitioner' because the BMA would see this as advertising. Instead he should highlight the sex educational and medico-sociological aspects of his work. Haire also sent his photograph, taken from a portrait painted by Cathleen Mann, Marchioness of Queensberry, but he said he was unsure how she spelt her title and advised Macmahon Ball to check her details in *Who's Who*.

Complaints began *before* the broadcast, including a telegram from the Reverend David J Knox in Sydney to Prime Minister Curtin on behalf of Moore Theological College's Public Morals Committee:

> Strongly oppose Doctor Norman Haire speaking over national network on birthrate question Wednesday – refer you to his published writings on subject also NSW Government's Police Report of his sex lectures here. (NAA. Series M1415, 21 August 1944)

Curtin, who had rejected his Catholic upbringing, stood firm and sent the Protestant theologian a strong reply, informing him that 'Macmahon Ball had made enquiries of leading members of the medical profession in Sydney' and in their opinion Dr Haire, who was a member of the BMA, 'would be the most competent man available in Australia to put the case [and] that under the provisions of the Australian Broadcasting Act both National and Commercial broadcasting stations are permitted almost complete freedom in the selection of their programmes'.

Dame Enid Lyons, the key speaker against birth control, was a Catholic convert and mother of 11[2] who began her parliamentary career in 1943 after the death of her Prime Minister husband and was to become one of Australia's most admired women. In her autobiography (1972, 172) she said she had made her maiden speech while 'knee-deep in shawls and feeding bottles'. She had also considered the population question and was alarmed by 'the movement for sex education in schools'. In 1942 she was one of the conservative experts who served on the National Health and Medical Research Council's inquiry into the decline of the birthrate.

Her autobiography included a chapter about the ABC debate which gave this account of her involvement after a 'chance encounter' with Macmahon Ball outside Melbourne's General Post Office:

---

2 She had 12 children but, like the Zions, one child had died in infancy.

The ABC population debate

'Dame Enid', he said, 'I wonder if you would help me?' (this was the type of bait to which I invariably rose). He was arranging a new program feature for the ABC... It would take the form of debates on questions of current interest, the more controversial the better. Would I be prepared to take part on a program to be called 'Birth Rationing?' 'Well, not under that title', I said... 'But you would debate the subject'? 'Yes, I think so'. 'Well, what title would you suggest?' After a moment's thought I said, 'What about Population Unlimited?, would that do?' Mr Macmahon Ball thought it would, and then and there the matter was settled; in the space of a few minutes in... a throng of shoppers I had committed myself to one of the most disturbing experiences I was to know as a Member of Parliament.

She said she began her preparations when she arrived in Sydney. This could not be true because the speakers had to submit their speech to the ABC (to comply with the security constraints of live broadcasts) and the ABC sent a complete set of these speeches to the participants a week before the debate. While she might have forgotten some things, she captured the drama that began shortly before the debate when she received a message asking her to return a phone call as 'a matter of great urgency'. The caller was a friend of her late husband's who wanted her to withdraw because 'Haire was not his real name'; he was an alien who was possibly under security surveillance; he was also a familiar figure in King's Cross where he lectured to audiences 'composed largely of young men of a type whose social acceptability had not yet reached its present permissive position'. This use of euphemisms and innuendo was typical of the slurs on Haire's reputation: he *was* born in Australia, there was nothing sinister about his name-change and he was often in King's Cross because he lived in the area and gave lectures there.

Lyons did not withdraw for two reasons: she trusted Macmahon Ball who reassured her and the program had been advertised for weeks and she did not want to be unfair to the ABC. The flyers had described 'birth rationing' as being Australia's most drastic form of rationing and promised that the problem would be debated frankly by speakers with outstanding qualifications:

Dame Enid Lyons will insist on the urgency of a new attitude towards motherhood among Australian women, a new readiness to subordinate other interests to the supreme interests and obligations of family life. Dr Norman Haire, gynaecologist and sexologist, of London and Sydney, will counsel caution in any schemes for encouraging large families. Mr Colin Clark, economist and head of the Queensland Bureau of Industry and Statistics, will reinforce Dame Enid's case with a series of arresting facts and figures. Mrs Jessie Street will deal particularly with the social and economic problems facing Australian mothers today (NAA. MP 298/4, N/17/1, 8 August 1944).

The two main opponents Haire and Lyons were evenly matched and Figure 13.1 cleverly summarises the issues:

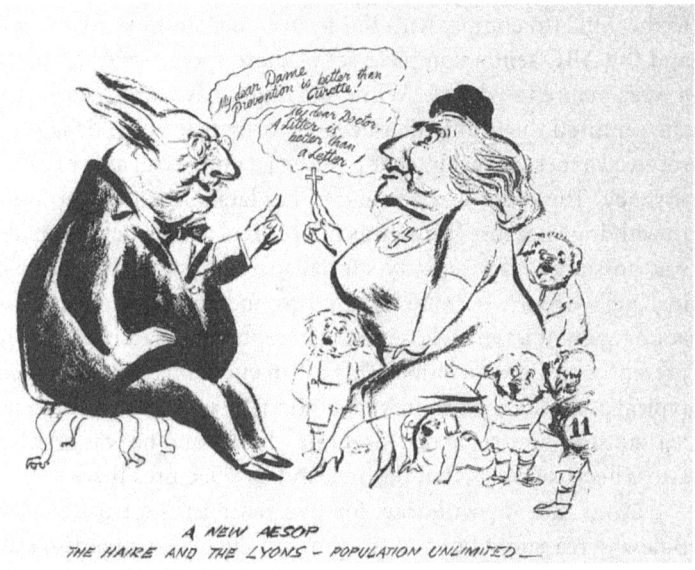

Haire: 'My dear Dame, prevention is better than curette!'
Lyons: 'My dear Doctor, a litter is better than a letter!'

Figure 13.1. Cartoon of Haire and Lyons in the ABC's population debate.

THE ABC POPULATION DEBATE

'A new Aesop: the Haire and the Lyons – "Population unlimited"' was the caption; Haire with ears sits opposite Lyons who has a crucifix in her hand and is surrounded by her eleven koala-faced children.

Cartoonist Les Tanner told me in 1998 that it was anonymous for political reasons because Thomas Challen, who did it, 'worked for many socialist newspapers' and 1944 was 'a bitter time in Australian politics'[3]; Tanner worked with Challen at *The Daily Telegraph* and said he was 'a sad man who felt he had sold himself' and died in a fall from a bar room stool. Haire met Challen at Mona van Wein's 'at homes'.

Figure 13.2 shows the group standing in front of a microphone: Jessie Street is in the centre speaking from notes, Enid Lyons is facing her, Norman Haire is in a bow tie and the tall man in the overcoat was probably there to enforce wartime censorship. Clark spoke from Melbourne by telephone.

Lyons did not like Haire's views but said the debate was friendly. They were well matched because Robert Menzies said her oratory could make him weep even if she was talking about the state of a railway.[4] When Lyons met Haire, shortly before the debate, she was appalled by his fatness but thought his voice was the most beautiful she had ever heard, surpassing that of the Shakespearean actor Sir John Gielgud 'whose voice is famous for the music of its tones' (Lyons 1972, 85). He had received similar tributes as a schoolboy and, as an adult, his speeches made such an impact that 'you might go to see Bernard Shaw on a platform with Haire, but it is Norman you'd remember' (Hesling 1960, 13). Sadly it is now impossible to hear his voice and John Spence, from ABC Radio Archives Sound Recording, gave me the reason in 1998: 'Unfortunately, the ABC Archives does not have the broadcast itself because the ABC only started keeping sound recordings in the 1970s'. In her keynote address to the Forum on Australian Library History 2007, Carmel Maguire said the failure to keep 'early broadcasts merits a black mark on our cultural bottom line'.

---

3   The cartoon included a note from Les Tanner to Mrs (Patricia) Ranald MacDonald: 'The cartoonist in question was Thomas Arthur Challon [sic] who drew under the pen name 'TAC' (HC – 7.30).
4   Steketee (2008) quoting Henderson.

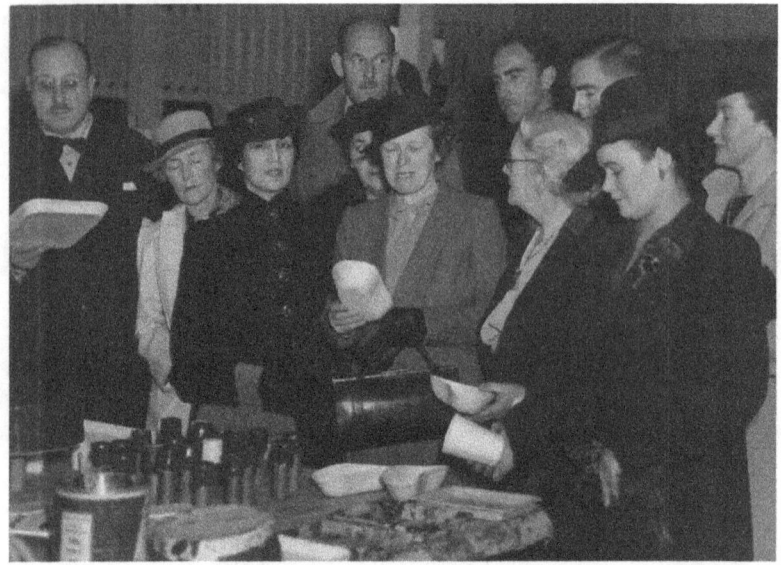

Figure 13.2. Speakers at the ABC's 'Population unlimited?' debate, 20 May 1944.

Lyons said Haire had used 'rounded phrases' and developed the argument 'logically and with oratorical skill', making 'full use of his mellifluous and persuasive voice. He was carrying the crowded audience with him' until he said that his mother was 'always either pregnant or suckling, usually both at the same time'.

> For eighteen years she had scarcely a night's unbroken sleep. At the age of forty she, who had been an exceptionally strong and healthy young woman, had through her excessive and uncontrolled fertility become a devitalised, irritable, cantankerous, prematurely old woman. Only then, too late, did she attempt to prevent conception. *For all that she got out of life she might as well have been a prize cow.* (ABC 1944, 9)

Haire was pilloried for this comment, and his last sentence (an emotional expression of his concern) was deleted from the ABC's threepenny pamphlet but fortunately a transcript has survived (NAA. SP 369/3, vol. 1/2, 1944). The extra words in italics are in the transcript but not in the published pamphlet. Journalist Robert Pullan (1984) discussed Clement Semmler's long censorship battles with the ABC to publish his book *The ABC – Aunt Sally and sacred cow* (1981) which was an apt title because mothers in the 1940s, particularly those with large broods, *were* sacred cows. Haire was accused of having mocked motherhood, and the pro-natalist bulls were in full roar in parliament claiming that he had said his mother 'lived the life of a prize milch cow'. Senator James McLachlan called him despicable and said, 'such remarks should not be broadcast' and Senator O'Flaherty yelled, 'He is not human.' Politicians pounced on Haire's alleged comment but ignored his contentious proposals – for instance, that governments should fund a 'No-Baby Bonus' for childless couples of 'bad stock', because having good 'migrants from the womb' was as important as choosing suitable migrants from overseas (ABC 1944, 8). Haire advocated contraception as part of the Malthusian creed: 'Not quantity but quality: It is not the number of children born that is important but the number which survive to become healthy, happy and useful adults and to produce children in turn.'

A strong moderator might have kept order but the elderly chair, a 'modest and unassuming' judge (Ward 1988), had no control over Colin Clark who was supposed to travel to Sydney by air but was 'off-loaded from his plane' two hours before the broadcast *in the interest of high military priorities* (ABC 1944, 3, 10). Clark was speaking by telephone and the moderator did not try to stop his tirade about the 'perversion' of preventing childbearing by 'unnatural' practices. The deletion of the transcript words (shown in italics) softened the impact of Clark's crude remarks:

> What Dr Haire described as contraception *means in plain language preceding intercourse by covering up the sexual organs by pieces of rubber or metal or by chemicals or by the interruption of co-habitation. Such acts are filthy, vicious and disgusting. They* constitute one of the worst forms of sexual immorality. The practice being so widespread does not make it any more moral; rather the reverse, and I think we look pretty foolish when we stand round solemnly and learnedly discussing whether people should commit such acts or not. The only moral act by which the births may be restricted is by partial or complete abstinence. (ABC 1944, 10)

Clark was a Catholic convert and father of nine who claimed that contraception had been 'condemned by all religions' and this embarrassed his debating partner Enid Lyons who said he used the words such as 'moral turpitude' (which he didn't) but she was right to say that he sounded like 'an old-time Redemptionist missioner.' She claimed that, after hearing him, 'Haire could barely restrain himself and when the moment came he sprang to his feet in fury.' She was severely 'rattled' and was later rebuked by 'a middle-aged woman' – Miss EA Mackay the official stenographer – who said, 'I am a Catholic like you and I think you should be ashamed of yourself. It has all been thoroughly disgraceful'. Haire was a polished performer and the speakers were standing so he could not have jumped up in fury, although he *was* very unwise to respond to Clark's taunt by criticising his religious views (the italics show the phrases omitted from the pamphlet):

> It is quite evident that Mr Clark's views on birth control are determined *by the peculiar religious superstition of the Church to which he belongs.* The rules of his particular religion are valid for him ... but there is no reason why he should try to persuade or enforce them on other people. He may find some one or other modes of contraception filthy and disgusting, but it is ridiculous to say that they are considered so by all decent people, because the majority of people in our civilisation are decent and they practice birth control. He says that these methods are condemned by all religions. That is not so. The Lambeth Conference in 1930, composed of Anglican bishops, approved of birth control where there was a good reason for limiting a family, and numerous other religious bodies in America and elsewhere have given their approval in the same way. *You must not be misled by the religious prejudices of Mr Clark.* (ABC 1944, 19)

Macmahon Ball sent a letter of thanks to the speakers and enclosed ten copies of the pamphlet. In a second letter to Haire, he apologised for not speaking to him 'more fully' after the broadcast because he had wanted to thank him 'very sincerely': he was really grateful for all the trouble Haire had taken and for the 'considerable restraint' he had 'showed under provocation. The case you put was extremely logical and must have had very great persuasive power to all that heard it. It was the more effective because you put it with such quietness and restraint' (NAA. MP 298/4, HA/11/3).

The ABC's efforts to implement innovative programs and to encourage free speech had been a public relations disaster but Chair WJ Cleary and General Manager Charles Moses bravely defended the program despite the flaws which Macmahon Ball listed for the General Manager in this *post-mortem*. He felt that it was 'seriously marred by certain unexpected features': Dr Norman Haire showed some lack of verbal tact in two passages of his opening speech where he referred to the 'cow-like' quality of a woman with a large family, and where he emphasised the very satisfactory qualities of modern contraceptive methods. His serious breach of discretion, however, was his reference in reply to Colin Clark, to the 'religious superstitions' which determined Clark's views. Macmahon Ball had made it very clear to Haire in a long interview on the previous day that he must avoid any references that would arouse bitterness between Protestant and Roman Catholic, and he was very disappointed that he should have forgotten himself to this extent. However, it should be remembered that Haire spoke under extreme provocation.

Macmahon Ball described Mr Clark's contribution as 'calamitous'. He had been trying hard to arrange a meeting with him for weeks and they had still planned to meet for a careful discussion before the broadcast but when he was off-loaded from the plane it was impossible. Macmahon Ball had sent him written advice about the line he should take and felt 'there was no possible excuse for the tone and content of his broadcast. The bitter and militant religious note and the crudely realistic description of common contraceptive methods were the worst features of a generally bad broadcast'.

Macmahon Ball 'felt that Mrs Street did not define her position with any clarity' and the chair did not create the atmosphere needed for the meeting. He concluded: 'These things have caused me very great regret and disappointment since I feel that I am directly responsible to the Commission' (NAA. MP 298/4/0, N/17/3, WOB3 25 August 1944). Curiously, he said nothing about Lyons.

Haire's comments about Clark's religious prejudices suited his enemies who wrongly claimed that Haire spoke about Clark's 'filthy religion' and ignored the fact that Clark had used the word when he said that contraception was 'filthy'. Charles Moses made a diplomatic concession to a critic: 'In the actual heat of the debate these plans did not work out exactly as we expected.' Calwell had telephoned him to complain after having first tried to contact the Chair and the Vice-Chair; he said the ABC should not have arranged the discussion and that 'Dr Norman Haire should not have been engaged to broadcast'. Calwell planned to discuss the matter in a Cabinet meeting and wanted the ABC's assurance that Dr Haire would never be permitted to broadcast over national stations again.

Moses parried the politicians' questions on 14 September 1944 (NAA. MP 298/4). He replied to Senator Nash's questions to the Postmaster-General, confirming that the ABC was aware of Dr Norman Haire's views on sex before it engaged him to participate in the 'Population Unlimited?' broadcast. Moses said it would be a matter of opinion whether Haire's 'views on sex were offensive to decent living citizens or were calculated to undermine family life'.

When asked if the Postmaster-General (PMG])or the Commission had received protests against the action of the Commission in giving Dr Haire 'nation-wide advertisement for his propaganda on sex', Moses said the ABC had received only ten protest letters after Dr Haire appeared in 'Population Unlimited?'. Moses was also asked

> In the national interest as well as in the common interest of the good of the community will the PMG seek the assurance from the Commission that it will refrain from any future engagement of Dr Haire to broadcast in any capacity whatsoever?

Moses replied, 'the Commission will give consideration to the request by the Honourable Senator.'

The Commission gave a similarly non-committal reply to a supporter, the Fellowship of Australian Writers: 'You may be sure we will keep in mind your suggestion that Dr Haire should be included in our programs again when a suitable opportunity occurs.'

In a confidential exchange of letters, Haire said he had 'loyally' observed Macmahon Ball's wishes and had only departed from the rules when Clark made his 'rather silly' and 'very insulting speech' and mentioned the two 'ardent Catholics' who attacked him in parliament – 'Mulcahy has one child, and Calwell two'. He implied that by having so few children they were ignoring their Church's teaching to have many. Macmahon Ball sent a joking reply: 'Apparently both gentlemen are more restrained at home than they are in parliament' (NAA. MP 298/4, HA/11/3).

Senator Ashley, one of the few politicians who spoke in support, said in the Senate that the ABC received many letters supporting Haire and all 32 (plus ten letters of criticism) have been kept in the broadcaster's press clippings file. 'FWC' of Toorak wanted to know why Haire had been attacked for his frankly spoken part in the ABC broadcast and said the ABC's *The nation's forum of the air* was 'good' and pleaded, 'let it continue unhampered by those adverse to free speech.'

Things got so muddled that on the following day *The Daily Telegraph* called the debate 'an ABC broadcast on sex' and reported that the Minister for Information (Mr Calwell) said in the House of Representatives that the Postmaster General was considering action to prevent similar broadcasts in the future. Mr Calwell was answering Mr Mulcahy (Labor, NSW) who described Dr Haire's remarks as 'offensive to the community and damaging to the future of Australia'. A reader took issue with *The Daily Telegraph*'s assertion that Dr Haire's part of the debate was 'objectionable':

> As one who listened to the whole of the debate, may I say that the only statements which were, to my mind, grossly offensive were those made by Mr Colin Clark. To brand, as he did, the majority of his fellow countrymen as guilty of 'filthy, vicious and disgusting' practices and of 'sexual immorality' is both an insult to, and a libel on, people who, in the vast majority of cases, are decent, responsible citizens (NAA. SP 15558/2).

Moses told the commissioners that some complaints about Haire's role came from people who had not heard the broadcast. This was true of Senator Foll (United Australia Party, Qld) who was 'glad' to hear that Senator Amour and others had deplored the views expressed by Dr Norman Haire in advocacy of birth control. He 'did not hear that broadcast' but had 'heard sufficient about it to endorse the criticism uttered by those honourable senators'. In the midst of this furore, Commissioner John Medley sent Enid Lyons this verse he had scribbled during a board meeting discussion:

> How can you preserve decorum
> At the meetings of a forum
> If a Haire can breathe defiance
> At a family of Lyons? (Medley, quoted in Serle 1993, 62)

He was alluding to a Latin proverb *Mortuo leoni et lepores insultant* which means 'even hares strike (or insult) a dead lion'. Haire courageously challenged the lions throughout his life but after his death some mean-spirited opponents disparaged the dead Haire by lying.

Clark, Lyons and Street all escaped parliamentary censure; Haire and Macmahon Ball were the liberal heroes and Jessie Street's mediocre contribution is surprising in view of her status as a feminist icon. Macmahon Ball had first wanted to select Dr WGK Duncan, the Director of Sydney University's Tutorial Classes[5] but, to provide gender and political balance, the ABC chose Jessie Street, who had stood unsuccessfully for Labor the previous year in a strongly conservative seat. She privately supported birth control but said ambiguously in the debate: 'I believe that the people who practise birth control today do not really feel that they are doing anything wrong'. She and Haire were debating in favour of population control but instead she argued for the birthrate to be *increased*: she praised the Soviet Union for glorifying motherhood and doubling its birthrate and suggested that Australia should do the same.

---

5 Dr Duncan, Mr WD Borrie and Dr A Grenfell Price were speakers in the ABC's 29 November 1944 debate (NAA. SP 369/3, Vol. 1.9).

Few mentioned her role and one man wrote to the ABC General Manager to praise Haire's 'outstanding contribution to the debate.' He was silent about Street and succinctly assessed the others: 'Dr Haire – Humanitarianism, Dame Enid Lyons – Sentimentality, Mr Clark – Bigotry.' He opposed 'any move which might be made to silence the voice of Dr Haire or of any other speaker whose views may not be acceptable to intolerant sectional groups.'

Catholics and Protestants were embroiled in bitter feuds in the 1940s and Canon Thomas Hammond was feared, loved and influential in Sydney as 'a Northern Irish evangelical' who led an 'ardent crusade against the "errors" of the Church of Rome' (Gill 1998). He was principal of the Moore Theological College and Secretary of its Public Morals Committee which, in a telegram to the Prime Minister, had tried to prevent the population debate. After the debate Hammond complained that the ABC had shown bias in selecting two Roman Catholics to represent one side of the discussion. Although his religious lobby group opposed Haire and contraception, he perversely complained about Lyons and Clark on religious grounds even though they *agreed* with the group's views.

Moses replied: 'I hope you will accept my assurances that the selection of these speakers was not in any sense based on religious grounds. Dame Enid Lyons was selected for her skill as a speaker, for her public reputation, and for the fact of her outstanding example as a woman who had been able to combine heavy family responsibilities with success in public life. Mr Colin Clark was selected because it was felt that as an economist and statistician, he would be able to give solid intellectual backing for the case put by Dame Enid' (NAA. 298/4, N/17/1).

The debate's chair, Harold Nicholas, was praised by John Ward (1988) in the *ADB* for being the first editor of the *Australian Quarterly* but did not mention his role in the ABC forum. To be fair, Clark was not in the Sydney studio and even a strong chair might have been ambushed by Clark's shift from his agreed statistical speech to a religious diatribe. Macmahon Ball's comment about Mrs Street not defining her position was chivalrous, but he may have been having a private joke when he told her on 11 September: 'Amongst the many listeners who expressed their appreciation of your talk, Mr Colin Clark was one of the most enthusiastic'.

Haire's sex education and birth control advocacy was vehemently denounced by Catholics, some Anglicans and the Women's Christian Temperance Union. Haire said that, as a result of their pressure, in 1943 the ABC had 'politely dropped' him after five appearances as an expert on their 'Army wants to know' sessions. The ABC was intrepid to risk more controversy by choosing him to lead the forum debate, and Haire (who was ill) was brave to accept. Fortunately, the ABC did not buckle under pressure – the issue went far beyond Haire and concerned the right to use contraception and the broadcaster's right to be unfettered by outside interference.

ABC historian Alan Thomas commented (1980, 111): 'The ABC's defence of Haire was a brave act and indicates that the Commission was more willing to challenge government interference on matters of morality and taste than it was on items more obviously political'. A second debate on *The battle for population* (ABC, 29 November 1944) was not contentious, perhaps because the moderator was the former NSW Premier, Sir Bertram Stevens. Haire wrote in *Woman* on 18 December that he found it refreshing to hear 'at least two speakers took a more rational view' and did not attribute Australia's low birthrate to the selfishness of married women and had 'pointed out that the enormous increase in population which took place during the last century was due less to a rise in the birthrate than to a fall in the death rate'. Haire had made similar points in the debate three months earlier (ABC, August 1944, 8).

In early 1945 Macmahon Ball returned to his position at the University of Melbourne in charge of the Department of Political Science and Haire returned to England in August 1946. While the ABC successfully resisted religious and political pressure in 1944, its independence became increasingly threatened soon after and it had to operate within various constraints: in 1946 laws were introduced to ban the ABC and commercial radio stations from broadcasting 'talks relating to sex matters or venereal disease' and in 1948 the ABC's discretion over 'political or controversial broadcasting' was limited by three additional provisions.

Colin Clark became obsessed with population and food supply; in the 1960s he became a member of the Pope's Commission on Population and contradicted the forecasts of his former employer, the Food and Agriculture Organisation of the United Nations, by stating that 'the earth can feed its people' (Peters 2001). He castigated researchers such as Dr Paul Ehrlich (1969) who warned about global starvation; and he opposed Germaine Greer at the Sydney Town Hall in a 1972 abortion debate that the ABC recorded but did not broadcast which began with this exchange:

> Clark: 'I don't know what to call you: Miss Greer or Mrs'.
> Greer: 'Call me Doctor' (Ryan 1989).

Clark's rude and rule-breaking performance in the ABC's 1944 debate was ignored in his 1989 obituaries and one claimed he was 'without doubt Australia's most renowned economist'. *The Age* (quoted by Arndt 1987) was less sycophantic, noting this British-born academic 'was perhaps best known for his eccentricity'. *The Times* called him 'a most engaging controversialist, completely happy to be in a minority of one, taking defeat in a good cause with modesty and good humour'.

The fact that most politicians supported Clark, despite his offensive behaviour, indicates the political power of the church and that policies to increase the birthrate were the norm in Australia in the 1940s. It also shows how brave Haire and the ABC Board were to defy this by taking a progressive, humanist stance, withstand strong criticism, and work to change these powerful conservative norms.

Haire was to spend his final years in London where he continued to fight for sexual reform.

14

Final years

Haire left Australia on 24 August 1946 as ship's surgeon on the SS *Port Macquarie* which, by coincidence, was the name of the district where he had inherited a 20-acre property. In mid September the ship made a brief stop in Capetown and continued on to London. He must have spent months settling in because it was not until 27 January 1947 that *The Times* announced he had 'returned to 127 Harley Street which is his permanent address.' London was chilly when he arrived, just as it had been in 1919, but this time it was different: the first time he was unknown and then welcomed but the opposition to him had grown in Britain and Australia, and the social climate towards him was now chilly.

In February he sent his résumé to 20 lowbrow British tabloids[1] and described his *Woman* articles in the hope of writing a British equivalent. None of them offered him paid work although they were happy to accept his letters and he kept one from *The Daily Telegraph*. It was by 'Mother of Four' who said that his letter was 'a message to the world and contains the wisdom of a Saviour!' She had been left destitute with several small children and felt that the government's 'miserable pittance' would 'only tempt people of inferior intellect' to breed. But if the government would help healthy unmarried women to rear their 'unwanted' babies, 'Britain would soon become an A1 nation' because a small healthy population would be better than 'a lot of inferior beings filling our lunatic asylums and hospitals'.

Haire had a chance meeting with Alan John (Jock) Marshall in a London street in early 1947 when Marshall was seeking a divorce,

---

1 These included: *Evening Standard, Evening News, Sunday Graphic, News of the World, People, Sunday Express, Sunday Dispatch, Empire News, Sunday Chronicle, Sunday Mercury, John Bull, Daily Mirror, Daily Express, Daily Herald, News Chronicle, Daily Sketch, Daily Graphic, Daily Mail, Daily Record* and *Daily Worker*.

recovering from malaria and about to start postgraduate studies at Oxford. He was also working as a correspondent for *The Mirror* and was very grateful to be paid in sterling. Haire sent Lotte Fink this news in October after Marshall led an Oxford University expedition to the 'Polar Regions' and said he sounded 'very subdued' when he spoke on the radio. In her memoir, Marshall's second wife said her husband 'heard a Rolls Royce coming to a purring halt beside him' and Haire emerged from the back seat beaming at his cleverness in having spotted him in the crowd. Marshall called Haire 'a medical practitioner and journalist who was flourishing in London as he had flourished in Sydney'. This was unlikely in these postwar years but perhaps Haire felt that success would follow if he looked the part and his extravagant car was a prop. Haire asked, 'was he feeding himself, was he worried, was his sex life normal?' He told Marshall that he looked ten years older than when he they last met in Sydney and Marshall promised to drink lots of milk and go to bed earlier and eat regular meals (Marshall 1998).

Haire was a bibliophile with a splendid library who fought for many years to safeguard sexology collections and in 1923 went to see Havelock Ellis about his 'invaluable and almost unique' collection. Haire discussed it with him again in 1930 and said that 'it would be a boon to humanity' if it was suitably housed but if it went to the British Museum it would 'almost certainly be unavailable for even the most serious student'. Haire wrote to Lafitte-Cyon after Ellis died and asked about the fate of his collection which could throw 'a flood of light on his contemporaries, both famous and obscure' for future generations. Haire's concerns were justified. In 1938 Havelock Ellis asked Alec Craig to help him to dispose of 'some hundred volumes' of his rarer sexological books.[2] Craig carried out his request and called it a 'collection' not a 'library' and said Ellis was not a bibliophile and cared little for them as books, they were not in any order and he relied on memory to find them. Books and other items were thrown out every time he moved house and 'the chief thing' left was the manuscript of his autobiography and some other items in his father's old sea chest. Although his will

---

2 An obituary to Havelock Ellis in *The Eugenics Review* (April 1938–January 1939, 112–13) included Alec Craig's description of the book disposal.

stipulated that his personal papers should be kept, these wishes were flouted by his three executors: Lafitte-Cyon, Edie (one of his sisters), and Mneme Kirkland, a lover. Lafitte-Cyon was to receive half of future royalties and the other half was to go to his sisters. However, the sisters burned everything in the chest and Mneme had 'stalked out with' the letters he had sent her (Grosskurth 1985, 445–47).

After hearing this Haire was determined to safeguard his own library which contained many rare books[3] and considered leaving it to the National Library of Australia (NLA). However, in response to Haire's 14 June 1947 offer (now missing[4]), the NLA Librarian Kenneth Binns replied that the idea 'had interested him considerably' and that 'works on sex' would be 'available in the library to any person with a serious study interest.' Haire adamantly opposed these restrictions because 'ordinary' people had great difficulty in obtaining books on sex which made it very important that people aged 18 and over could access them freely in the NLA or in other libraries such as New South Wales' public library. He did not want them limited to 'students' only, because sex affected the health and happiness of all adults, and even books on abnormal sexuality could be of 'strong interest' for many people, because of their own 'anomalies' or those of other members of their family. Haire remembered the searching questions he had been asked at Sydney's old public library on the corner of Bent and Macquarie Street nearly 40 years earlier, when he wanted to read books by Havelock Ellis or other similar books; and Ellis had often spoken to him about the formalities that he had had to go through, some decades earlier still, when he went to read

---

3   It included Margaret Leonora Eyles' *Commonsense about sex*, which was banned in Australia and, apart from his copy, 'has not survived in any other library in the country' (Moore 1975, 337).

4   On 17 September 2006 Dr Marie-Louise Ayers, Curator of Manuscripts at the National Library of Australia, replied to my query about this 14 June 1947 letter: she had searched NLA files and could not find any reference to it. She would forward the query to the Records Management Unit but felt it unlikely that it would be found. By chance, a former member of staff 'with a prodigious memory' was visiting and she searched through additional files which she suggested. Ayers thought it quite likely that the letter exists 'somewhere' in NLA files but they have exhausted their searching options.

there. Haire was making a very important point; libraries and librarians become *de facto* censors when they set limits on access to material, but surprisingly 'no library historian has ever researched librarians' role in censorship' (Moore May 2005, 297–98). Under the Literature Censorship Board's system, books with scholarly or other merit that were considered to be obscene were placed on 'restricted circulation' and could only to be accessed by persons who could demonstrate their credentials as psychologists, medical practitioners or tertiary students. Binns joined the Censorship Board in 1937 and Nicole Moore told me in 2007 that he employed their restrictions in the National Library. When Haire stipulated that *all* readers should have free access to his material, the NLA's enthusiasm vanished and Haire withdrew his offer. Binns helped improve the intellectual life of Australia's capital during Canberra's early years and he was the first Australian librarian to be awarded a Carnegie travelling fellowship but, while he helped turn the NLA into a national institution, he didn't lobby to acquire Haire's collection.

Binns' letter in August to the librarian at Australia House in London showed that the negotiations were over because Haire had not said anything further about donating his collection but suggested instead that they should send him a list of 'all our books on sex' so that he could liaise with the London librarian about book purchases for the NLA. Before Binns could authorise him 'to buy even moderately in this field' he needed to refer the matter to his Library Committee. But he would only consult the committee if 'Mr Haire was prepared to make any gift' that the committee 'would probably accept and, as a result of the gift, the obligation to continue in this field would be accepted'. However, Binns would not approach the committee about their 'buying in this field' because he did 'not think such a suggestion would be warmly received'. It was a very tortuous rejection. Binns did not respond to Haire's offer to help select books and used the committee as an excuse for his inertia but it could have been a face-saving silence because the list of 'all their books on sex' was probably a complete blank.

Haire detected hints of malevolence towards him soon after he returned to London. The nature of this malice was revealed in letters sent by two men he regarded as friends: AP Pillay, an Indian doctor who ran a pioneering contraception clinic in Bombay, and Norman Himes. Pillay was the editor-in-chief and financial backer of a quarterly journal called *Marriage Hygiene* which had been published in Bombay from 1934 to 1937 and was being resurrected. Himes was chosen as the American editor and called it 'the only scientific journal in the world devoted to advancing our knowledge of conjugal hygiene'. The editors' correspondence in 1947 and 1948 shows their priority was to promote the journal and block Haire's involvement with it. Himes told Pillay in March 1947 that he understood 'Haire had gone to Australia years ago' and suggested either Dr CP Blacker or Dr Maurice Newfield as a better choice of editor than Haire.[5] They refused and Pillay said it was a case of 'Hobson's choice', suggesting Haire for the role, possibly with assistance from Clifford Allen, the author of *Modern discoveries in medical psychology*. However, Haire became the English editor by default. Haire knew nothing of these machinations when he contacted Margaret Sanger who was in London and invited her for a meal but warned that he could not give her anything elaborate because of the austerity conditions. He asked if Pillay had told her that 'we are starting the *Marriage Hygiene* journal again next month' and that he had asked Haire 'to act as the editor for England.' They would welcome anything she wrote but Pillay said to make sure there was nothing about abortion or birth control which could cause difficulty with the US mails (2 July 1947, MSP – Smith S27, 244).

A few months later Pillay complained to Himes that 'someone with influence in England' was working against *Marriage Hygiene* and he guessed that it was either because Haire was editor or an excuse 'for crying down *Marriage Hygiene*'. He believed 'the stiffening opposition' was 'penetrating the USA as well' and reminded Himes that *The Eugenics Review* and *Marriage Hygiene* used to exchange advertisements and said he had just received an official letter from Lord Horder, the Eugenics Society President, informing him that this practice would 'not be

---

5 Blacker (1926) and Newfield had sound publishing credentials. Newfield had been an editor of both *The Eugenics Review* and *The British encyclopaedia of medical practice* and wrote under the pseudonym 'Michael Fielding' (1928).

advantageous to either journal as the contents of both were entirely different'. Pillay was very worried because:

> You can see that this is a mere pretext and the letter coming from Horder and not from Newfield (whom I know personally) or Blacker (whom I know well by correspondence) is ominous. I have written a confidential letter to explain the cause of this *volte face* to Newfield. I personally would very much like to get rid of Haire but how to do it gracefully and to find out a successor are the two problems (NHA. 11 October 1947).

The influential 'Tommy' Horder was the Royal family's doctor, senior physician at St Bartholomew's Hospital, president of the National Birth Control Association, president of the Eugenics Society, chair of the Joint Committee on Voluntary Sterilization, president of the Council for the Disposition of the Dead, vice president of the Cremation Society, chair of the Anti-Noise League and he also belonged to the society to suppress London's smells (*Time*, 4 May 1936). If Horder was disparaging *Marriage Hygiene* to silence Haire, this may have been to block a vocal outsider, or because they disagreed about sterilisation and Britain's population size – Haire had resigned from the Eugenics Society over their position on voluntary sterilisation and he had contradicted this powerful medical figure in a book review, writing: 'Lord Horder is concerned with what he calls the "declining population" of Great Britain. But the population of Great Britain is not declining'.

Haire sent Pillay a long letter in confidence on 16 October about the increasing resistance to the journal. Haire's trust was misplaced because ten days later Pillay forwarded this letter to Himes with a cover note: 'You will see Haire's version of it from the confidential letter I enclose'. Haire told Pillay that he 'did not think there has been any *volte face* at all' but it followed from much earlier events. He remembered Pillay telling him that a certain person had been too 'busy' to see him when he was in London. Haire said 'that group' [the medical establishment] is run by a small number of people with an 'authoritarian, not to say Fascist, outlook'. They are obsessed with power, convinced of their infallibility and knowledge and believe that anybody who does not agree is a heretic and should be suppressed, lest they harm the 'true Church!' – like the Roman Catholic Church but in a different province. It had been easy for them to subjugate most people, because while they were obscure and poor, approval by those higher up was necessary if they wanted their status and income to climb, while non-conformity meant being ignored or facing positive disapproval, often accompanied by a whispering campaign. Very few had either the guts or the money to withstand the 'suggestions' of the hierarchy. And so it had gone on, absorbing more and more individuals and even groups, and gaining power.

Haire said that initially they 'flirted with' him but soon found that he was too 'independent-minded' and too financially successful to accept their dictates. For a while he was tolerated, then ignored and for a long time they had worked against him 'in every possible way'. But, because it was not gentlemanly to publicly abuse or condemn, it was 'all done behind the scenes'. He said Pillay was 'much in the same boat' because he had a mind of his own and would not 'bow the knee'; it was obvious that, if he was rich enough to start the journal, money could not be used to 'tame' him. Control had been difficult because he was 'far away' where they had 'no local *satraps*' [rulers]. But while Pillay was in London on a visit, their attitude began to take shape: they did not actively cooperate with him but maintained just enough 'frosty cordiality to prevent an open breach' in case he 'might prove amenable to discipline later on'. But Pillay's editorial comments in the first issue of *Marriage Hygiene* dashed any hopes that he would accept their dictates: 'So down the drain you must go'. In Pillay's case, there was the added 'sin' of being 'a black man' – he was not white and ought to 'know his place!' They would indignantly deny this and give evidence to show that they worked on very cordial terms with 'coloured' people. Haire agreed that they did, if they 'knew their place'. Haire warned that Pillay should be prepared for the breach to grow and that the journal would either be ignored, or criticised. It would be probably be rumoured that Pillay was a transvestite because of an article he published in the first issue: if he wrote about sadism, he was a sadist or an abortionist if he wrote about abortion and that he himself had been called 'everything in Krafft-Ebing, and a good deal more'.

Haire asked if Pillay knew that Margaret Sanger 'was snubbed very badly' when she arrived in England to attend the Family Planning Association Conference on Infertility at the Nuffield Institute from 26 to 27 July 1947. She had told Haire about this when she came to his house to meet the Flügels. Haire was not telling the whole story about an episode which had happened during a dark period when she was sick and mourning the deaths of her husband and several friends who had died in the war or shortly after.

Haire's ostracism was unfair but Sanger, by her very public *faux pas*, was largely responsible for hers. Britain's mainstream press ignored her but her bizarre plans were picked up by American newspapers with the *Los Angeles Times* quoting her 21 July comments as she boarded a plane to attend the FPA conference in Oxford from 21 to 26 July 1947: she would advocate a ten-year moratorium on births in the hungry countries of Europe, including Britain, and urged people 'not to bring children into the world to starve.' *The Washington Post* reported that she also planned to seek United Nations help to sterilise 'people of low mental ability, morons and imbeciles.' *The Chicago Daily Tribune* reprinted two editorials from London's *Daily Mirror* 'which supports the Labor government'; one newspaper described the American gift-loan as a 'shabby deal' and urged the British government to 'get very tough' with the United States, and the other 'pitched into' Sanger after she arrived in Britain to advocate 'a birth moratorium.' Britain's *Daily Graphic* contrasted her views with those of Arthur Calwell, the Australian Minister for Immigration, who invented the 'populate or perish' slogan and was eager to receive Britain's 'surplus' population (Suitters 1973, 23). Sanger was misguided to think that couples would agree to remain childless and, after the Nazi horrors, her sterilisation proposal was unbelievably insensitive. *The New York Times* felt she would not get far after she 'dropped her controversial bomb' by proposing that cradles should 'stay empty for the next ten years' since the British government was 'spurring the birth rate by paying parents five shillings ($1) per week for each child except the first'. The Pope indirectly criticised her proposals.

In his confidential letter Haire offered to give Pillay examples of people 'who had to conform, or else' although he thought 'that group' (the medical fraternity) was doing good work in its own peculiar way and he had no wish to hamper its general activities. He sometimes challenged their views but was mostly content to go on working on his own, and thought that Pillay should do the same. He had written twice to the anthropologist George Pitt-Rivers who promised his article was coming, but it had not arrived. Kenneth Walker, professor of surgery and secretary of the British Social Hygiene Association, had written to him on another matter and in his reply Haire mentioned *Marriage Hygiene* but he did not reply either, nor had Professor Crew, a 'very old friend of more than 20 years' standing'. He felt there had been a 'suggestion' from 'higher up' that cooperation with Pillay was 'regarded with disfavour'. Pillay was a captain in World War I and had an OBE so Haire was naïve not to realise that *he* was the target of this disfavour.

Haire had several phone conversations with Françoise Lafitte-Cyon and they corresponded about her Havelock Ellis reminiscences, *Friendship's odyssey*, which she wrote as Françoise Delisle. Haire wished she had been explicit about Ellis' 'anomaly' (urolagnia, the fetish of gaining sexual pleasure from watching women urinate). She was offended by this remark and by his suggestion that others should also record their memories of Ellis. He had mentioned Margaret Sanger, 'Andrew Scott' [perhaps Mneme or Faith Oliver who had an affair with him in 1926] and Marjorie Ross who 'could contribute a strange and interesting chapter in his life – a love-affair between a man and a woman who had never actually met'.[6] This was as much an 'affair' as those he had with other women and Haire speculated that there was seldom or

---

6 Havelock Ellis treasured the photograph Marjorie Ross took of Sparkes Creek and featured it in his autobiography and kept it beside his bed. She had travelled to the area near Scone where he taught in a bush school and had captured the 'soft rounded sandstone boulder that lay, a little mass of brown, on the dull green slope' in which he had his erotic awakening. It is also the frontispiece of his book *Kanga creek: an Australian idyll*.

never anything which could technically be described as 'a breach of the Seventh Commandment'.

Haire replied briefly to Françoise, knowing that any letter would annoy her and he did not want to upset 'such a dear friend' of the man he greatly admired and owed a deep debt of gratitude. In response, she sent a subscription for *Marriage Hygiene* and an article she had written for it, both of which he acknowledged and forwarded to Pillay in Bombay. Haire told her they did not pay contributors and explained that he was 'not only writing articles' but arranging all the secretarial work in England to be done and paying for it 'even though he could ill afford it'. When she asked to see his review before publication he sensibly refused because 'one should review a book on the book's own merits'. He submitted his review of *Friendship's Odyssey* to *Time and Tide*, a respected British weekly which supported literary talent, and explained to Françoise that while he was interested in what she wrote, if he had to 'refrain carefully from saying anything' that might hurt her feelings, it would be quite impossible to make 'any sort of frank criticism'.

Haire wrote again to assure her about her book's historical importance and said that, although its publication might cause embarrassing complications during her life, posterity would benefit. Haire thought he 'did not over-rate the importance of the anomaly' and would thank God for it (if he believed in a God), because he doubted that, if Havelock Ellis had been perfectly 'normal', that he would have chosen his lifework and brought relief to hundreds of thousands, perhaps millions of unhappy men and women. The same applies to the link between Haire's work and his 'anomaly'. Haire was sure that Marjorie Ross would never write about Ellis because she was 'a shy retiring little thing, rather like a nice mouse'. The friendship was the love of her life, 'her *secret* glory' and no one else knew her secret. Ellis had mentioned Haire's name in some of his letters to her, and, when she discovered that he went to Sydney's public library regularly, she grasped the opportunity of speaking to somebody who knew him. Haire asked if 'another woman' Françoise mentioned was the one whose 'maliciously witty' accounts were 'more like a clever caricature than a photograph'. He meant Ethel Mannin.

Lafitte-Cyon was riled by Haire's foolish comment that Ellis must have been 'a pain in the neck to live with'. Perhaps in the hope of calming her, Haire described himself as being hard to live with and, in a comment which sheds light on his relationship with Willem van de Hagt, said he preferred the everyday company of 'phlegmatic, bovine persons' while 'reserving highly complicated and neurotic people for an occasional, though essential, stimulus'. In verbose rage Lafitte-Cyon denied any incompatibility and said that she and Ellis 'fitted each other'; the 'way was always certain and easy'; she said that Haire was 'too intellectual, too Freudian'; he analysed 'negatively' and that he could not 'synthesize positively, which is the way of love'. She agreed there might be a valuable story about the 'distant loves of an old man' but Ross was only 'one of three' and Ellis destroyed all her letters and she wanted to spare her this knowledge. Only she could write the story despite the lack of Marjorie's letters, many of which she had read. The 'affair' was of little importance to her because Marjorie was at the antipodes and she had been at his side. 'However, author should not write to critic (though you started it). This is the last'. Although she dreaded going to London, she 'might' see him for a talk in the second week of September.

After this petulance, Françoise was forced to be civil when she wanted to beg a favour: she wanted him to suggest a good gynaecologist for her son and his wife who lived in Melbourne. Haire replied that 'there was no hatchet to bury' on his part and pointed out that as Melbourne was 600 miles from Sydney he 'wasn't in close touch' with gynaecologists there but suggested that her son should ring Dr Wallace, mention his name and ask Wallace to give a recommendation. This was her final letter but she continued to clash with him and sent Dr Pillay a stinging criticism of Haire's obituary for Havelock Ellis. She said Haire was 'not hampered by false prudery' and 'his interpretation was out of focus'; she was 'amazed' by his 'audacity', although 'one is grateful' to him 'for making it plain that Ellis was not a Freudian.' She kept her sharpest barb till last: 'an article such as Norman Haire's, for all its good points (and there are several) causes me fully to understand Ellis' lack of congeniality [with Haire]'.

Haire also asked Hugh de Selincourt to write about Havelock Ellis but this novelist and cricket commentator declined. He explained to Margaret Sanger who was a lover:

> I can't do that; it would merely get poor Françoise on her tragic silly warpath and raise an unseemly squabble and queer the pitch for the book. But he wants to meet me, and says he will gladly drive down here, so along he is colossally coming. As I am fascinated by difference in people, and there is no doubt of his reverence for Havelock, though his physical presence was intensely distasteful to him. (14 March 1948. MSP – Smith S28)

His note stressed Françoise's irrationality and gave the reason why Ellis disliked Haire. If he was repulsed by Haire's bulk, others probably shared his gut reaction and, although few would admit to this prejudice, it often expanded into a dislike of his body and soul. But had he been slim, his apologia for sexual reform would still have enraged many people. De Selincourt sent a more charitable note to Sanger after Haire visited him in Sussex, saying that what she said about Haire strongly appealed to him. 'There is something simple and dear about him' and he enjoyed their talk about Havelock Ellis, although he 'could not help being wildly tickled by a whole lot of his attitude'.

Haire was sufficiently broad-minded and generous to publish Françoise's anti-artificial insemination diatribe later in the *JSE* but, after it appeared and Françoise sent a letter to correct the people who disagreed with her views, Haire responded pointedly in a footnote that the letter was her personal view and that the journal was 'in no way committed' to such a view; it was 'apparent from her stigmatisation of artificial insemination as "crazy" that she approached the matter 'emotionally, and not objectively' but those familiar with her *Friendship's odyssey*, or her other writings would not 'expect objectivity from her – Editor'.

Pillay informed Himes that Haire's statement about articles being held up for comments was false and that it had only applied when Haire's review of *Friendship's odyssey* had been sent to Françoise for comment. Pillay's action, in sending Haire's review to her, was either misguided or a deliberate attempt to undermine him. Pillay told Himes that many people would contribute if Haire was not the British editor. Pillay ended melodramatically: 'If he can't get on with me, he and I must part.' This was hypocritical because Pillay was trying to sever his links with Haire.

Pillay's letter from *Marriage Hygiene*'s Australian editor, Dr Wallace, in May warned him to 'drop' Haire as editor and that Dr Babbage told him that Haire's association with it was 'the real reason' why he had refused to join the editorial board in Australia. A friend of Wallace's (a consulting physician in Sydney) said he didn't think the journal would go down well in Sydney because Haire was associated with it and 'his name stinks in Sydney'. Various people had written to Wallace, including Blacker, making references to Haire in 'strictly confidential' terms and he thought that if Pillay had a 'highly respected' English editor they would receive many more literary contributions from Australia. Ironically, a decade earlier Wallace had suffered from the same kind of character assassination that he was now applying to Haire.[7]

The man who declined to be involved with the journal because of its links with Haire was Canon Stuart Barton Babbage, a former Dean of St Andrew's Cathedral who later helped run Billy Graham's Sydney evangelical crusades. When Babbage published his memoirs in 2004 he was described as a 'loose cannon' and a 'wayward dean' who was 'fiercely committed to social justice and the acceptance of the dignity of all minorities in society'. In 2008 I asked Babbage about the 1948 discussions and he said he 'did not know Dr Haire personally' and did not remember Wallace but knew that Haire had 'a mixed reputation'. His only recollection was the report of a young man who was sent by his mother to Dr Haire for sex education but then alleged that Haire had masturbated him. The young man was homosexual and was 'later in trouble for sex offences' and so his report should be 'taken with caution'.

This indicates that a whispering campaign was at work to oust Haire and the reply Himes sent Pillay in May 1948 shows that he too had

---

7 When Dr Wallace asked for help from Britain's Eugenics Society to start a eugenics society in Victoria in 1938 they asked members to spy on him and 'Informant C' [Sir James Barrett] said he was 'a sincere and ethical, but rather unstable enthusiast. Rather neatly, saying that his character is conveyed by his Christian names, which are Victor Hugo!' (Wyndham 2003, 128–29).

no qualms about accepting these rumours and spreading them. Himes imagined what Babbage said about Haire was true and commented that he had 'a lot of enemies' which might not be deserved but felt there must be some fire with 'all that smoke' because RL Dickinson, who was not 'squeamish', would have nothing to do with him in the 1930s. Perhaps this was in retaliation to Haire's comments to Himes that Dickinson 'was not the man for detail' which Himes had relayed to him.

Himes thought Haire had 'raised a furore in Australia' and imagined that 'personality' was the trouble: 'ego drive and perhaps a certain lack of refinement plus a marked lack of tact in dealing with sexual questions'. In 1940s Australia it was easy to create moral outrage because sex was a topic that should not be discussed in polite conversation. Despite the help and hospitality Himes had received from Haire, he distanced himself by saying, 'I hardly knew him intimately'. He also tried to blame Pillay and told him, if he looked over their correspondence, he would see Himes had never had approved the appointment of Haire – 'but you had to go ahead on your own and did not consult me'.

Himes said that he liked the 'tactful and appreciative' letter Pillay sent Haire in which he explained his 'very painful' decision to close the journal's London office because it had not been sent any original articles except for Haire's 'brilliant contributions'. Pillay acknowledged Haire's generous help during the previous 14 months but said he had to consider finances and the journal's survival and he hoped Haire would 'understand [his] side of the question and forgive'. He knew that, 'as far as energy, efficiency and professional knowledge' were concerned, Haire's place could not be filled and that was why he was not making any effort to do it. Pillay signed it with his grateful thanks and warm personal regards. His appreciation was totally insincere and he added in his letter to Himes: 'even Haire's best friends advised me that *Marriage Hygiene* would be better in the British Isles and even elsewhere without him'. Pillay then contradicted himself by saying, 'He has no friends in England now and is practically a stranger. He himself has asked me to announce that he is resigning due to pressure of work!! That problem has therefore solved itself'.

Haire had many good friends but he may have become a stranger to Pillay after the *Marriage Hygiene* rift. Haire was also unwell, living outside London and busy establishing *The Journal of Sex Education (JSE)*. When the first issue appeared in August 1948 it included a eulogy for the WLSR which had served as a coordinating body for various associations working for sexual reform. The WLSR was mainly involved in the fields of education and it was an intellectual and scholarly organisation which did not exert pressure on governments in petitions, demonstrations or press campaigns (Tamagne 2004, 115). It had multiple aims and an amorphous structure, which explains why it failed, whereas Sanger's successful one-theme birth control strategy led to the founding of the International Planned Parenthood Federation in the early 1950s (Dose 2003, 11).

After the WLSR disbanded, the League's national sections agreed to continue independently: the British section became the Sex Education Society (SES) and continued its activities until the outbreak of the World War II. It was dormant for eight years and then 'came back to life in the autumn of 1947.' Haire gave a disingenuous disclaimer: 'The Journal has no official connection with the Sex Education Society, though the Editor of the one at present happens to be the President of the other'. In reality, both were dependent on his drive and financial backing and both ceased with his death in 1952. Ralf Dose (2003, 5) blamed the complex nature of their objectives as another factor in the WLSR's failure: 'It offered something for and by everyone'.

Two American academics reached a similar conclusion in their study of 'Sex as a scholarly discipline' which 'began in the last years of the 19th century'. They found that sexology journals had 'an ambiguous audience' and although Hirschfeld, Havelock Ellis, Haire and Bloch 'could perhaps be called sexologists', most researchers were also known in other fields, for instance in biology (Alfred Kinsey), psychoanalysis (Sigmund Freud), law (Ben Lindsey) or philosophy (Bertrand Russell and René Guyon). Sexual studies were multidisciplinary and the rewards mainly went to those who published in their own professional journals. Many did not want the stigma of being called a sexologist. Their one common bond was their 'recognition of the need for sex education', but they could not agree whether to aim at the professional educator or the general public (Elcano & Bullough 1981, 75, 77).

In addition to the *Marriage Hygiene* strife, a letter to Margaret Sanger revealed that Haire had financial worries. He hoped she might help her old colleague Edith How-Martyn who was terribly ill when he saw her while he was in Australia and was still sick and poor. Edith 'had no suspicion' he was writing, although if his finances had been as good as they were before the war he would have sent her regular assistance. Unfortunately, his 'practice had all but disappeared' while he was in Australia and, although it had 'picked up far more quickly' than he expected, his expenses were 'two or three times as great as they were before the war, and repairs and replacements ran into many thousands of pounds'. He was talking about 127 Harley Street and Nettleden Lodge, both of which were requisitioned during the war and had been extensively damaged. He would get a 'small part of this back' as compensation but until then he had to cut down his expenditure (9 September 1948 – Smith S28, 754).

Marriage Hygiene also had problems; it was revamped as *The International Journal of Sexology* in August 1948 and ceased altogether in May 1955. Haire's review of Pillay's book (*JSE*, February 1949, 162–65) suggests that he knew what had been happening when he wrote that 'in view of the paper shortage' and publishers' backlog it was 'deplorable that good material and labour' had been wasted on the book. He said it was impossible 'to indicate more than a fraction of the defects and errors of Dr Pillay's book' and his comment, 'his attitude towards sexual matters is tolerant, liberal and enlightened', was code for 'he means well but...'

Haire, in his role as president of the Sex Education Society, continued to lobby for abortion and sterilisation law reform and, in *The Lancet* on 23 October 1948, discussed the distressing example of a pregnant 31-year-old 'mentally deficient and unstable' woman: the family doctor and two psychiatrists had testified that she was unfit to raise a child and recommended both abortion and sterilisation. Although Haire agreed with them, he wanted to be sure he was not risking a criminal charge or a civil action and asked the Secretary of the Medical Defence Union for advice. After exhaustive discussions they had 'very reluctantly' decided that neither of these operations would be safe for them to carry out from a legal point of view and that nothing could be done for the woman because the laws forbidding abortion and sterilisation were 'far from clear'. Haire pleaded, 'is is not time that the profession should move for the alteration of laws relating to abortion and sterilisation?'

As well as editing and writing articles and reviews for the *JSE*, Haire ran his practice, chaired meetings of the Sex Education Society, wrote his weekly column for *Woman* and maintained his links with friends. When the progressive educator AS Neill mentioned his interest in a book that George Ives had written in 1939, Haire arranged for him to get a copy of it although it was ten years since it had been published. Neill thanked Ives for the gift of his book which was waiting for him at Haire's house and said that Ives' erudition was 'wonderful' and that he had been engrossed in the book on his train trip home (Croall 1983, 331). Between 1892 and 1949, Ives had filled 45 scrapbooks with press-clipping reports of crimes, punishments and homosexuality; Haire did the same on a more modest scale[8] and a similarly voyeuristic collection, made from 1832 to 1869 by a Scottish Laird, forms the basis of Thomas Boyle's 1990 book with a wonderfully melodramatic title *Black swine in the sewers of Hampstead: beneath the surface of Victorian sensationalism*.

Haire's interests were wide-ranging and he gave his views about Britain's publicly funded National Health Service (NHS) which was launched in July 1948. He told his Australian readers of *Woman* that, 'as a specialist of 30 years' standing', he could afford to stay out of the NHS but most general practitioners and many specialists had to take part in it or face financial ruin. He said reports of the scheme's operation were gloomy; the NHS doctors were 'frightfully overworked' by the 'free' (tax-supported) scheme; it encouraged people to visit with trivial complaints and disadvantaged really sick patients. Although Haire stayed out of the scheme as a doctor, he had to go into it as a patient which meant that he no longer had to pay for the insulin, needles and syringes for his diabetes. The NHS also paid for the treatment of his chronic winter-long colds – 'medicines to be taken internally, mixtures to be inhaled, drops to be instilled into the nose' – but he was soon to place demands

---

8   Press cuttings from English newspapers on birth control, sexual crimes and deviations. London. Bulk 1913–1949. 13 vol (HC – Related Materials).

on the service as a seriously ill hospitalised patient; he had suffered from angina since 1944 and his heart problems were becoming worse.

Once more, he used his column in *Woman* to describe his experience as a hospital patient and recommended it as something every doctor should experience. He had a serious heart attack in early 1950 and, although he praised the accommodation and the treatment, he hated the food: he said the meat was usually overcooked and tasteless; there was very little fruit and the vegetables, and it was often swedes and turnips, which he loathed and called 'animal food'. He lost weight because the food was revolting but felt there was no excuse for such poorly cooked and unappetising food. For the next 14 months he maintained a very restricted diet and dropped from 19 stone 4 lbs (124 kilograms) to 15 stone (95.25 kilograms) because he had to reduce the load on his heart by 20 percent. He said he felt better but lacked energy and needed to rest frequently.

When Betty Roland (1990, 149–50) visited him in London, she was shocked to see he was 'reduced to a ghost of himself' and looked pale and haggard, with his clothes hanging loosely and his collar several sizes too large. Despite this, he still had the same zeal when he bounded into lecture halls to deliver his public lectures. He maintained an actor's bravura but he sometimes overstated his credentials; for instance, in the 1950 edition of *Who's Who in Australia*, as well as giving his qualifications and achievements, he listed such mundane credentials as being a Freeman of the City of London (available for a fee); a Fellow of the Royal Society of Medicine (available to doctors, dentists and vets); and a member of the BMA (the professional association for doctors) and the Harveian Society of London (a history of medicine group which commemorated William Harvey). It was not hard to join the clubs he mentioned in London (The City Livery Club) and Sydney (the Masonic Club and the Royal Automobile Club of Australia). He may have deliberately exaggerated his credentials in a bid to persuade people to come forward and finance his lecture tours or request him to lecture.

He continued his association with Allen & Unwin and, in early 1951, sent them a report about a German book *Schule der Liebe* (*School of love*) by 'Diotima', which in Greek means complete woman or love goddess. Haire strongly advised them not to translate the book because it was too old, showed no outstanding merit or value and because, instead of using terms such as vagina and penis, the author chose words such as 'love-muscle' which Haire said was like calling the female genitals 'pussy'. He felt it was 'extremely likely that the book would be prosecuted on account of the combination of unsuitable language, frankness and sentimental style'. He described it as inaccurate and old-fashioned and said America had produced many better books which they might consider reprinting.

A few days later Haire sent them an indignant letter because they had sent him a cheque for £1.11.6 as a reading fee. He returned it and was 'not sure if it was an error or an insult' because he could not get an ordinary typist who knew German to read a book of that length for such a small sum. He argued that it should have been at least ten guineas and said he would rather have nothing than the amount offered. The publisher said they could not pay that amount to the people they employed as readers of the thousands of books they received each year and still remain solvent. Then the publisher capitulated and asked Haire, 'May we amicably settle this unfortunate business by sending you five guineas with our apologies?'

Haire once received a friendly letter signed 'Member' complaining about his short-comings when he chaired a Sex Education Society meeting about the sex lives of unmarried adults. Haire said it started late and was derailed by speeches about animal copulation and married people's sex life. Surprisingly, Member wanted Haire to be more assertive:

> The chairman has the right and the duty to cut short any question or statement that is irrelevant. He should make the different speakers STICK TO THE POINT! You don't . . . Also you are naïve indeed if you do not realise that 'moralists' and so-called religious people, especially the Catholics, send along people to your meetings whose job it is to obstruct and prevent us getting the enlightenment we so sorely need. [Knowing] how easy-going you are [they] come with long speeches and questions that are outside the subject and take up a mass of time and divert our thoughts from the real subject. We admire your courage and your will to help us but please let us have another chairman or woman of decisive

action. One can be perfectly courteous while being firm – Stick to the point. Keep up the good work – but get the right assistance. (5 April 1949. HC – 3.25)

The complainant said Haire was 'easy-going' and so he was – with his friends. Haire was always interested to hear his opponents' views and would listen politely even if they were filibustering, but while he may have been an exasperating moderator he was never timid. Patrick O'Connor told me a story about Haire's kindness to his father, Paddy O'Connor. The men had met in the 1930s, as members of the Abortion Reform Society, and in the 1940s, encouraged by Haire, Paddy started a publishing company.[9] Patrick knew from the way his father talked that Haire was a fine man who believed in the right of every human to live in freedom, according to his or her own choice. Patrick's mother had been unwell for several years in the 1940s – one pregnancy had to be terminated and a baby had died a few weeks after birth. Haire became her obstetrician and Patrick was safely delivered during a London heatwave in September 1949. During her pregnancy, Haire had sent his chauffeur round to the O'Connor's place with a delicacy made by his Viennese cook; it was a *dobosh-torte* (a multi-layered Hungarian sponge cake with chocolate, cream, nuts and topped with toffee), a real treat and a triumph to produce in the midst of postwar sugar rationing. This gift to an anxious couple became a family legend. Haire was very practical and, as there was no refrigerator in the house, on the day of the birth, he ordered blocks of ice to be delivered and put in the bath so that he could have cold drinks while he worked: at that time home births were common but refrigerators were rare (O'Connor, 8 September 2006).

In 1998 Haire's niece Gloria Savill told me about a secret act of generosity when her father 'Bertie' was a farmer in Queensland during the 1940s. She was about ten years old when Haire 'sent an underprivileged boy' to their farm. As far as she could remember, he was about 14-years-old and had been very sick. Haire told her mother to 'fatten him up and cook him a rabbit every day.' The 'boy would eat a

---

9   The company was moderately successful and its main publication was a journal called *Medical Digest* whose editorial board 'probably included surgeons and physicians of Haire's acquaintance' (O'Connor 2005).

whole baked rabbit every day by himself', and when he went back to the city he was so fat she didn't think his mother would have known him'. She guessed 'Dr Haire had another side to him'.

In London Haire lent his Rolls Royce, complete with his chauffeur dressed in livery, so that Averil Fink (Lotte Fink's daughter-in-law) could make an impressive appearance at a Buckingham Palace garden party.[10] He also calmed her during her first pregnancy after a doctor in a National Health hospital said that her baby had two heads. When her husband phoned in panic, Haire scolded them because 'you can't expect anything better than that in a NHS hospital' and then ordered an X-Ray which showed a healthy baby. His generosity, in giving a set of fish knives and forks with ivory handles to this couple, who were at the time living in shared accommodation and eating on packing cases, could be seen as either gauche or as an encouragement to aspire to better things.

A timid person would not have tackled the Archbishop of Canterbury and Haire did this – twice. Reports of assisted pregnancies had appeared in medical journals in the 1940s and, in response, the Archbishop of Canterbury set up a commission on artificial insemination, and the *British Medical Journal* reported on 11 September 1948 that they had called for the procedure to be made a crime. Haire felt that artificial insemination was preferable to adoption and wrote in rage to the journal after the commissioners had reported that 'the evils necessarily involved in artificial insemination (donor) are so grave that early consideration should be given to the framing of legislation to make the practice *a criminal offence*' (Haire added the italics). He described their suggestion 'as a monstrous impertinence'; he did 'not question the right of any Church to lay down rules for the conduct of its own members.' However, he found it 'intolerable in a free community' for any Church to compel citizens who were *not* members to conform to its standards of behaviour. 'We inveigh against the tyranny of totalitarian States, Nazi, Fascist, or Communist. The tyranny that the Churches would exercise, if they had the power, would be no less totalitarian. It is for all thinking men and women to be ever on watch that the Churches do not obtain

---

10   Ruth Latukefu showed me the translation of her mother Lotte Fink's 20 July 1948 letter from Haire which mentioned this.

such power.' The journal published four letters of religious outrage and one which challenged the suggestion that AI was adulterous. The British government did not ban AI but stated that it was 'undesirable and not to be encouraged'.

Haire gave steely support for condom-vending machines outside chemist shops, despite the pandemonium their installation had caused. The Archbishop of Canterbury stated that 'the uncontrolled purveying of contraceptives' from slot-machines 'had caused the greatest horror and indignation' (*The Times*, 13 October 1949). The following day the Association of Municipal Councils sent the Prime Minister and members of parliament their resolution that such sales were 'harmful and dangerous to the individual and the State and especially to young people.' A week later the Home Secretary Chuter Ede (who became Baron Ede for his humanitarian services) was cheered when he announced in the House of Commons that a 'model by-law', making it an offence to sell contraceptives from street vending machines, would be circulated to all country and county borough authorities and it was duly proclaimed. *The Times* did not publish Haire's protests and it also pointedly ignored the campaigns of Marie Stopes, Margaret Sanger and Alfred Kinsey.

The Washington Post was more liberal and reported on 21 October that Dr Norman Haire 'regarded the proposed ban on the sale of prophylactics from automatic machines with dismay. The articles are sometimes used as contraceptives, but are used much more frequently as preventives against disease. We need increased productivity and productivity can be adversely affected if venereal disease increases'. He was also quoted in the 21 October issue of *The Chicago Daily Tribune* which shied away from mentioning VD and omitted the final sentence.

At least Haire had the opportunity to give a full and funny account in the *JSE* and said that the 'wowsers' had been making a great fuss about the sale of condoms from automatic machines and that Mr Chute Ede had 'capitulated to them'. Many of his readers may not have been familiar with this Australian slang for 'a censorious person; a killjoy' but they would have sensed Haire's annoyance at his disapproving opponents' insistence on describing condoms as contraceptives which was the truth, but not the whole truth. The condom frequently was used as a contraceptive but just as often it was used to prevent venereal disease. During the war wowsers had 'foamed at the mouth and screamed shrilly that the authorities were encouraging immorality by providing "contraceptives" for the troops'. But the government put national security first and declined to forbid the issue of condoms. Now 'Archbishops and lesser fry' were again foaming at the mouth because condoms were being sold from automatic machines, so that the public could buy them when the ordinary sources of supply were shut. If their efforts persuaded many local authorities to ban the sales, 'an alarming increase in the incidence of venereal disease' would follow.

He was absolutely certain about one thing: 'The majority of men and women cannot be rendered sexually abstinent by force' and, although from puberty at about the age of 14, people were ripe for marriage or mating, most people could not marry till five, ten or more years later. But it was just during adolescence and early adulthood that the natural physiological sex urge was at its strongest and as Professor Kinsey's recent researches have shown, sexual activity is greatest at this period, too. Young people cannot, or will not, remain sexually abstinent for long years and it was not desirable that they should. However, if they engaged in sexual activity, it was desirable that it should not harm society; 'if illegitimate children are considered undesirable, then the production of illegitimate children may be avoided by the use of contraception'. The 'true patriot' would press for the multiplication of these automatic machines. 'It is only those who pay allegiance to some Mumbo-Jumbo in the sky who will prefer to see men and women, who break an outworn taboo, pay for their "sin" by acquiring venereal disease'. Haire continued 'it must be remembered that, the more the healthy adults abstain from moderate heterosexual intercourse, the more they will indulge in substitute sexual activities – auto-erotic, homosexual, or of other kinds condemned by conventional standards. Do the wowsers think these substitute activities more desirable than ordinary heterosexual intercourse?' They would have been riled by Haire's comments and outraged by the wit and irrefutable logic of his final paragraph.

Australia seemed to be replaying Haire's 1949 battle for condoms in 1999, after the Victorian premier allowed condom-vending machines in state high schools. Opposing views were debated on ABC Radio and Professor Gabor Kovaks, representing the Family Planning Association, reminded listeners there had been uproar when condoms were first sold in supermarkets but 'now you don't look twice at them.' In his opinion, 'Contraception should be as freely available as possible. Contraception does not lead to sexual activity. And the lack of contraception does not prevent sexual activity. So if we accept the fact that young people are going to be sexually active, let's do our very best to have them practising safe sex, not having unplanned pregnancies, and not catching sexually transmitted diseases' (ABC Radio National, 25 October 1999). His irrefutable logic resembles Haire's comments such as 'Men and women cannot be rendered sexually abstinent by force' and 'Women over the age of consent should not be condemned to sexual starvation against their will'. However, Kovaks could speak freely without having to fear that his words would bring retribution.

Britain's Abortion Law Reform Association began campaigning in 1936 and was invigorated by the historic 1938 legal decision in favour of Dr Bourne, but things moved more slowly in Australia. Haire received a plea in 1948 for help in setting up a similar group and sent this sensible reply from London, reprinted in *Everyday sex problems* (1948, 75):

> I think it would be an excellent thing if a Society for Reform of the Abortion Law was founded in Australia, but I feel that such a society should be started by women themselves. I have done quite enough pioneering, and borne[11] quite enough of the heat and burden of the day. Now, in my middle fifties, I feel that somebody else can take on part of the ungrateful task. I should be very happy to do what I could to help.

Haire wrote an article on abortion in Australia in the February–March 1950 issue of the *JSE* stating he had performed an abortion

---

11 Dr CW LaSalle commented (2001) that Haire's choice of 'borne' was probably a word-play reference to the abortion hero Dr Aleck Bourne. Australian feminists did not take up the challenge for reform; in the wake of Britain's liberalising 1967 Abortion Act, the Humanist Society of NSW established the Abortion Law Reform Association in 1968.

once during the six years he was there, on a woman whose life was at risk because rheumatic fever had badly damaged her heart. Even so, her heart specialist had only reluctantly provided Haire with the written certificate he needed to operate. In Britain he performed many abortions which he mentioned when the *BMJ* published a series of letters about abortions and psychoneurosis in 1949. Haire, in response to Aleck Bourne's letter, said he had only seen one fatality in 34 years and 'in his 19 years' experience of injecting paste into the uterus under a general anaesthetic' he had never before seen any sign of shock. He was referring to the death of a 19-year-old woman who was about 28 weeks pregnant and was referred by her doctor and a psychiatrist who stated she was mentally disturbed and suicidal. Haire followed his usual abortion procedure but she died of shock about 15 minutes after the operation. He reported her death to the coroner and, following an inquest, a jury returned a verdict of death 'by misadventure.'

When Haire looked back on the crime- and health-related consequences of illegal abortions in Australia before World War I, he said these were exacerbated after World War II by the anti-abortion laws which aimed to increase the birthrate. Because of them, well-qualified doctors dared not operate and women were forced to take abortifacients or make clandestine visits to nurses or doctors who were often incompetent or drunk and sometimes both. Haire called for abortions to be performed by competent persons under better conditions. The 'Haire was an abortionist' rumour was rejected by two doctors I spoke to in 1999 who were in practice in the 1940s: Dr Lachlan Lang, who in the 1970s helped to set up Preterm, a legally sanctioned abortion clinic in Sydney, and Dr Rod Bretherton who ran a pioneering medical clinic in Melbourne and wrote a book about the abortifacient *RU 486*. Since the medical profession was very parochial, these two 'abortion-friendly' men would have known if Haire *had* performed abortions in Australia.

Haire included a book review by Ivor Montagu in the *JSE* but distanced himself from his old friend by calling him 'one of the most prominent and distinguished Communists in this country'. He explained that the reason for having it reviewed by 'an avowed Communist' was to show readers the Soviet point of view. He considered his words carefully and wondered if the reviewer's explanations were rationalisations, and 'whether the explanation, or part of it at any rate, may not more easily be found in the USSR's fear (whether that fear is well or ill-founded) of conflict with the Western Powers' (*JSE*, August–September 1949, 1).

However, there was nothing coy about the question and answer section of his subscription-only *The Journal of Sex Education* which gave him licence to tell people everything they wanted to know about homosexuality but were afraid to ask. One woman asked detailed questions about the mechanics of homosexuality and wanted to know if a woman could 'unwittingly marry one' and whether homosexuals were born or made. He provided lengthy clinical descriptions of homosexual sexual activity and said some homosexuals were effeminate in manner, speech, or gesture but others did not excite suspicion about their sexuality. Some homosexuals were women haters but others felt more at ease with them and it was quite common for women to feel that such men 'understand' them and so fall in love with them. It was quite possible for a woman to marry a homosexual man unwittingly and 'unfortunately this happens quite often and the outcome is usually unhappy'. Lesbians were female homosexuals and mild degrees of homosexuality were probably more common in women than men because physical endearments between women attracted less attention than it would between men. Also, the criminal code makes male homosexual acts a punishable offence, but takes no notice of homosexual acts between females. He asked, 'have you never read *The well of loneliness* by Radcliffe Hall?' (*JSE*, December 1949–January 1950, 125–26). Few people have read this wordy novel which became famous after it was prosecuted for obscene libel.

Haire reacted strongly when a woman complained that 'queries from homosexuals sound so terribly apologetic! Do homosexuals *never* have the courage of their own convictions! Do they never stand up for themselves?' He was a little bewildered by her outburst because he had never said that homosexual activities were immoral or unnatural; although any sexual activity might be immoral if it infringed another person's sexual rights, but that was also true of heterosexual relationships. To him the word *unnatural* had very little meaning and she seemed to consider the 'use of contraceptives as unnatural!' He said these were no more unnatural than such things as reading glasses which many people used in our 'unnatural' civilisation. She had commented that sexual activities with her friend *would* be unnatural, if they had not restricted them to fondling the bodies which 'God gave' them. Haire said her implied condemnation of dildos seemed 'very narrow-minded' but he was used to this and that most people approved of their own sexual activity but found other people's sexual activity immoral or unnatural. She claimed that they only started their relationship because they could not find marriage partners and because heterosexual intercourse outside marriage was too risky. He dismissed this as a rationalisation and said they were 'inclined to homosexuality' and, if they wanted to publish their homosexuality 'from the housetops', they should do so. But this would cause 'a good deal of inconvenience and unpleasantness' because there were 'very obstinate prejudices' about this and it would be very disagreeable, and perhaps even disastrous, for them to wantonly challenge public opinion. He was outlining his own strategy when he suggested that it would be 'much wiser to do what you can, gradually and carefully to alter public opinion' to counteract these prejudices in a gradual process of re-education on sex problems in general, and homosexuality in particular. He said they would be wise to support all movements with this aim and ended with the sarcastic suggestion that she might like to become a subscriber to the journal or 'even make a donation' (*JSE*, December 1951–January 1952, 134–36).

He was *very* supportive and his journal reprinted the ten-page transcript of an 'historic moment' when a panel discussion of homosexuality was sponsored by Saks, the department store, and broadcast in 1948 by a private New York radio station. The sympathetic discussion was led by Professor J Raymond Walsh (an economist and radio commentator) and the five eminent panel members came from the fields of law, psychiatry, politics, religion and sexology. It was the medium not the message that provided the radical breakthrough; Haire commented that there was 'nothing very profound, and nothing very new in what the speakers said about homosexuality itself' but 'what is important and surprising is that it was possible to make such a broadcast at all'. It was made possible by the 'courage and vision' of Josiah P Marvel who was the 'moving spirit' behind the Quakers' rehabilitation service for young homosexual prisoners. Haire praised them and said that 'Here, in England, where no Commercial stations exist, where the BBC has a monopoly, and where broadcasting suffers under the dead hand of the Churches, such a broadcast would at the present time be unthinkable' (*JSE*, November 1949, 49). Nor could it have been made in Australia.

Shortly before his death Haire discussed British hypocrisy about homosexuality. He agreed it was understandable for people to pretend to know nothing about a prominent person's homosexuality while the person was alive, but 'we continue the practice long after they are dead. Even though they themselves have made the truth quite plain, between the lines, in their writings, biographers and critics carefully refrain from any reference to the existence of a sexual variation which may have exercised a predominating influence on the writers' works'. He acknowledged that people were beginning to admit that 'Swinburne's sexual life was not completely orthodox'. He refrained from mentioning some equally striking examples, among persons recently deceased, because many had been his patients. Haire attempted to lift this embargo in a six-page review of a biography of Florence Nightingale.

He reviewed three books for the April–May 1952 issue of the *JSE*.[12] The first two reviews appeared but not the third one about Nightingale which was apparently too shocking to publish. She had died in 1910 so sufficient time had elapsed and, because of her importance in English history, he felt that a sexologist was 'justified in dotting the i's and crossing the t's' of the implications in the 1950 biography about her written by Mrs Cecil Woodham-Smith. He thought there was no doubt that Florence Nightingale suffered severely from guilt and feelings of inferiority due to her sexual fantasies and her worry about masturbation. Her 'anxiety' and 'feeling of sinfulness' brought her to the 'verge of insanity' after her realisation, quite early, that she was attracted

---

12 HC – 2.16 includes this note: 'April: pages 1–12, *How to improve your sexual relations* (Hirsch); *Chose the sex of your children* (Benedict); *Florence Nightingale* – sent to Mr Wood 14.12.51'. The first two reviews appeared in *JSE* April–May 1952, 233–35, but not the Nightingale review.

to other women. 'She was unmistakeably homosexual' although there was no evidence whether 'she ever carried out homosexual *acts*'; but 'no experienced sexologist, after reading this book, can possibly doubt that she was homosexual'. He knew that his diagnosis would produce indignant repudiation from the biographer and many others because 'we English are hypocrites'. Most people prefer to 'shut their eyes to the facts' about Florence Nightingale, as they did in the case of Lawrence of Arabia, Field-Marshall Lord Kitchener, AE Housman and many other important figures in the past century. The suppression of Haire's well-argued review shows that homosexuality in the 1950s was still 'the love which does not dare speak its name'. Haire remained silent about his homosexuality because he could not risk 'coming out' or being seen as 'gay-friendly'. He was speaking from experience; for 40 years the fear of exposure and ruin had forced him to mask his Jewish origins and his sexuality. He could never be himself, he had to act a 'normal' role, onstage and off, and this enforced concealment took a heavy toll.

Throughout his life homosexuals were hounded and the situation became worse after the 1951 Cold War spy scandal in which two Cambridge-educated homosexuals, Guy Burgess and Donald Maclean, defected to the Soviet Union. As a result, many people linked the word 'homosexual' with 'spy' and, when the CIA exerted pressure on Britain to 'take steps', the police obliged by entrapping and arresting men in public places. The postwar period was an anxious time for homosexuals; Jewish homosexuals were doubly stigmatised as thieves and traitors and had even more cause for fear (Loftin 2007, 577). As history professor Nicholas Edsall noted in his excellent survey (2003, 292): 'By mid-1950s the number of arrests and prosecutions for various homosexual offences – sodomy, indecent assault, gross indecency – was five to seven times greater than just before the war.' He discussed the 1953 trial of Lord Montagu of Beaulieu and film director Kenneth Hume on charges of indecently assaulting two boy scouts and the 1954 prosecution of Montagu, his cousin Michael Pitt-Rivers and journalist Peter Wildeblood, for homosexual acts with willing partners, as 'the most notorious case, and ultimately the most important in the anti-homosexual campaign of the early 1950s'. The police leaked details to the press and it was widely believed that 'the real reason for the prosecution was to catch someone with a title, thus making an example and ensuring publicity' (Ferris 1993, 157 and *The Times*, 25 March 1954). The vindictive nature of the case and the subsequent publicity[13] and public outcry led to political action and in September 1957, after a three-year inquiry, the 13-member committee chaired by Sir John Wolfenden concluded that 'outlawing homosexuality impinged on civil liberties' – but their proposals to decriminalise homosexuality were rejected.

Although the aggressive hunting-down of homosexuals ceased, the underlying position remained the same and no one dared say they were homosexual. It took another ten years of intense lobbying before the law permitted sexual relations between adults over the age of 21 – 'in private' but not at all in the Merchant Navy or the Armed Services – and it was not until February 2000 that the British parliament passed a law lowering the age of consent for gay men to 16, the same as for heterosexual adults. Haire had been a quiet catalyst for this reform.

Despite his deteriorating health, Haire was making excited plans for a four-month American lecture tour. Unlike his tours in 1925 and 1934 which were unpaid, in 1951 the Bank of England's monetary restrictions limited his freedom outside New York (where he would be 'the guest of a grateful patient') unless he received fees for his lectures. He told Margaret Sanger on 5 November that both the Chicago and the Montgomery, West Virginia people were going to pay him $150 per lecture and asked if she could suggest him as a speaker at branches of the Planned Parenthood Federation and the Department of Veterans Administration. Haire planned to speak to rationalists, secularists and freethinkers, he might also give radio talks or write for magazines and he would lecture in New York, Chicago and West Virginia and also visit Baltimore and Florida before going to Bloomington, Indiana, to see Kinsey's institute. His talks would cover 'Sex in relation to psychiatry, Contraceptive methods sterilisation and abortion, Sex problems in

---

13 This case inspired a bawdy limerick, sung to the tune of *The twelve days of Christmas*, which includes the line 'Four Boy Scouts' and ends, 'And my Lord Montagu of Beaulieu'.

adolescence, Prostitution, Sex delinquency, Banning of books, Sex variations, Masturbation, A rational attitude towards sex, Sex, sin and sanity, Homosexuality, and Mother or baby? – the Pope's Recent Edict.'

The edict was the directive by Pope Pius XII which banned abortion, sterilisation and artificial insemination, plus another part of his speech aimed at all Catholics, which Protestant countries interpreted to mean that the life of the unborn child was valued more than that of the mother. Haire protested: he had a letter published in *The Lancet* on 9 November 1951 suggesting that NHS patients should choose non-Catholic doctors; he travelled north to speak at a rally of over 800 people in Bradford; and he wrote an editorial in the *JSE* about the global shockwaves from this harsh edict and it was discussed at the Sex Education Society's December meeting. Haire had an unlikely ally in *The Church of England Newspaper* which denounced the edict as 'inhuman, callous and cruel.' Vatican officials said that the Pope's speech 'had been misrepresented because of faulty translations' but the Pope's ambiguous clarification was not reassuring – 'it is the mother who must decide whether she wishes her child to be born at the cost of her life.'

Haire suffered from asthma, an enlarged liver, diabetes, angina and other heart-related ills, and Samuel Oram, his King's College Hospital heart specialist, warned him not to overdo things on his trip because he 'did not have the cardiac reserve to stand a strenuous time' (HC – 3.25). Curiously, Oram did not tell him to cut down on cigarettes which he always bought in bulk. Haire arrived in New York on New Year's Day and his 1952 diary listed a busy schedule with the highlights being his lecture on 11 January 1952, celebratory dinners, the theatre, and meetings with such eminent Americans as the psychoanalyst Franz Cohn; Herman Wells, the President of Indiana University and Kinsey's benefactor; the Benjamins; the Lehfeldts; and Edward Sagarin, who under the pseudonym Donald Webster Cory wrote *The homosexual in America*. On 21 January Harry Benjamin hosted Haire's 60th birthday party and the guest list of sexologists included Hugo Gernsback (who founded the journal *Sexology*) and seven men who later founded the Society for the Scientific Study of Sexuality.[14] The following day Haire

---

14 Benjamin, November 1969. The founders were Hans Lehfeldt, Albert Ellis

was admitted to hospital with acute heart failure and stayed there for eight days; on 7 February he delivered the lectures he was paid for in Montgomery, West Virginia and then travelled 1200 kilometres north to Chicago where he gave afternoon and evening lectures on 19 February to the Department of Veterans Administration. He was to have gone to Florida but was readmitted to hospital instead and had to cancel the rest of the lectures and return home as quickly as possible. Understandably, there were gaps in his diary but on 1 May there was an entry after he landed in Liverpool which itemised the cost of luggage, boat, haircut and a telegram.

Haire's overtaxed heart could not stand the strain and he wrote in the June–July issue of the *JSE*: 'my lecture tour in the United States ended in catastrophe'. He was keenly disappointed about the cancellation and regretted not visiting Alfred Kinsey and his institute in Indiana. However, he was cheered when Kinsey and Benjamin came to see him in hospital. His American friends and colleagues were overwhelmingly hospitable and he was especially indebted in New York to Robert Kronemeyer,[15] a clinical psychologist who had Haire as a house guest, Harry Benjamin, Hans Lehfeldt, Albert Ellis, and Robert Sherwin and, in Chicago to Edwin Hirsch. He also thanked Hugo Gernsback, Donald Webster Cory and Mr RF Stettenheim and 'many others too'. Haire kept copies of their get well greetings, including this one from Alfred Kinsey on 18 July:

> Dr Benjamin writes to me that he has recently heard from you. Unfortunately he reports that you have been very much handicapped, but I want to join him in admiring you for sticking to it. I wish there had been more time to become acquainted. You have done a good job through these years in approaching these problems of sex. I still hope that sometime somewhere we may be able to discuss things more and in greater detail.

(cognitive physiologist), Henry Guze (physiologist), Robert V Sherwin (lawyer), Benjamin and Hugo G Bengel. See sexscience.org.

15 Kronemeyer subsequently developed syntonic therapy delivery of light to the eyes and in 1980 wrote a book which pleased religious groups by claiming that homosexuality is a learned response which can be unlearned.

Robert Kronemyer and his wife reminisced fondly about him and extended an open invitation for his next visit and begged him to 'stay out of that urn, because I'm coming over next summer or BUST. As always, Bob.' Berta Ruck sent a warm-hearted but muddled hand-written note saying she was 'too sorry' to hear what had happened. Like him, she had thought that the USA tour would be such a worthwhile venture, and said how 'Bitter!' it must have been 'to have it crashed by a heart-attack'. She expected they had over-tired him and hoped he would 'soon regain ground in every way'. She gave him news about her brother and made a strange comment: 'I expect you have his biography of Hugh Walpole, I know he was a good friend of yours'.

She was right about their friendship – Walpole lent Haire $1000 in 1940.[16] They were rich ex-patriots (from Australia and New Zealand respectively); had unhappy childhoods; preferred male company; collected books; each owned a Rolls Royce and slept with their chauffeur; were involved with art, theatre and the literary world; spoke German; gave lecture tours; liked eating; were overweight and had diabetes. But she was wrong about the author of *Hugh Walpole: a biography*. In 1998 Sir Rupert Hart-Davis told me her letter was 'a mass of nonsense' because his biography of Walpole 'is the only one there has ever been.' Jeremy Lewis (2004) called it 'a masterpiece of discretion in which his hero's homosexuality was hidden from the old ladies who read Walpole's novels' but allusions to Turkish baths providing 'informal opportunities for meeting interesting strangers' were obvious to those in the know.

Ernst Gräfenberg sent Haire a note dated 4 March 1952[17] expressing his sorrow about Haire's sickness and his disappointment that they could not keep their dinner date in New York. He was glad that Haire felt much better after returning home but he didn't agree with his view that sexual life diminished in old age. Gräfenberg repeated an anecdote about Oliver Wendell Holmes who, as an 80-year-old judge, was walking

---

16 Rupert Hart-Davis (1952, xii) noted in *Hugh Walpole: a biography*, 'I am most grateful to the following friends of Hugh's, to whom I have talked, and who have lent me his letters to them and given me permission to quote from their letters to him: [the list included] Dr Norman Haire'.

17 The letter probably should have been dated 4 July (not March) since it refers to a book review which was published in *JAMA* on 28 June 1952.

with an octogenarian colleague when a pretty girl passed by and Holmes said: 'Oh how wonderful it would be to be 70 again!!' This story has been around since Roman times[18] but it was a good joke to link with Gräfenberg's belief that 'there is no borderline!' when sexual activity ceases, and he mentioned old ladies in his Berlin practice who discussed their sex lives. What Haire said in his letter is unknown but, given his impending death, Haire may have had no sexual desire or ability and felt better if he imagined that others felt the same way, like Sophocles who at 80 rejoiced, 'at last I am free of a cruel and insane master'.

It would be interesting to know what Haire asked about a book written by Hermann Stieve, a German anatomist whose sinister activities were concealed for many years. Gräfenberg said that he had not read the book itself, only the 28 June 1952 review in the *Journal of the American Medical Association*. It described the book as 'well written' and based on an 'intensive study of men and women who were killed in air raids and other serious disturbances' which showed that 'strong emotion, such as fear, can lead to uterine bleeding in sensitive women'. *The Times* praised Stieve in August 1949 as a hero whose scientific freedom was under threat. The horror of his barbarity under the Third Reich is now known but after the war he continued to work in Germany as a university professor, a bust was made in his honour although, in his 1952 book, Stieve described his studies of executed women (who were told of their impending deaths) to see what impact this stress had on their menstrual cycles (Seidelman 1999).

Just as there are two accounts of the meeting between Norman Haire and Aleister Crowley, there are disputed claims about *Sexual anomalies and perversions* which was supposedly written by Magnus Hirschfeld's 'pupils'. Arthur Koestler said he was the sole author. In the 1940s he became famous, then rich, after writing *Darkness at noon* so Haire, in his introduction to the 1952 edition, was rude to say 'it was evident that the text was compiled by a foreigner' who 'was not completely familiar' with English. Haire said for this reason he carefully revised the text, amended the language and punctuation where necessary, deleted some

---

18 Milton Lomask (1987, 35) quoted Catherine Drinker Bowen who omitted this anecdote from her study of Holmes after discovering it was a myth.

passages, inserted some, corrected some statements, and brought the text up-to-date. Koestler (1969, 271) got even by claiming: 'I have never met Mr Haire, but I have looked him up in *Who's Who* for 1946, where he occupies more space than either Winston Churchill or George Bernard Shaw. I am told that he died in 1952'. The preface to the second edition of *Sexual anomalies* included the preface to the first edition and perhaps Haire kept it because it flatteringly referred to the WLSR's Copenhagen and London congresses being held 'under the chairmanship of the famous English sexologist Dr Norman Haire.' He was a *delegate* in Copenhagen and Hirschfeld was the president of the London congress but neither Haire nor Koestler would have liked the publisher's claim that the pupils' contribution was 'only that of a plasterer who puts the final touches to an edifice that is otherwise complete.'

Allen & Unwin wrote to Haire in June 1952 and proposed to reduce his royalties for *Birth-control methods* from 15 percent to 12½ percent (in order to keep the sale price at six shillings). He found this very unsatisfactory and suggested they should keep to the terms of the contract, and, if necessary, raise the price of the book. Haire had kept on working after Ernest Jerdan's suicide and Conchita Supervia's death and he showed the same courageous determination and professionalism when he was faced with his own death. This final dispute with his publisher was a metaphor for his whole life and showed that no matter what difficulties he might face, he always battled for what he thought was right.

He remained an iconoclast and in the month of his death he wrote a long, thoughtful preface to Albert Ellis' book *Sex beliefs and customs* in which he applauded the work of the Society for the Prevention of Venereal Disease while he ridiculed its rival, the National Council for Combating Venereal Disease, who claimed that preventive measures such as condoms would encourage vice: Haire called them 'the Society for the Prevention of the Prevention of Venereal Disease.'

In early September Haire was admitted to hospital and died three weeks later.

15

Conclusion

Norman Zions had a burning ambition to be an actor during his Sydney boyhood and although he made his brilliant career in medicine – as Dr Norman Haire – his acting talent and speaking eloquence helped to make this possible. At the age of 26 he became the Medical Superintendent of Newcastle Hospital but after he was unfairly held responsible for a patient's death during the influenza pandemic he left his homeland. On his arrival in London in 1919 he adopted a new name and soon changed from being an unknown, poor foreigner to a celebrity with a gynaecology practice in Harley Street, a chauffeur-driven Rolls Royce and a country house. He was a feeling, thinking and doing man, equal parts hedonist and humanist; a tall, fat and flamboyant rationalist who was secretly homosexual and said blunt things in a beautiful voice.

He had loyal supporters and irate denigrators who hated the way people flocked to his lectures and eagerly bought his informative books about birth control and sexology. In 1922 he took a leading role in the world's first international conference on birth control which was held in London and he also starred in conferences and lecture tours in America and in Germany, France and Spain where he lectured in German, French and Spanish. He was among the first to provide the poor with free birth control clinics and he convinced Britain's medical profession of the need to learn about contraception and provide it. Haire was a superb administrator and with Dora Russell he organised the WLSR's highly successful 1929 congress in London which many of the world's intellectual avant-garde attended. Illness struck in 1932, and in 1933 his books were amongst those destroyed in Hitler's book burnings. In 1940 he returned to Australia where he faced stiff opposition from the time of his arrival until he left in 1946: the security service tried to silence him, the ABC Board was criticised in parliament for choosing him as the key speaker in a population debate and his weekly advice column in the magazine *Woman* was strongly opposed by the Catholic Church. Most of his final years were in Britain where he bravely persevered in his quest to finetune sexual morality so that individuals and communities could live as harmoniously as possible.

Many people saw him as a passionate and quick-witted extrovert but he was also a thoughtful, complex and intensely private person and in 1935 he told Berta Ruck, 'we shall all be much better dead for I believe in *Nothing after death*'. He may have been joking but perhaps he suffered from depression or his health and money worries and the worsening situation in Germany had made his life meaningless, a sad irony for a man who campaigned to help eradicate sexual anxieties so that others would have a much better life on earth. His death notice specified his unsentimental, secular wishes:

> Norman Haire of Sydney, Australia, and of 127 Harley Street, aged 60. Cremation at St Marylebone Crematorium, East End Road and North Circular Road, East Finchley ... No religious ceremony and no flowers. (*The Times*, 13 September 1952)

The New York Times described him as an 'Australian-born gynaecologist, active in the birth control movement in Great Britain since 1919' who had died in a London hospital three weeks after being admitted with heart trouble. He was 'an author and one of Britain's leading authorities on sex, he was president of the Sex Education Society and a member of the British Society for the Study of Sex Psychology'.

From the 1940s *The Times* refused to publish Haire's letters or mention his work and wrote a grudging obituary, calling him 'a physician who courted unpopularity by his determined advocacy of birth control and sex education'. This makes as little sense as saying that Galileo and van Gogh courted unpopularity because of their devotion to science or art. Haire aimed to enlighten people and end their sexual misery and, as Clive James (2007) said of another man with a noble ambition, 'sometimes it takes an obsessive person to do great things.' *The Times*' hostile obituarist underscored the pettiness of Haire's opponents:

CONCLUSION

Working as he did in a domain open to the blasts of bitter controversy, it was to be expected that Haire should not only meet opposition but incur a certain degree of personal enmity – the more so because of his extreme outspokenness and because in the matter of theology he was to be found in the rationalist camp. Yet those who were admitted to his friendship (and they were many, drawn as often from artistic and literary as from sociological circles) found him a charming companion, light-hearted, witty, sympathetic, cultured, and loyal. The theatre was one of his passions, and he was a connoisseur of acting and stage craft. A big, massively made man, he somewhat oddly combined teetotalism with a nice gastronomic palate.

Haire was more than 'a connoisseur of acting' – he was a consummate actor – and *The Times'* obituarist also disparaged Haire's 'unconventionality', saying his 'opulent' Chinoiserie furnishings 'did not always find favour', and concluded with the standard opaque phraseology to suggest homosexuality – 'He was unmarried'.

The Lancet's obituarist was more generous and, after listing his postgraduate study at the *Institut für Sexualwissenschaft* in Berlin, said that in 1921 he was a founding member and medical officer in charge of the Walworth Women's Welfare Centre, 'the first welfare centre in Britain to offer contraceptive advice to its patients', and listed the conferences he attended. Haire's interest in sex education was not confined to his large clinical practice; he was known on five continents as an author, lecturer and editor. He edited 'The international library of sexology and psychology' series and *The Journal of Sex Education* and was a member of the editorial committee of two others: '*Le Problème Sexuel* and *Anthropos* and wrote articles under the name of Wykeham Terriss.'[1] They occasionally overstated their praise: Haire did not run the first birth control clinic in Britain, although it was the first *medically*

---

1 Haire's three-page résumé for his US tour noted: 'Dr Haire is an Honorary Associate of the Rationalist Association of Australia, and has written for the *Australian Rationalist* and the *New Zealand Rationalist*. He was for many years a member of the Council, and a frequent lecturer, at the Rationalist Society of New South Wales. He has also contributed to the *London Literary Guide* and the *London Freethinker*' (HC – 3.27).

399

staffed one, and Haire did not organise the 1929 congress alone but did it jointly with Dora Russell.

Not surprisingly the warmest tributes were written in his own journal – *The Journal of Sex Education* – by Robert Wood, the editor, Harold Avery, Haire's celebrity doctor whose patients ranged from dockland labourers to royalty, and Harry Benjamin an American disciple of Steinach who lived to be 101 and was Haire's colleague and close friend. Wood called Haire's death a blow to sexology and sex education and said it had been his 'great privilege' to work with him on the journal for four years. He said Haire read most of the books before he sent them out for review and added characteristically 'direct and terse' comments in the margins. Success was often followed by 'safe' views, and many radicals become 'Grand Old Men' but Haire never compromised or modified a 'soundly based opinion to court popularity'. He was an eminent authority on sexuality and its persuasive advocate. His attitude 'was affirmative rather than negative – a very rare thing in our sex-negating culture'. He was obviously dying when he returned from his American tour but he insisted on providing the Sex Education Society with his 'American impressions'; he feared he might break down during the lecture but he managed two hours of talk and discussion. It was 'his farewell, and his friends knew it' and would remember him with affection and gratitude. He was 'witty, amusing, courageous, and blunt in his speech, and carried his vast learning lightly'. Wood said he would never forget Haire's 'kindness, generosity, and stimulating personality' (*JSE*, September–October 1952, 1).

Harry Benjamin lamented that sexology and sex education had 'suffered an almost irreparable loss in Haire's death'. His tireless energy and capacity for work were the envy of his friends and he devoted this to advance the cause of sexual enlightenment. As a result, 'innumerable people, patients, and readers' owed him an enormous debt of gratitude. 'The combination of a brilliant mind with an enormous store of knowledge was unique' and his experience as a sexologist and gynaecologist was so great that it seemed that he was irreplaceable. 'Through his many writings he has let us all share generously in his knowledge, his humour, and his philosophy of life. His publications are his lasting monument. Let us be grateful for having them'.

Conclusion

Harold Avery said Haire was 'a man who stood steadfastly by the truth as he saw it, who hated nothing but ignorance and human misery, and who sought unfailingly to free mankind from a legacy of prejudice and superstition'. He caught rheumatic fever in 1932 and was never fit again but his practice and work came first and he was a 'dedicated servant of humanity'. Avery said that he never complained even when diabetes 'put an end to his enjoyment of rich and exotic foods'. Although Haire was stoic about his health, he *did* complain about 'the famous specialist' (Avery) who 'for some reason' did not want him to start injections of insulin for diabetes and, while he followed this advice, his energy was so drained that he had to restrict his work to a third of a day, three days a week (*Woman*, 11 July 1949).

Despite Haire's altercation with the Drysdales over the Walworth Women's Welfare Centre, CV Drysdale[2] was warmly generous in the June–September 1952 issue of *The Malthusian*, saying that many in the birth control movement shared the Neo-Malthusian 'deep regret' at his death, 'after thirty years of devoted service to these causes and to the spread of sex enlightenment'. He outlined Haire's early career at the centre which opened in November 1921 with Haire as its chief Honorary Medical Officer who ran it 'with great success' and revised the League's practical leaflet while he was there. He kept in touch with other birth control societies in Britain, attended many international conferences and became recognised as a leading authority in the field. He was a remarkably clear thinker, lecturer and writer, and his 1936 book *Birth-control methods* was very valuable because he drew from wide personal experience of the methods and devices and described them clearly and objectively. His great courage, energy and devotion was shown by his views on abortion, sterilisation and the need for sex enlightenment which he expressed in *The Journal of Sex Education* and by the determined way he carried on his numerous activities up to the eve of his death, although his heart was weakened by rheumatic fever in 1932 and he was a diabetic. The 'Neo-Malthusian Crusade' had always

---

2 In its 1961 obituary for Dr Drysdale, *The Times* was still coy about birth control, praising his work on electrical measurements and briefly mentioning his 'considerable regard for the theories propounded by Malthus'.

been 'distinguished for the large number of its zealous, self-sacrificing adherents, and among them Dr Norman Haire will hold a distinguished place.'

Margaret Sanger sent Haire a very strange letter on 18 September, almost a week *after* his death notice was published in *The New York Times*. She showed some sympathy that his trip ended in illness and he spent his time in a hospital and she commented 'of course you have wonderful friends everywhere, and it is quite possible that you will try to come over another time'. However, the letter was really about her and it was triggered by page 273 in the June–July issue of *JSE*; she was very pleased to see Haire's comment about his work in London as medical adviser in 1920 for the Malthusian League and also to see that he had denied 'the ridiculous stupid statement that Marie Stopes continues to make that she opened and founded the first birth control clinic in the world'. Sanger said her letter was 'just a word to congratulate you that you have done this' but she 'would prefer that these comments are for you personally and not to be given publicity'. Sanger was outdoing Stopes in self-promotion and she was so concerned to tell Haire all her good works that she had overlooked the fact that he was dead.

On 31 October 1952 *The Times* advertised the sale of Haire's house 'and the Chinoiserie therein' and published this Wills and Bequest Notice on 10 December: 'Dr Norman Haire of Harley Street, W and Sydney, Australia, left an estate in England valued at £31,365 (duty paid £2886). He left the library of books and other publications to the University of Sydney, and, after other legacies[3] and bequests, the residue of his property to the university directing that it be paid to the Vice-Chancellor to be applied in such manner as the Senate of the university determines for the study of sexology'. Nettleden Lodge, Ashridge Park, Hertfordshire was advertised for sale privately or by auction in July 1953. It was listed as a 16th-century country residence set in 46 acres with four reception rooms, eight bedrooms, three bathrooms, central heating, mains electricity, garages for four cars, stables for six horses,

---

3   Haire left £1000 to his 'his life-long friend' Willem van de Hagt who was also entitled to £8000 in Haire's safe deposit (University of Sydney. Letter from PR Kimber to the Registrar, point 4, 13 November 1952).

CONCLUSION

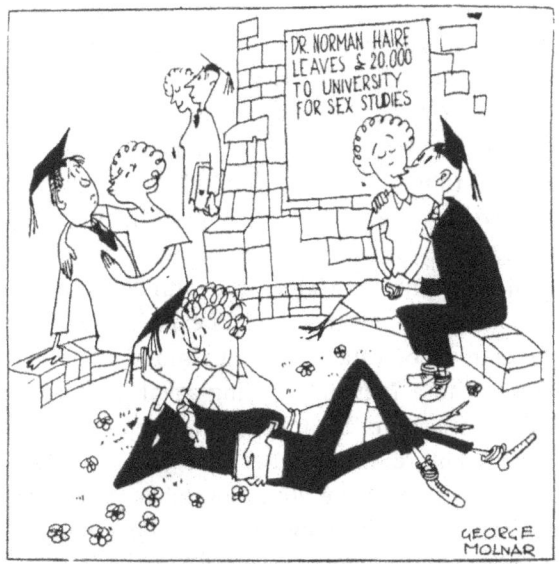

"*And when will we get the money?*"

Figure 15.1. Cartoon by George Molnar, *The Daily Telegraph* (Sydney), 3 December 1952. Reproduced with permission of Katie Molnar.

two modern bungalows and a cottage (*The Times*, 8 and 13 May 1953). In 1954 it was sold for £9600.

George Molnar (1952) responded to the news with a cartoon. It is fitting that by leaving his money to the University of Sydney for the study of sex 'to annoy the wowsers'[4] Haire had made a final posthumous curtain call with consummate theatrical skill.

The sale of Haire's assets was finalised after the University of Sydney sent a 29 March 1957 letter to his solicitors, Lionel Dare & Reed & Martin, instructing them 'to put a reserve land valuation of £400 on Haire's property at Port Macquarie, with the proviso that if a bid is made in the vicinity of £282.10.0, that the auctioneer be instructed to accept it'. The *Australian encyclopaedia* (1963, 9: 83A) listed Haire as one of 40 benefactors who gave £20,000 or more to the University of Sydney.

---

4 Haire's comment to his friend AS (Paddy) O'Connor was quoted by RF Foster in *WB Yeats: a life. II: The arch-poet 1915–1939* (Oxford: Oxford University Press), 2003, p 497, fn 4.

Haire's executors were his solicitor Philip Kimber and Lloyds Bank Ltd and they felt it was in the public interest to ignore his will and destroy his papers. They decided that since he was a sexologist and there was correspondence from a number of distinguished persons which might have caused embarrassment if it fell into the wrong hands, they would burn everything and did so (Kelly 2001). They also burnt the Sex Education Society's records.[5] After the University of Sydney's Senate informed Kimber they would accept the bequest, on 13 November 1952 Kimber supplied the university's Registrar with details of Haire's library of 'about 6,000 items', larger than he had expected, which would 'cost a substantial sum' to be catalogued. Two months later, after Kimber handed the items to a London shipping agent, the packers itemised a much smaller collection: '2,700 books and a quantity of papers and drawings.' The agent's covering letter of 8 January 1953 continued: 'As [Kimber's] telegram of the 20th November stated that you were arranging to catalogue all the items we have not made any list whatever, but have just packed the books as received'.

Unfortunately, Haire's heirs were cavalier about their inheritance: despite Kimber's telegram, the items were *not* catalogued and there is no way of knowing whether the whole consignment arrived in 1953 or if any material was lost during the move to the University of Sydney's new Fisher Library which opened in 1962. Haire's books, records and correspondence have been deliberately destroyed in the 1930s, 50s, 60s and 70s. Frank Forster, then a Norman Haire Fellow, wrote to Dora Russell on 27 July 1978, informing her that 'seventeen very large tea-chests had remained undisturbed in store until about three years ago'. He spoke about 'going through' Haire's collection in the Fisher Library and said he had found large gaps 'on the personal side' although the record of his life until he reached England in 1919 appeared to be 'intact' and 'all that appears to be missing is the file on the London congress, 1929'. He was mistaken because the Dora Russell Papers in Amsterdam contain the archives of the WLSR's 1929 congress with

---

5 Weeks (1977, 262, fn 9). 'According to information supplied to me by Haire's executor, the records of the Sex Education Society, which had about six hundred members, were destroyed after his death'.

the extensive correspondence between Russell and Haire and there are also many other sexology and birth control archives that contain Haire correspondence which are listed in the bibliography.

Forster mentioned two great collections of correspondence during the 1920s and 30s – letters to and from Havelock Ellis, Magnus Hirschfeld and Karl Giese – and a very extensive accumulation of papers from Haire's 1940–46 stay in Australia. He commented, 'I guess no one in London thought that these warranted incineration although some would have here'. Forster and his assistant then culled Haire's collection which had been estimated to be about 6000 items in 1952 and threw away so much that Haire's papers now fit into eight standard archive boxes. If an art historian tried to dispose of art works, curators would have prevented it, but, in the case of these sexology treasures, Forster was given permission and then profusely thanked. On 30 June 1978 Forster wrote to Pamela Green, the Fisher Library's Rare Book and Special Collections Librarian, saying that he had 'returned to Melbourne pleased with what [his assistant and] he had achieved last week – thanks to your help'. Green replied:

> I must also thank you both very much for the gallant work you undertook in exorcising one of our nightmares, namely the Hare [sic] duplicates on Floor 8. Mr Bryan joins me in the thank yous. I wish some of our other nightmares could be disposed of as easily.[6]

The British Museum had tried to acquire some of Haire's sexology collection but they were refused because the Fisher Library had been named as the beneficiary. Unfortunately, the university where Haire studied did not treasure his gift. In her first letter to Forster, Green said they were 'still tracking down bits and pieces of the Haire Library' when in June 1976 her memory had been 'jolted' by the discovery that 'some volumes had been transferred to the WH and Elizabeth Deane Collection'[7]; Haire's library had been 'deliberately broken up over the

---

6   FFA. Green's unsigned, undated, letter in response to Forster's 30 June 1978 letter; Harrison Bryan was the University of Sydney librarian from 1963 to 1980, then director-general of the National Library of Australia.

7   The collection of William H Deane, the Rare Books and Special Collection

years to place the usable materials where it was best suited' but if staff 'gradually kept checking the Haire catalogue' against the main Fisher Library catalogue they would 'eventually have a reasonable picture of the dispositions.' She said in her 3 June 1976 letter to Forster that she did not know if the cards they had were 'for the complete collection' and that some of Haire's material might have been added to the erotica in Deane's collection.

Green's description of the Haire collection as a nightmare to be exorcised shows that library staff were either unaware the collection existed, uncertain about the collection's size or did not know where to find it. However, despite this, they were prepared to judge which parts were 'usable'. The lack of custodial care is clearly evident: the material was never fully indexed, it was never stamped to demonstrate ownership (making it hard to prove ownership), some of it is in Melbourne, and Haire's diary for 1906–1914 has been lost. There were rumours that a Rare Books librarian had been an alcoholic[8] but, even if this was false, these examples show a lack of professionalism in the 1970s among senior library staff. Ironically, there is a full inventory of the Norman Haire papers in the archives of the Frank Forster Library in Melbourne's Royal Australian College of Obstetricians and Gynaecologists. Forster died in 1995 but the Haire biography he undertook to write was never published. The college archivist explained this was 'due to bouts of ill health in his latter years' (Winspear 2004, 4) but the reason he gave me in 1988 was that he had approached a publisher in the 1970s 'who had not been very enthusiastic' and that some people spoke about approaching their solicitors when he had mentioned Haire's name.

Library's largest benefactor, comprises the remainder of Deane's private library after it was partly destroyed by fire and the materials purchased from the Deane funds. Its strengths are material on the history and philosophy of science, witchcraft, demonology and significant Australiana. It also includes a large collection of erotica as well as the Deane business archives. See www.library.usyd.edu.au/libraries/rare/3.2spec.html.

8 In an attempt to verify this rumour, I asked a former University of Sydney professor, who asked a senior colleague of his who 'knew of only one alcoholic librarian who was there for several years in the late 1980s'. The academic felt it was inappropriate to give the name because the person had resigned and then joined AA and was working as a drug counsellor.

Conclusion

Three vignettes of Haire, written in 1958, 1990 and 1998, paint evocative pictures of him. The first is by author William Plomer who gave this account of their meeting in 1935: Haire was 'dark with a longish, whitish, rather flabby face, with the alert expression of a trained observer who had seen a lot of life, in this instance, largely below the belt'. He had a 'notably pear-shaped' figure and was wearing a black coat and striped trousers and seemed to be 'entirely without puritanical prejudices'; he had great experience of the 'dreadful physical and psychological muddles, fears, frustrations, and pains into which men and women are dragged by the sexual instinct' and had devoted his hard-working life 'to easing or preventing' these things. Plomer believed he was 'a benevolent and beneficent man' whose specialised view of 'human life and human nature was uncommonly clear and direct'. Plomer noted Haire's strange combination of 'indiscretion and trustfulness' but considered these were 'part of his method' and character and that it was this directness and candour that helped make him a fine specimen of 20th-century man – scientific; seemingly untroubled by racial, social or professional conventions; functioning independently and well in advance of public and medical opinion; unspiritual, materialistic; inclined to proselytise for what he believed would save or improve human life and to oppose those tendencies that have caused complex and widespread suffering (Plomer 1958, 37–40).

The second account was written in 1990 by Professor Hans Lehfeldt, a German gynaecologist who, with Haire's help, had established a birth control clinic in Berlin. Lehfeldt at the age of 99 had fond memories of his 40-year friendship with Haire and called him 'a gourmand as well as a gourmet' whose cooking reflected his special recipes collected from around the world. He once advised an acquaintance, 'from housewife to housewife', how to cook a special sort of ham and he *was* a good housewife. He was also a very generous host and meals in his house were an event, whether he was entertaining scientists during an international congress or having an informal dinner with friends. The Lehfeldts attended several of his parties in the 1920s and met 'an Australian friend of Norman' (Ernest Jerdan) who lived there. A few months before Haire's death, Lehfeldt and his wife visited London and, although he was seriously ill, Haire insisted on holding a lavish party in their honour, paying special attention to the food and décor in the large dining room which was sparingly lit by candles in the corners, placed so that the light filtered through large water-filled containers. Haire would not let staff serve dinner but, with a flourish, ladled food from enormous silver containers to plates and, using special metal holders, placed them in front of each guest. The large room in the basement was festively decorated and the buffet was spread with delicacies such as eggs and other farm products which were very hard to get in England in 1952 and came from Haire's country property.

I heard the third story from Gloria Savill in 1998 who said she remembered her uncle Norman's letter about geese he was breeding as a hobby and 'for the table' at his country estate. She said he took food *very* seriously and there is an example of this nostalgia for his food-producing activities in rural England when Haire listed 'mixed farming' as his recreation in the 1941 edition of *Who's Who in Australia*. Such entries are always interesting because they are written by the subjects themselves and reflect the way they want to be seen.

Two articles, in 1974 and 2002, show that the importance of Haire's work has not diminished. The first was written by Roy Lewis, an economist and feature writer for *The Times* who in 1974 evaluated the futurology forecasts made by 100 eminent scientists and social scientists in 1925.[9] They had made mistakes and no one had predicted the Great Depression but Norman Haire and Anthony Ludovici were on his list and, more significantly still, Haire was one of the few to prophesy correctly that effective contraception 'would be the cornerstone of women's freedom' and to forecast that there would be 'widespread trial marriage, easy divorce, some polyandry, and final liberation as the result of ectogenesis late in the century.' He was wrong about polyandry, in which a woman is married to several men, but he was partly right about ectogenesis in which babies are developed in artificial wombs. Haire made this prediction in *Hymen* and it was repeated by Aldous

---

9 Lewis (1974) did not name the authors of these forecasts which Kegan Paul published in their To-day and to-morrow series. The first was *Quo vadimus? Some glimpses of the future* by EE Fournier d'Albe.

Huxley in *Brave new world* and, while it has not yet happened, IVF and surrogacy are the first steps. The accuracy of most of his predictions show how advanced his thinking was.

The second article was written in 2002 by Katharine Viner, a reporter for *The Guardian*, who 'discovered' Haire while browsing through birth control materials exhibited in London after 75 years of being 'underused, undervalued'. The first gem she found displayed in the Women's Library (formerly the Fawcett Library) was Haire's 'forward-thinking book' *The comparative value of current contraceptive methods*. Although written in 1928, she found it 'startling for how little has changed', as most of those methods he mentioned are still in use. She said his only omission was the 'female sheath', which she called a '1990s discovery', but goat's bladder sheaths had been used for this purpose in ancient Rome. She was impressed with Haire's conclusion that withdrawal 'is certainly a very reliable preventive, but interferes with sexual satisfaction so greatly that it is quite unsuitable for general use.' She praised Haire for extolling the benefits of orgasm for women, and his warning that 'a great many gynaecological problems are due to lack of sexual satisfaction in women and could be avoided if men and women were taught early enough that a woman should have complete sexual satisfaction' but she thought he had been 'too squeamish' to mention the 'straight pleasure' of orgasm. Haire's silence made sense; while it was acceptable to argue that orgasms could prevent illness, the wowsers would have pounced if they thought he was encouraging women to enjoy sex. Viner called her article 'Look back in awe' and Haire topped her list of birth control pioneers because his work remains 'awe inspiring'.

Surprisingly, despite the success of the WLSR's 1929 London congress in which Haire played a key role, Ivan Crozier (2001) made an extremely negative appraisal of him in a 30-page article about his role in the congress and again to a lesser degree in 2003. In the first article he questioned the sincerity of Stella Browne's warm tribute to Haire, implying that she meant exactly the opposite of what she had said and suggested that 'we might want to think about Browne's own reasons for supporting her enemy against Dora Russell!', but it is his hypothesis which should be questioned. In his view (2001, 223), the need to suggest a united front 'got Haire the support for the 1929 WLSR congress, even from those who might not have wished to have anything to do with him personally'. This showed Haire's consummate skill: he overcame strong opposition with tact, drive and skill and, by co-ordinating the factions, enabled the congress to go ahead and ensured its success. This was even more remarkable in view of the strident opposition Haire faced from Havelock Ellis and his painful duty of having to defy the wishes of his mentor and England's 'sage of sex'. Russell's 1983 tribute echoed Stella Browne's warmth when she described Haire as a man 'who deserves to be remembered in the Sex Reform movement as a whole' and she called the 1929 congress the peak of the progressive movement which began in 1918 and 'included virtually every man or woman in Britain of what might be called the intellectual avant-garde'.

Crozier also criticised Haire for his private comment to Havelock Ellis on 21 September 1930: 'I do not know of anybody else who has both the knowledge and the courage to make him a better leader than myself in the movement for sex reform'. This was a realistic observation but Crozier (2001, 306) said it 'typified Haire's blundering, egocentric style' and that Haire, when he was unable to achieve success by 'pugilism and belligerence alone', sometimes 'had to be obsequious' and achieved this 'by establishing a ring of contacts'. Crozier gave no examples of Haire's pugilism or belligerence, and ignored the fact that having contacts – today called 'networking' – was essential not obsequious, and that keeping the medical profession on side was a prerequisite for survival. He questioned Haire's motives and disparaged his generosity in giving free treatment to poor women at birth control clinics and called him 'an objectionable, grandstanding sycophant'. This lacks the objectivity of a historian and has an odd tone, as though he knew Haire personally.

Crozier dissected Haire's 'dubious character' for three pages and his 'other troubles and scandals' for four and then concluded disingenuously: 'Lest we be too hasty to condemn, we should note that Haire's personality was not completely unpalatable; he did offer much help to Jewish sexologists escaping the Nazi regime'. Crozier said he hoped to 'illustrate' Haire's career as the first sexologist in Harley Street by examining his networks and the part he played in organising the first

CONCLUSION

major conference in London on sexuality and sex reform. However, this was a crude caricature, not an 'illustration', and his portrayal of Haire as a buffoon and villain started with his choice of epigraphs. The first portrayed him as a lightweight celebrity:

> The correct answer to 'Do you know who Norman Haire is? is 'Oh, good Lord, who doesn't'. (Mannin 1930, 194)

The second one portrayed Haire as a criminal and comes from John Webster's macabre 17th-century play, *The Duchess of Malfi*, whose central character is conscienceless, cunning and hates good:

> Indeed he rails at those things which he wants:
> Would be as lecherous, covetous, or proud,
> Bloody, or envious, as any man
> If he had means to be so.[10]

Crozier's attempt to present Haire as a flawed character failed just as it did in the previously discussed attempt to belittle Haire's acting ability. Crozier concluded his second article (2003, 37) with the claim that 'having made little impact in London, Norman Haire moved back to Sydney and took up the cause on his home ground. He died in 1953, still in his sixties, leaving his papers to Sydney University but otherwise disappearing from public view'. In fact Haire died in London in 1952 at the age of 60; Crozier's subjective comments were equally wrong.

Haire correctly judged that his articles in the magazine *Woman* from 1941 to 1951 'had a considerable effect in moulding Australian public opinion, in making people realise that it is not only desirable, but possible, to make sex knowledge available in a simple and inoffensive form to the public'. He worked with groups such as the New Education Fellowship and the Workers' Educational Association; the Parents and Citizens' Association was beginning to hold sex education lectures; and the YWCA had engaged a 'well-known clergyman to run marriage preparation courses'. This was a remarkable achievement because for many years his fiercest opposition came from conservative Christians

---

10 Crozier (2001, 299) quoting from *The Duchess of Malfi*, Act 1, Scene 1.

and there is evidence that he made a convert: John Crowlesmith (1949, 4), the secretary of Cambridge's Methodist Society for Medical and Pastoral Psychology, 'found little to complain about' when he reviewed Haire's *Everyday sex problems* and in most instances he could say a hearty 'Amen'. He thought that Haire was playing 'the devil's advocate' and was really 'on the side of the angels' and suspected that Haire was 'tilting at windmills' and liked to shock people. Haire underlined his conclusion in red pen:

> But taking it all in all, this is a wise, courageous and constructive book, full of sane counsel, shrewd advice, and practical goodness. It truly combines profit and pleasure. The author knows what he wants to say, and what is more, how to say it, and possesses both the expert knowledge and the experience necessary to drive home his points.

Another reviewer applauded Haire's aim to 'achieve a form of society in which the sexual relation is not regarded as sinful, and only to be indulged after half a lifetime of inhibitory training. The best compliment one can pay Mr Haire is that if such a society should eventually come about, he will have helped to make it possible' (*JSE*, June 1949, 251–52).

Haire's zeal and tenacity and *Woman*'s civil libertarian stance allowed it to survive for a decade in a puritanical period: he was not exaggerating in the October–November 1950 issue of the *JSE* when he wrote this valediction for *Woman:* 'No such articles have ever appeared in any Australian paper before, and the public, who found it difficult to obtain simple informative popular-scientific articles about sex, apparently considered the articles so helpful that the circulation of the magazine doubled within five months.'[11] However, after they had been appearing for five months, a deputation of Roman Catholics demanded that the articles should be stopped. When the editor refused, a second

---

11 Haire was exaggerating when he claimed in *Honi Soit* on 6 May 1943 that his articles caused *Woman*'s circulation to double and he was corrected by Guy Natusch on 14 and 17 May 1943: while Haire 'had a good influence on circulation, so did ... Margo Parker'. In 1940 *Woman*'s circulation was below 100,000 and climbed to 304,080 in 1944, still half that of the *Australian Women's Weekly* (statistics quoted by Griffen-Foley 1999, 299).

deputation repeated the demand and threatened to put *Woman* on the list of books that Catholics were forbidden to read, that sermons would be preached against the magazine from every Catholic pulpit in Australia, and that efforts would be made to persuade advertisers to withdraw their advertisements. They carried out their threats and Elizabeth Riddell told me that she and Haire used to laugh on hearing about priests fulminating that 'Wykeham Terriss would burn in Hell'. The articles were discontinued for a few months but the circulation of the paper fell. He was invited to resume his column and the circulation increased again rapidly: '*Woman* appeared every Friday morning and within an hour or so it was sold out'. There were reports that Catholic girls in offices begged non-Catholic friends to buy the paper and lend it to them. They were not even supposed to *read* it, but many of them did. Haire and the articles were regularly attacked by Dr Leslie Rumble, a priest whose show *Question box* was broadcast on Sunday evenings from radio station 2SM which was owned by the Catholic Church and controlled by the Catholic Archdiocese of Sydney.

Peter Coleman (1962, 82), in his pioneering review of Australian censorship, called Haire 'one of Australia's most famous freethinkers and sex reformers' and said the column in *Woman* was 'probably the most free-thinking series of articles ever written for a mass circulation magazine'. Robert Pullan (1984, 13) wrote in his account of Australia's fight for free speech: 'The impulse to censor is deeply rooted in human sexuality and in the instinct of self-preservation', explaining that government suppression of the words and pictures it considers citizens are not mature enough to read or see is analogous to the universal anxiety parents experience about their children's sexuality as they make the transition to the autonomy of adulthood. In the history of sexual censorship, our laws and restrictions are a product of this 'loss of control' anxiety. The corollary is in Shakespeare's words 'we hate that which we often fear', which explain why many people who feared Haire's message hated him.

A less flattering story surfaced in response to George Munster's 1983 profile of Haire in the *Sydney Morning Herald*. Peter Ryan (not the priest who hounded Haire in the 1940s but a newspaper columnist and former Director of Melbourne University Press) sent him this note:

Bill Cook (Secretary of the Australian rationalists) stayed as Haire's guest in Harley Street in 1950. He asked Cook to bring back in his hand luggage a parcel containing a precious possession 'of great sentimental value'. Cook agreed, but when he got the valuable article to the office of Haire's Australian solicitor, it proved to be currency (or securities) in breach of exchange controls. It could have drawn a couple of years in jail for Cook, if Customs had searched his briefcase. What a mate!

This story feels bogus, starting with the incorrect date: Cook stayed as Haire's house guest and received help from his host to travel to Rome as the Rational Society of Australia delegate to the 9 September 1949 International Freethought Conference. Cook was again in London on 21 November to give a 'Sex and rationalism' lecture to the Sex Education Society. The allegations make no sense because Haire was rich and did not plan to return to Australia and, if the parcel *had* contained contraband, Haire's solicitor would have been unlikely to have opened it in Cook's presence or described the contents. I contacted Gwen Hause, Bill Cook's daughter, but as she was very young then she referred me to Lois Sweet (1998), 'a good friend of her parents'. Lois Sweet felt it might be significant that Cook and Ryan were not friends, Ryan's letter was sent after Cook's death and Cook had never told the story to his four closest friends – her husband Hyde Sweet; historian Brian Fitzpatrick; 'Pansy' (Sir Roy) Wright, Chancellor of the University of Melbourne; or psychiatrist Dr Bill Orchard who said, 'He couldn't be such a fool as to take something without knowing what it was.' She added that it would have been completely out of character and, if Cook had been fooled, he would have either said nothing or 'exploded and had it out with Haire'.

Munster thanked Ryan for his comment and noted that 'about ten people' had contacted him, chiefly by telephone. He found this level of interest was 'inexplicable in terms of its merits. Haire must have left a strong impression on people'. Anthropologist Les Hiatt asked if there was enough material for a more substantial biography, adding that Ethel Mannin had called Haire 'a repulsive glutton.' It was strange that he felt that this spiteful, trivial example would contribute anything to a picture of Haire. She had volatile tastes and her admiration of Haire soured after he wrote a sarcastic review of one of her books in the *JSE* in

December 1948 and said she was 'warm-hearted but often sentimental and muddle-headed' and her views, although never dull, were 'utterly at variance with those of her early period'. She switched from Marxism to anarchism and then tried pacifism, and made these changes 'so rapidly' that he found it was 'difficult to keep up with her.'

When she admired him, Ethel Mannin (1930, 191, 194) called Haire 'the one completely rational person' she had ever met and his opponents responded to the challenges he posed: on 18 May 1952 *The New York Times* featured a display advertisement for a religious academic's *Manifesto on sex standards* which was written 'to challenge and answer Norman Haire and other freethinkers'. There was even a hoax Wykeham Terriss whose nuisance phone calls made *Woman* warn its readers to hang up on this 'person of dubious character'. Dame Enid Lyons (1972, 88) felt 'he was merely ahead of his time. He did not live to see television in Australia. With what gusto he would have joined in today's impassioned arguments for the abolition of censorship! He was almost the first bright harbinger in Australia of the permissive age.' When we spoke in 1998, Elizabeth Riddell, who was the 1940s editor of *Woman*, said, 'today Haire would be a sensation – he'd be another Derek Llewellyn Jones'. She meant the 'compassionate obstetrician, radio doctor and academic who became famous in Sydney from the 1970s after writing *Everywoman* which sold more than two million copies and helped thousands of women'. These were some of the generous words the Hon Elisabeth Kirkby, Llewellyn Jones' ex-wife, read in parliament on his death in December 1997.

Haire's name has sometimes prompted hints about his politics, sexuality and the source of his wealth. Most of the money speculations have their origin in gossips' belief that 'where there's money there's muck'. Probably the strangest of them is the claim that he made his money from two embezzlement schemes. Haire had been an enthusiastic member of the Eugenics Society (now the Galton Institute) but had resigned in disgust in 1934, so a story by its treasurer John Peel (not Sir John, the Queen's Surgeon-Gynaecologist) in the March 1994 *Galton Institute Newsletter* might be recycled retaliatory gossip. Peel called Haire 'one of the many colourful characters in the English birth control movement during the 1920s' and a stalwart of the Eugenics Society who 'operated a private nursing home in East Sussex' for women during the early months of pregnancy for treatment to ensure that they had babies 'of the desired sex'. His 'treatment' was wholesome food and placebo tablets 'saucily coloured pink or blue'[12] and he was never short of patients because he offered a money-back guarantee. This meant that the disappointed couples lost nothing and might even return while the happy couples praised the clinic to others. Haire had 'profited nicely from an actuarial certainty of a 50 percent success rate'. He improved his odds by using excuses to refuse potential patients who had already had a number of births of the same sex. In 2007, Betty Nixon, the institute's secretary, said the late John Peel had 'an encyclopaedic knowledge' but neither she nor his son Robert Peel, the institute's librarian, could provide further details. This 'deep-rooted belief' that diet or exercise could influence the child's sex 'until the twelfth week of pregnancy' was ranked as the most popular old wives' tale in *The encyclopaedia of sexual knowledge*. Haire was the editor, and referred in a footnote to Dr Felix Unterberger's efforts to 'determine' the sex of a child by changing the chemistry of a woman's vaginal secretions at the time of fertilisation. In 1940 *Time* discussed this possibility in an article on 'Baking-soda boys' and in 1948 Haire believed that progress was being made in the 'mastery of sex determination'.

The implausible story of an East Sussex nursing home in the 1920s seems to have merged with an equally implausible one about a Hertfordshire nursing home in the 1930s which was told by local historians (Dickson 2007, quoting Senar 1983). Haire may have taught patients sex-selection techniques to try *before* conception but it would have been futile and fraudulent to have offered such 'treatment' to pregnant women at Nettleden Lodge. He was rich and famous so there was no motive for such a scam and there were compelling deterrents; it would have been detected and he would have been denounced and

---

12   Pink and blue pills had featured in a scam by three brothers, Richard, Edward and Leonard Chrimes, who sold pills for 'female complaints' to more than 10,000 women in London and then tried to blackmail them for attempting to 'commit the fearful crime of abortion'. Angus McLaren (1977, 380-87) gave details of the affair and their 1898 trial and sentencing.

struck off the medical register. Haire was a rationalist and a humanist who aimed to reduce sexual ignorance, so the idea of deceiving gullible women in a sex-selection fraud was not in keeping with his beliefs.

In Australia one of Haire's nephews heard a story which was being spread by a Catholic priest called Father Peter Ryan that Haire had made his money by selling contraceptives. When he reported this gossip to his uncle, Haire laughed because 'unfortunately, this was quite untrue'. Haire wrote a disclaimer in a 1937 book to set the record straight: 'I have no financial interest in any of the substances, or in any of the firms, mentioned'. Haire devoted many hours of unpaid time giving lectures, helping people, providing free services in inner-city clinics and writing, and his critics were disconcerted by his ability to do this and run a thriving practice; some jealously claimed that he must have become rich dishonestly. Mannin did not suggest this in her third autobiography but mistakenly claimed that 'a great part of his considerable income' came from fitting the Gräfenberg intra-uterine ring which 'was to the Twenties what the Pill is to the Seventies'. In fact his money came sporadically from clandestine artificial inseminations but it flowed once he tapped the lucrative rejuvenation market.

Haire said little about his politics, the sources of his wealth or his sexuality but others were less reticent. Some said Haire was a hypocrite or coward to say nothing about his homosexuality but they forgot that it was a crime and homosexuals had to be discreet to survive. Munster made an oblique reference to this in 1983, calling it 'a subject about which he knew most from personal experience, but on which he said least in public and about which he was guarded in private'. Haire *was* homosexual but Lotte Fink told her daughter Ruth it was 'totally taboo', 'never acknowledged' and 'only the inner circle of his friends knew'.

Magnus Hirschfeld had been more forthright in his book *Sexual anomalities and perversions* (1938), a second edition of which Haire edited in 1952. There are five sections on homosexuality, a term coined by Karl Maria Benkert in 1869.[13] Havelock Ellis conceded the meaning

---

13 This Austro-Hungarian writer, using the pseudonym Karoly Maria Kertbeny, coined the hybrid term *der Homosexuelle* (homosexual) from the Greek word *homos* (same) + the Latin root *sexus* (male or female sex, gender).

was 'fairly clear and definite' and non-judgemental but disliked its 'awkward disadvantage of being a bastard term compounded of Greek and Latin elements'. When Haire edited the tribute to Hirschfeld by his students in 1928, he said Hirschfeld was 'persecuted and slandered on account of his championship of scientific truth' which is an extremely discreet way of saying he was homosexual. In the book itself Haire vehemently disagreed with Hirschfeld's assertion that 'a homosexual who marries condemns a healthy woman either to barrenness, or to bearing mentally defective children.' Haire made this comment in a footnote, adding that he thought it 'most unwise of predominantly homosexual men or women to marry.' In later life Haire gave a eugenic explanation for his own childlessness, saying that as a child he had seen a relative having an epileptic fit and later, after discovering one of his grandfathers had epilepsy, he felt it 'wiser not to have children and run the risk of passing the taint on to them'. Some relatives thought he was 'over-scrupulous' but it made a convenient cover. Ironically, Hirschfeld's biographer said that a reception given by 'Dr Haire and his wife' [sic] made Hirschfeld's stay in London 'memorable' (Wolff 1986, 388).

Quentin Crisp, a gay 1970s icon, recalled that 'men of the twenties searched themselves for vestiges of effeminacy as though for lice'. Reasons for this are given by John Ayto (1993) who argued that 'euphemisers' were given unprecedented opportunities when *homosexual* entered the English language in 1892.[14] Taboos prevented direct reference to it for at least the first two-thirds of the 20th century and most synonyms are derogatory and based on the notion that it is 'unusual' or strange. George Ives agreed when HL Mencken defined it as 'one of the worst taboos in civilized man.'[15] In *Australia's birthstain: the startling legacy of the convict era*, Babette Smith claimed that the 'stain' of homosexuality had made many people deny their convict roots, and even in the 1980s homosexuals were forced to follow the 'don't ask, don't tell' rule to survive the disapproval by family and friends, beatings, blackmail, police entrapment, exposure, job loss, arrest, public disgrace and humiliation. Many were murdered or driven to suicide.

---

14 In CG Chaddock's translation of Kraff-Ebbing's *Psychopathia sexulis*.
15 Ives (WLSR 1930, 340) quoting Ishill (1929, 60).

Conclusion

Frank Foster gave a strange reply to my question in 1993, saying, 'No, I do not consider him homosexual! He sought his sexual pleasures in more deviant play'. When Forster interviewed Dr Helena Wright in London in 1978, she described Haire as being like a 'great neutered cat'. Forster recollected Christopher Isherwood's suggestion that Haire 'got a thrill from having boys pee in his mouth' and said it was 'just gossip'. Then he mentioned a 'very memorable dinner-party which had been arranged by Phyllis Grosskurth'; two of the other guests were notorious homosexuals who had been jailed in the 1930s and he said they 'laughed at the suggestion of Norman Haire being a homosexual'. Forster did not make it clear if he had attended the dinner party or had only heard about it or whether the homosexuals were laughing because Haire was homosexual or because he wasn't. Forster was similarly vague when he recycled this gossip in his biographical profile of Haire: 'Some considered him homosexual, but he was never clearly active; others thought him a "neuter."' Foster and Grosskurth have different recollections about this party and there seem to be flaws in both accounts. She felt that Havelock Ellis 'must have known that Haire was homosexual although many people were not certain'. She had asked Anatole James who 'once worked for him' if Haire was homosexual and he responded, 'Heavens, yes! But he was an old humbug'. Anatole James was the pseudonym of Geoffrey Evans Pickering, a solicitor who was struck off the roll for gross indecency and jailed (*The Times*, 25 July 1918), and it is unlikely that he would have sought work as Haire's chauffeur, cleaner, cook or surgery nurse, and Haire, who had enemies waiting to catch him out, was unlikely to have employed James who was perhaps one of the 'notorious' homosexuals who attended Grosskurth's party.

Jeffrey Weeks' ground-breaking *Coming out* (1977) included Haire in a list of homosexuals who contributed to the British Society for the Study of Sex Psychology from the 1920s. Historians Roy Porter and Lesley Hall said Haire was homosexual in *The facts of life* (1995) and quoted Weeks as their source. In February 2001 Weeks told me he had not done any work on Haire since writing the book but thought that 'Haire had been anxious to keep his case histories confidential and no doubt to keep his own sexuality quiet'. Perhaps Plomer and others who said that Haire was 'notoriously indiscreet' were wrong. Weeks interviewed 'a couple of people' in the 1970s who knew Haire and they 'made it clear' that he was homosexual with a 'slightly dubious reputation as someone on the make' but Weeks didn't follow that up.

Grosskurth had little recollection of Haire in January 2000 but told me that Helena Wright shuddered at the mention of his name. Perhaps Wright was reacting to Haire's 1949 response to her assertion in *Sex fulfillment in married women* that a woman 'was never intended by Nature to have an orgasm at all.' He said it did not enhance her family planning reputation and urged people to throw the book away. In view of Dr Wright's missionary work and her interest in the paranormal, Haire, as a rationalist and atheist, may have shuddered at the mention of *her* name. It could have been a family antipathy because Wright's sister, the Polish-born Margaret Lowenfeld, a pioneer of child psychiatry, informed the British Society for the Study of Sex Psychology in 1933 that she did not 'personally wish to have any connection with Dr Norman Haire'.[16]

Ralf Dose, who in Berlin was for many years the secretary general of the Magnus Hirschfeld Society and the managing director of the Society's Research Unit on the History of Sexual Sciences, told me in November 2000 that he dimly remembered an interview that Manfred Herzer (a leading German gay historian) had with the birth control pioneer Hans Lehfeldt. When Herzer asked about Haire's homosexuality, Lehfeldt said, 'it was known, but he never talked about it.' Dose said that Lehfeldt, 'as an ardent admirer of women, never had access to the inner circles of homosexuals.' In the early 1930s homosexuality was Germany's 'national perversion' and significantly, to quote Christopher Isherwood, 'Berlin meant boys'. Haire could relax there or in the theatrical world; one of his friends was Brian Desmond Hurst, an openly homosexual Irish film director who was never arrested despite his penchant for boys who were 'pretty, witty or rich.'[17]

But there was a limit to this liberality even among bohemians where 'theatrical' was a code word for homosexual and everyone remembered

---

16 Hall (1995, 673, fn 27) quoting BSSSP (1933).
17 Attributed to the 1950s sex goddess Diana Dors (Griffiths 2006, 43).

how swiftly Oscar Wilde's foolish libel charge had rebounded on him and destroyed his career.[18] The severity of his sentence to two years' hard labour and his humiliating exile in France made homosexuals very fearful. Self-censorship and circumlocution were their protective responses, which explains why Haire called Wilde 'one of these unfortunate sexual psychopaths who went to prison for his offences against the sexual code.'[19] Ironically, he criticised a Wilde biographer for paying 'insufficient consideration to his sexual life, and any book which does this, in the case of Wilde, whose sexual life was so important, leaves much to be desired.' He had similar misgivings when a Sarah Bernhardt book gave scanty attention to her 'rich and varied' sexual life, saying that it was 'like Hamlet without the Prince'.[20] This did not mean Haire was a hypocrite or that he lacked insight. Far from it: he showed caution, not cowardice, and he had to seem to be detached or else face professional suicide. The popular song 'Anything goes', did *not* apply to homosexuality and in 1921 Haire called it 'one of the most unfortunate disabilities from which any individual can suffer.'[21]

Professor Nicholas Edsall (2003, 294), whose analysis of the Montagu–Wildeblood case was discussed earlier, made perceptive comments about Haire's role in the fight for homosexual law reform: 'Against this legal onslaught the homosexual subculture had no defense. There were no organisations in Britain comparable to the Mattachine Society in the United States, Arcadie in France, or even the Society for Human Rights in Germany, let alone the Dutch COC' – the Dutch acronym for the gay rights Center for Culture and Recreation. 'The last, tenuous link with the British Society for the Study of Sex Psychology' was broken when 'its post-war successor, the Sex Education Society, died following the death of Norman Haire'. The Sex Education Society was small, not exclusively concerned with homosexuality and it provided

---

18 Angus McLaren (2007, 608) noted Noel Coward's careful concealment of his sexuality to protect his livelihood.

19 *Woman* (19 August 1946, 39).

20 Wild review (*JSE*, 1949-1950, 144) and Bernhardt review (*JSE*, 1950, 193).

21 From a paper Haire read to the BSSSP on 28 November 1921, published as BSSSP Publication 11, 1923, Paper 2, p. 29.

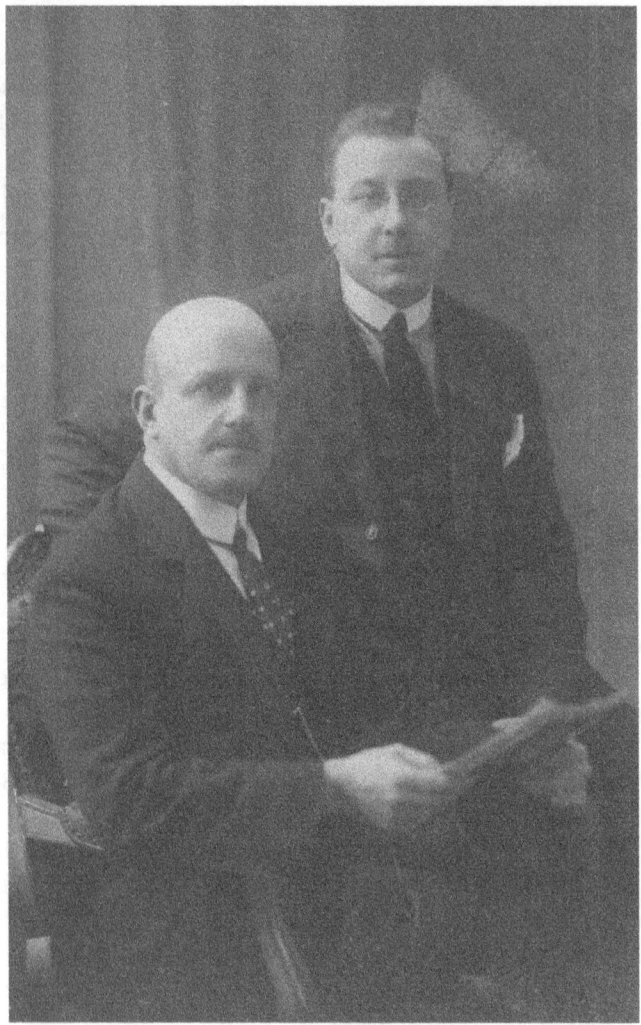

Figure 15.2. Norman Haire and his partner, Willem van de Hagt.

CONCLUSION

information, not support, but it had provided a 'front, a forum, and contacts'. Edsall paid this tribute to Haire: 'More than anyone else it was he who had kept the issue of sexual reform alive, though only barely, through the lean years of the 1930s and the post-war years in Britain. But following his death there was no organisation with even the limited agenda and membership of the Sex Education Society until near the end of the decade. Luck, a degree of discretion, or good connections were the only protections available to the individual homosexual'.

At the age of almost 85 EM Forster expressed his anger at the limitations imposed on homosexuals during his lifetime: 'How *annoyed* I am with Society for wasting my time by making homosexuality criminal. The subterfuges, the self-consciousness that might have been avoided' (Moffat 2010, 18, 319). Forster stipulated that because of its homosexual theme his novel *Maurice* should be published posthumously and, in the 'terminal note' he added in 1960, commented that he had not used the word homosexuality when he wrote the novel in 1913 but, since then, public attitudes in Britain had changed 'from ignorance and terror to familiarity and contempt.'

As an established middle-aged writer, he sent this comment to Christopher Isherwood: 'Dr Norman Haire has tittered to William [Plomer] that if my novels were analysed they would reveal a pretty mess, and that the works of H Walpole and S Maugham would be even prettier.'[22] Such allusions would have escaped most readers who imagined homosexuality was rare and did not recognise even the most obvious examples. Haire concealed his own homosexuality so carefully that the identity of his 'life-long friend', Willem van de Hagt, was not made public until after Haire's death. Haire *was* gay but only very few people knew this and even fewer were invited into the closet; Ivan Crozier (2001, 308) was wrong to claim that 'Haire was known to be "gay-friendly."' In 2004 historians Alison Bashford and Carolyn Strange were also mistaken to claim that 'Haire's own homosexuality was an open secret' and the evidence they gave for this was his reference 'with some

---

22 Forster's letter to Isherwood, 16 January 1935, in *Selected letters of EM Forster*, Volume 2, 1985, 129-30. William Plomer, a novelist, poet and literary editor, was never openly homosexual.

regularity' in *Woman* to his own anxious adolescence and his mention of 'young men tragically "emasculating" themselves and even killing themselves because of the "guilt feeling" of being sexually abnormal'.[23] They also cited his 1946 book *Sex talks* as their reference but neither of these sources mention 'guilt feeling' or 'emasculating' or 'being sexually abnormal.' Haire said his reasons for writing on sex could be 'traced in the turmoil and unhappiness of my own adolescence', when, like most other people, he did not understand the disturbing new urges which our civilisation, with its postponement of marriage for many years after sexual maturity made it hard or impossible to satisfy. Once he mentioned a friend's attempted suicide having made a great impression.[24] In repressive societies, when masturbation was called 'the secret vice' and non-marital sex was seen as a sin, many adolescents felt anxious and guilty. It does not follow that sexual reformers are homosexual; no one would argue that campaigners to prevent child abuse *are* child abusers. Haire was homosexual but it was not 'an open secret' and, because he excluded papers on homosexuality at conferences, some might even argue that he was 'gay-unfriendly'.

Ralf Dose (2003, 11–15) emphasised that Haire's writing on contraception in the 1920s breached medical barriers and his advice to thousands of men and women helped to dispel myths and allay sexual fears and increase their happiness. Haire and the WLSR (with Hirschfeld and Haire as the unlikely midwives) were the catalysts for law reforms in such diverse areas as abortion, censorship, divorce and homosexuality. Haire also promoted and provided safe, effective contraception and non-judgemental sex education. Haire was in his late 20s when he arrived in London at the end of World War I; the intelligentsia was deeply influenced by 19th-century thinkers such as Karl Marx, Charles Darwin and Herbert Spencer whose grand visions seemed indifferent to individuals. In contrast, Haire always focused on

---

23   Bashford & Strange (2004, 83). Bashford received a University of Sydney grant for a project on 'The science of sex: an analysis of the Norman Haire Collection at the University of Sydney'. Available at www.usyd.edu.au/ro/performance/sesqui_2002.shtml [Accessed 24 November 2005].

24   Haire mentioned it in 'Why I write on sex' (*Woman*, 26 October 1942, 8).

Conclusion

individuals and this multidisciplinary 20th-century campaigner made an enormous difference by helping people to have satisfying sex lives and make choices about child bearing and he worked in the vanguard for these civil rights reforms. He was never self-centred and, despite his rejection of religion, his life's work exemplifies the Jewish *tikkun olam* concept of 'repairing the world'. He was brave and life affirming, in the words of historian Manning Clark, he was an enlarger who struggled with the straighteners of life, or wowsers, as Haire called them.

Norman was a shy, delicate child who was intimidated by his father and bullied at school; as a young man he was unsure of himself and wanted to 'sit at the feet' of others but he gained confidence, courage and stability in the 1920s once he started his lifelong relationship with an older man: Willem van de Hagt (1879–1961), the administrator of the Rotterdam Zoo, who also ran a contraceptive export business. They had a secret, often interrupted relationship and Haire mentioned making 50 visits to Holland in the first decade of their partnership. This calm, scholarly man, who wrote an archaeology thesis in Latin in 1903 (which is still in print),[25] was Haire's anchor and inspiration but he remains an enigma despite many attempts to find out more.[26] However, he should be acknowledged for providing the wisdom, serenity and support which enabled Haire to ring out his old, unhappy past and ring in his new one as a crusader. Haire wanted to uplift humanity, not by abolishing sexual morality but by providing a 'new sexual ethic' which would reflect

---

25   van de Hagt's *De urbe Agrigentinorum quae innotuerunt* [*What they have discovered about the city of Agrigento*](1903) is available from online booksellers including Amazon and Google Books.

26   Diligent searching found very little: Kees Moeliker, the current administrator of the Rotterdam Zoo, asked friends, placed queries on the internet and consulted archives; as did the actress Miriam Margolyes who is a friend of one of Haire's relatives; Ralf Dose passed my request on to Paul Snijders, a Dutch antiquarian bookseller, who found that M and EJ van Aaken van Schaardenburgh – probably his heirs – had signed Willem van de Hagt's death certificate in 1961. Paul checked local cemeteries and telephone directories and wrote to the municipal archives in the towns where they lived then but found that there is no van de Hagt archive in the Dutch State Archives and said that in the Netherlands it is impossible to obtain access to a relatively recent testament without the consent of the heirs and he could not find their address.

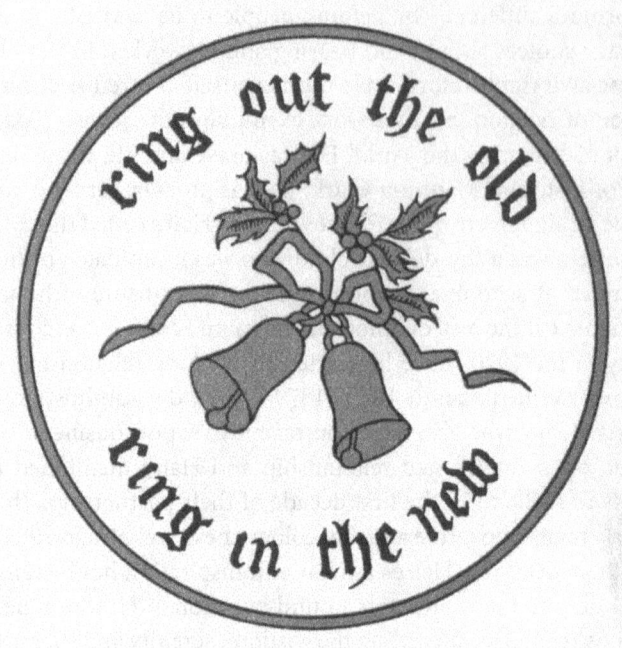

Figure 15.3. Haire's greeting card.

'scientific knowledge and social and economic circumstances' rather than an 'outworn' Biblical ethic.

Haire's greeting for the festive season reflects this uplifting aim and may also be a secret tribute to the man who helped him to ring in his new life. It makes an appropriate epitaph – he always used words precisely so his choice of an archaic typeface for his message seems like an intentional joke.

Abbreviations

AAMC	Australian Army Medical Corps
AASW	Australian Association of Scientific Workers
ABC	Australian Broadcasting Corporation
ADB	*Australian dictionary of biography*
A & R	Angus & Robertson
ALP	Australian Labor Party
ANU	Australian National University
ASIO	Australian Security Intelligence Organisation
AUC	Allen & Unwin Correspondence. Museum of English Life, University of Reading
BBC	British Broadcasting Commission
BL	British Library
BSSSP	British Society for the Study of Sex Psychology
BMA	British Medical Association
CofA	Commonwealth of Australia
DRP	Dora Russell Papers. International Institute of Social History, Amsterdam, The Netherlands.
ESA	Eugenics Society Archives. London: Wellcome Institute for the History of Medicine, SA/EUG.
FFA	Frank Forster Archives, RACOG, Melbourne
FPA	Family Planning Association
HC	Haire Collection
HE	Henry Havelock Ellis
IPPF	International Planned Parenthood Federation
JAMA	*The Journal of the Americal Medical Association*
JHP	Julian Huxley Papers. Houston, Texas: Fondren Library, Rice University
JSE	*The Journal of Sex Education*
LC	Library of Congress, Washington
LSE	London School of Economics

ML	Mitchell Library, Sydney.
NAA	National Archives of Australia
NHA	Norman Himes Archive, Frances A Countway Library, Boston, Massachusetts.
MSP – Smith	Margaret Sanger Papers. Northampton, MA: Smith College, Sophia Smith Collection
MSP – LC	Margaret Sanger Papers. Library of Congress, Washington.
MSP – NYU	Margaret Sanger Papers. New York University, New York.
NSW	New South Wales
RACOG	Royal Australian College of Obstetricians and Gynaecologists, Melbourne
RACP	Royal Australian College of Physicians, Sydney
RHA	Racial Hygiene Association
RMO	Resident Medical Officer
SMH	*Sydney Morning Herald*
SP	Walter J Henry Sprott Papers, Kings College Cambridge.
SUDS	Sydney University Dramatic Society
USRBC	University of Sydney. Rare Book Collection
VD	Venereal Disease
WLAM	Wellcome Library Archives and Manuscripts, London
WLSR	World League for Sexual Reform
WT	Wykeham Terriss (Norman Haire pseudonym)

References

Primary sources

Allen & Unwin Correspondence [AUC]. Reading: Museum of English Life, University of Reading.
——1922. Haire to Stanley Unwin, 22 April, AUC 3/2.
——1924. Extract of an anonymous letter sent to Dr N Haire, 30 December, AUC 14/12.
——1925. Haire to Stanley Unwin, 9 January, AUC 14/12.
——1925. Haire to Unwin, 13 January, AUC, 14/12.
——1925. Haire to Unwin, 16 February, AUC, 14/12.
——1925. Haire to Unwin, 19 February [date crossed out with 2 March 1925 inserted above], AUC, 12/12.
——1925. Haire to Unwin, 12 March, AUC 14/12.
——1925. Haire to Unwin, 17 April, AUC 14/12
——1936. Haire to CA Furth, 5 May, AUC 48/11.
Australian Association of Scientific Workers (NSW).
——1944. AASW (NSW) Annuarl Report NAA A6122, 2017 digitised copy. Barcode 4025162.
——1944. Five years of the AAWS.
——1943. Annual report, 20 June.
Australian War Memorial. *Roll of Honour*. Graham Leask. Died 20 July 1916. [Online] Available: www.awm.gov.au/cms_images/AWM131/029/029393.pdf [Accessed 19 December 2009].
Blue Star Line (1938). Australia brochure. Australian Service ANZ No. 5 1/1/1938-15 M, l - Fraser Darrah Collection. [Online] Available: www.bluestarline.org/Australia_brochure/Australia_brochure_front.html [Accessed 10 May 2008].
Bowler, John (Secretary, Royal South Street Society, Ballarat) (2005). Personal communication, 29 April.

British Library [BL]. Norman Haire Letters
——1920. Add 70540. Haire to Havelock Ellis, 31 May, f 8.
——1921. Add 70540. Haire, Letters to Havelock Ellis, 12 Jan, f 9.
——1922. Add 70540. Haire, Letters to Havelock Ellis, 7 Feb, f 10.
——1921. Add 5867. Haire to Stopes, 6 June, f 35.
——1922. Add 70539. Stella Browne to Havelock Ellis, 6 March.
——1922. Add 58567. Haire to Stopes 28 July, f 45.
——1922. Add 58567. Haire to Stopes, 2 August, f 46.
——1923. Add 70540. Haire to Ellis, 20 August, f 38–43.
——1926. Add 70540. Haire to Ellis, 4 November, f 44.
——1929. Add 58567. Haire to Stopes, 24 October, f 50.
——1930. Add 70540. Haire to Havelock Ellis, 21 September, ff 53–55.
——1930. Add 58567. Haire to Stopes, 22 December, f 55.
——1931. Add 70540. Haire to Havelock Ellis, [n.d.], f. 56.
——1931. Add 58567. Haire to Stopes, 16 February, f 57.
——1931, Add 58567. Haire to Stopes, 5 August, f.58.
——1934. Add 70540. Haire to Havelock Ellis, 29 May, f. 60.
——1934. Add 70540. Haire to Ellis, 9 July, f. 61.
——1933. Add 70542. Haire to Lafitte-Cyon, 14 June, f. 63.
——1934. Add 58567. Haire to Stopes, 14 March, ff 63–64.
——1934. Add 5867. Enclosed with 14 March letter: 'Report of a lecture at Cromer Welfare and Sunlight Centre, by Haire: 'Practical methods of birth control' (Illustrated by lantern slides) [undated], ff. 65–80.
——1934. Add 58567. Haire to Stopes, 14 March, f 74.
——1947. Add 70573. Haire to Lafitte-Cyon [n.d.], f. 182.
——1947. Add 70573. Haire to F Lafitte-Cyon, 9 August, f 183–85.
——1947. Add 70573. Haire to Lafitte-Cyon, 13 August, f. 187.
——1947. Add 70573. Haire to Lafitte-Cyon, 15 August, f. 188.
——1947. Add 70573. Haire to Lafitte-Cyon, 17 August, f. 190.
——1947. Add 70573. Haire to Lafitte-Cyon, 18 August, f. 191.
——1947. Add 70573. Haire to Lafitte-Cyon, 4 September, f. 192.
——1947. Add 70573. Haire to Lafitte-Cyon, 9 September, f. 193.
——1947. Add 70573. Lafitte-Cyon to [Pillay], 8 November, f. 195–96.
British Sexology Society Archives (1921). 83rd Management Meeting, 21 March. Austin, Texas. Harry Ransom Humanities Research Centre at the University of Texas, Austin. From notes supplied by Lesley Hall.

References

The British Society for the Study of Sex Psychology [BSSSP]

——1923. Paul, Eden. Steinach's rejuvenation experiments. Publication 11, (1) *Rejuvenation: Steinach's researches on the sex glands*. London: BSSSP, pp. 1–13. Read to BSSSP January 1921.

——1923. Haire, Norman. Recent developments of Steinach's work. Publication 11, (2) *Rejuvenation: Steinach's researches on the sex glands*. London: BSSSP, pp. 14–36. Read to BSSSP, 28 Nov 1921.

——1923. Minutes, 111th Management Committee, 10 May.

——1923. Minutes, 115th Management Committee, 4 October.

——1926. Minutes, 144th Management Committee, 8 April.

——1933. 'Letter received from Dr Margaret Lowenfeld's secretary, ML Stewart'. 22 November.

Brody, Stephanie (2010) (Harry Ransom Centre, The University of Texas at Austin). Personal communication, 17 February.

City of Sydney (1919). Letter of reference for Norman Zions, 30 May.

Cohen, Norman (1999). Personal communication, 7 December.

Coleman, Peter (2012). Personal communication, 30 July.

Cope, Ian (1998). Personal communication, 5 May.

Dalby, Alyson (Librarian, RACP, Sydney) (2007). Personal communication, January.

Dickson, Ken (archivist of Little Gaddesden, Hertfordshire) (2007). Personal communication, 15 March.

Dose, Ralf (2011). Personal communication, 4 July.

Dose, Ralf (2000). Personal communication, 10 November.

Eraso, Yolanda (2009). Personal communication, 5 February.

Eugenics Society Archives (1921). Letter from Hon Secretary Eugenics Society to Norman Haire on 5 March in response to his letter requesting membership information. London: Wellcome Institute for the History of Medicine, AS/EUG/C.139.

Fleming, Susan (Clinical Superintendent, King George V Hospital, Sydney) (1981). Letter from J Westone, Canberra, 16 March.

Forster, Frank MC

——1981. Susan Fleming, received a letter from J Westone, Canberra, on 16 March and forwarded it to Forster, who acknowledged the letter on 23 April. Melbourne: Frank Forster Collection, The Library, RACOG.

——1988. Personal communication, 5 August.
——1993. Personal communication, 29 June.
——1993. Personal communication, 24 August.
——1996. 'Norman Haire (1892–1952)', *ADB*. [Online]. Available: adb.anu.edu.au/biography/haire-norman-10390 [Accessed 23 October 2012].
Frischknecht, Beat (2008). Personal communication, 6 February.
Norman Haire Collection, Rare Books and Special Collections Library, The University of Sydney (HC)
——2.01 – Haire. Sex and the individual. Lectures 3–10. 25 Sept–20 Nov 1945. Typescripts. 15; 22; 23; 25; 22; 22; 26; 21; 21; 29 pp.
——2.03 – Haire. Radio talks, 1942. 2GB. Typescript. With listeners' questions and answers.
——2.04 – Haire. Lecture: the falling birthrate. Typescript.
——2.06 – Haire. Lecture: morals in wartime. 1943. Extracts, 4 pp.
——2.08 – Haire. *Hymen, or, the future of marriage*. Extracts. Typescript. 2 pp.
——2.09 – Haire. *Through a doctor's spectacles*. Typescript. [1941].
——2.10 – Haire. Sex education – Dr Haire's reply. Typescript with ms annotations. 10 pp.
——2.11 – Haire. Sex education in schools. Typescript. 4 pp.
——2.12 – Haire. Melodrama. Typescript 2 pp. + Holograph draft.
——2.14 – Haire. Music. Typescript. 2 pp.
——2.15 – Haire. The burglar. Typescript. 4 pp.
——2.17 – Scientific evidence. Typescript. 21 pp.
——2.18 – Haire's recipes. 1936.
——2.20 – Press cuttings. Bound volume. Cuttings. 1922–1923.
——3.01 – *Hurstville Propeller*. Typescripts. 5 pp, 7 April 1943 and 2 pp, 3 May 1943.
——3.02 – *The Daily Telegraph* (Sydney). 2 Items. Holograph Ms. 12 Nov 1940. 2 pp; Typescript. 18 May 1942. 2 pp.
——3.03 – *Sydney Morning Herald*. 5 items. Typescripts. 1 p, 26 August 1942; 2 pp, 31 August 1942; 1 p, 14 September 1942; 1 p, 11 December 1942 and 2 pp, 23 June 1944.
——3.04 – *Woman*, 19 March 1941 – 20 Sept 1951. 1 Folder.
——3.06 – Australian Cultural Society. 1942. Typescripts. 8 items.
——3.07 – Haire to Kegan, Paul & Co. Re publication of *Hymen: or, the future of marriage*. Typescript.

——3.08 – Haire. Biographical notes and references by various authors. Typescripts. 16 items.

——3.10 – NSW General Medical Council. Typescript and ms notes. [1 January 1926].

——3.16 – Ellis to Haire, 12 Feb 1924.

——3.17 – Dr Henry T Gillett. Typescripts 10 September 1925 to 11 February 1931.

——3.20 – Magnus Hirschfeld. Typescripts. 1923 to 1935.

——3.22 – Terrence Millen. Typescript. 1937.

——3.23 – Mervyn Findlay (solicitor) re court case: *McKenzie v Haire*. Typescripts. 1942 to 1947.

——3.24 – Nettleden Lodge, Hertfordshire. Papers relating to purchase etc. Typescript. Plans.

——Item 4 – Photographs. Norman Haire. Nettleden Lodge etc..

——Item 7.30 – [Cartoon] A new Aesop: the Haire and the Lyons – 'Population unlimited'

——Item 7.36 (and 7.37) – Norman Haire. *Comparative value of current contraceptive methods*. 1928.

——Item 8.03 – Haire's appointment diary, 1924. He also had diaries for 1929, 1931, 1933, 1950 and 1952 but many are blank.

——Item 12 – A doctor looks at life. Typescript. 4 pp. [1941].

——Item 19 – Haire, Norman. *Hymen: or, the future of marriage*. London: Kegan Paul, 1928.

——Item 26 – Rutgers, J *The sexual life in its biological significance*. Translated by Norman Haire. Dresden: RE Giesecke, 1924.

——1923. Letter from Haire to WJH Sprott, 17 June [SP].

——1923. BL Add 70540, Haire to Ellis, 20 August, f 43.

——1924. Ellis to Haire, 12 February. (HC, 3.16).

——1925. Haire to Ellis, 24 February. (HC, 3.16).

——1925. Haire to Unwin, 17 April. (AUC, 14/12).

——1925. Haire to Ellis, 5 June. (HC, 316).

——1926. Haire to Ellis, 12 September. (HC, 3.16).

——1927. Ellis to Haire, 15 February. (HC, 3.16).

——1927. Haire to Ellis, 16 February. (HC, 3.16).

——1927. Haire to Ellis, 18 July. (HC, 3.16).

———1927. Haire to Marjorie Farrer, North Kensington Women's Welfare Centre, 21 June. London: WLAM.
———1928. ES Daniels to Himes, 4 September. NHA, BMS, Box 34, Folder 385, from notes supplied by Lesley A Hall.
———1931. Henry T Gillett to Haire, 9 February. (HC 3.17).
———1931. Haire to Gillett, 11 February. (HC 3.17).
———1935. Letters and telegram of condolence about Hirschfeld's death from Norman Haire to Ernst Maass, 18 and 29 May (supplied by Ralf Dose).
Hall, Lesley A (2007). Personal communication, 26 May.
Himes, Norman. [NHA]
———1926 Haire to Himes, 25 August [NHA].
———1926. Haire to Himes, 30 September [NHA].
———1926. Haire to Himes, 9 November [NHA].
———1927. Haire to Himes, 19 January [NHA].
———1928. Haire to Himes, 19 July [NHA].
———1928. Haire to Himes, 19 September [NHA].
———1929. Haire to Himes, 18 February [NHA].
———1929. Himes to Haire, 14 March [NHA].
Horan, Ronald S (1998). Personal communication, 16 May.
How-Martyn, Edith (1929). Letter to Sanger. 3 January [MSP–Smith].
Huxley, Julian – Julian Huxley Papers. Houston, Texas: Fondren Library, Rice University. [JHP].
———1920. Letter from Blacker to Huxley, 24 February, 10.1. [JHP].
———1933. Letter from Haire to Huxley. 30 June. [JHP].
Kerr, AL (1919). Major Adjutant, pro PMO, 2nd M D, Military Forces of the Commonwealth, Victoria Barracks, Sydney. Correspondence, 22 July. (H C, 03.27).
Lafitte-Cyon, Francoise (1947). Haire–Lafitte-Cyon Correspondence. BL – Add 70542, 9 August, f 184.
Latukefu, Ruth (2003). Personal communication, 18 February.
Mancini, Renata (Archivist, University of Sydney), 1998. Personal communication, 27 March.
NAA Series A 367/1, Item C69409. Haire, Dr Norman (formerly Zions) 1940–1946. Digitised copy – barcode 782659.
———1940. Secret Memorandum for The Secretary, Prime Minister's Department, Canberra. Re: Dr Norman Haire (formerly Zajac – crossed out, Zions above)

References

from Office Secretary, Australia House. Copy to Departments of Attorney-General, Interior and Army, 27 May.

——1942. Letter from HR Jones, Director to Inspector-in-Charge, Commonwealth Investigation Branch, Sydney, 18 June.

—— 1942. Letter from Haire, 2 October.

——1942. Re Norman Haire, SC Taylor, Deputy Director of Security for NSW to Director General of Security, Canberra, 27 November.

——1946. Investigation Branch, Canberra. Reg no C69409 – Dr Norman Haire left Sydney … on the steamer 'Port Macquarie' on the 24th August.

NAA Series A461/1, Item H247/1/8.

——1944. Florence Kenna to Prime Minister, 8 February.

NAA Series A 472/1, Item W 1613. Dr Norman Haire, 1940-44.

——1942. Bohun telegram to Arthur Calwell, 8 October.

——1942. Dr Norman Haire – 'Sex "Education" racket should be stopped', press clipping from *The Daily Mirror*, 17 October, p. 6.

——1943. Selected statements taken from a lecture 'Morals in war time' delivered by Dr Norman Haire at the King's Cross Theatrette, 83 Darlinghurst Road, King's Cross on Sunday night April 11, 1943.

——1943. Letter from EJ Holloway to JM Fraser, 27 September.

——1943. Secret Memo. Ref. No. 10, 233 from the Director of Security, to the Deputy Director of Security in Sydney, 30 October.

NAA Series A 2910, Item 432/24/83/48. 'Publications – Dr Norman Haire'. Haire to Kenneth Binns, Librarian, Commonwealth National Library, 10 July 1947; Binns to Haire, 12 August 1947 Digitised copy, Barcode 231709.

NAA Series A6122, Item 2017. 1942–1953, Australian Association of Scientific Workers – Queensland – Vol. 1 – f. 23 in the AASW (NSW) 1944 Annual Report. Digitised copy – barcode 4025162.

NAA Series AWM 41, Item 1544. Australia's population problem, by Norman Haire. Digitised copy – barcode 5171816.

NAA Series BP 241/1, Item Q 25548. Haire, (formerly Zajac) – Queensland investigation case file.

——1943. Arthur Calwell's confidential letter to the Hon EJ Holloway, 20 September.

NAA Series D 596/2, Item 1936/9416. Importation of *Birth-control methods*, by Norman Haire. 12 February 1937 decision the book 'is not to be regarded as a prohibited import'.

NAA Series K 269, Incoming passenger list to Freemantle *Melbourne Star* – Dr Haire passenger in MV *Melbourne Star* from England. Arrived Freemantle, WA 1730 hours, 26 July 1940.

NAA Series M 1415. Item 453, 22 October 1943 – 2 January 1945. Personal Papers of Prime Minister Curtin – Correspondence 'P' including Public Morals Committee re Dr Norman Haire.

——1944. Telegram from Rev David J Knox, The Rectory, Gladesville to the Prime Minister, 21 August – digitized copy – barcode 1733382.

——1944. EW Tonkin (Private Secretary) to Rev DJ Knox, 12 October.

NAA Series MP 298/4, Item 52/21/1. Mrs Jessie Street [Forum of the Air]. 1944.

——1944. Macmahon Ball to Street, 11 September.

——1944. Moses to Canon TC Hammond, 18 September.

——1944. Mr AT Thielfall to the General Manager, 25 September.

NAA Series MP 298/4, N/17/1, Nation's Forum of the Air – General, 1944–46. Nation's Forum of the Air – Second Session,

——1944. Macmahon Ball to Molesworth, re draft statement of publicity, 8.

——1944. Press clippings in response to the debate.

——1944. Haire to Macmahon Ball, 8 June.

——1944. Macmahon Ball to Haire, 13 June.

——1944. Haire to Macmahon Ball, 10 August.

——1944. Moses to Commissioners, 14 September.

——1944. Moses to Canon TC Hammond, 18 September.

NAA Series MP 298/4/0, N/17/3, WOB3, Nations Forum of the Air, Macmahon Ball to Moses, 25 August 1944.

NAA Series MP 298/5, Item HA/11/3. Dr Norman Haire [Forum of the Air]

——1944, Macmahon Ball to Haire, 6 June.

——1944. Macmahon Ball to Haire, 11 September.

——1944. Macmahon Ball to Haire, 20 September.

NAA Series SP 42/2, Item C1946/10597, 1945–1946, Barcode 7464767: Dr Norman Haire – Application for Passport Facilities, 7 pp.

NAA Series SP 369/3, Item Vol. 1/2. *Nation's Forum of the Air*, 'Population unlimited?' Topical debate broadcast from the Assembly Hall. Transcript of the script by Miss EA Mackay, Topical debate broadcast from the Assembly Hall, Sydney on 23 August 1944. Speakers: Dame Enid Lyons, Mr Colin Clark, Dr Norman Haire, Mrs Jessie Street.

References

——1939. ABC, Office of the Federal Talks Controller. Memorandum to: The General Manager, Managers' meeting agenda: 1 March, from BH Molesworth.

NAA Series SP 369/3, Item Vol. 1/9. Nation's Forum of the Air – 'The Battle for Population'. Topical debate broadcast 29 November 1944 [Box 1].

NAA Series SP 1558/2, General Manager's correspondence with the States and the Commission, 1 January 1936 to 31 December 1948.

——1944. Moses to Macmahon Ball, 20 May.

——1944. Moses to all Commissioners, 24 August.

——1944. JM Martin, for the Director-General, Post-Master General's Department to the General Manager, ABC, with copies to Macmahon Ball, Molesworth and McCall, 3 October.

Nixon, Betty, (General Secretary, Galton Institute). 2007. Personal communication, 18 May.

Racial Hygiene Association papers, Sydney:

——1931. Executive Committee, 20 July. MLMSS 7173, Box 1.

——1932. Executive Meeting, 7 June. ML MSS 3838.

Registry of Birth, Death and Marriages (1919). File number 1919. Sydney.

Russell, Dora (1929). Dora Russell Papers. Haire to Russell, 1 January 1929. International Institute of Social History, Amsterdam, The Netherlands.

Sands, Lee (2009). Information Officer, Records and Archives, British Medical Association. Personal communication, July.

Sanger, Margaret (1921). Haire to Sanger. [MSP – LC], 15 September, 8:971.

—— 1921. Haire to Sanger. [MSP – LC], 1 October, 8: 967, provided by Lesley Hall.

—— 1923. Ellis to Sanger. [MSP – LC], 9 February.

—— 1923. Ellis to Sanger. [MSP – LC], 28 August.

—— 1923. Ellis to Sanger. [MSP – LC], 26 November.

—— 1926. N Himes asking for introduction to leaders of British birth control movement. In the margin 'AL: Dr Haire, Dr Drysdale, Dr B Dunlop, Edith How-Martyn, sent.' [MSP – Smith], 16 April. Sanger Reel S03.

—— 1929. Edith How-Martyn to Sanger. [SMP – Smith], 3 January.

Savill, Gloria. (Bert Hare's daughter) (1998). Personal communication, 24 October.

Sengoopta, Chandak (2006). Personal communication, 25 July.

Shenfield, Gillian (1999). Personal communication, 20 November.

Singer, Charles. Charles Singer papers, Wellcome Library. PP/CJS/A6/Box 1. Charles Singer to Dr Norman Haire, 15 February 1939.

—— Norman Haire to Professor Charles Singer, 21 February 1939.
Sprott, Walter J Herbert (SP).
—— 1928. Letter from Harie to Sprott, 21 December.
—— 1927. Letter from Haire to Sprott, 20 September.
—— 1923. Letter from Haire to Sprott, 17 June.
University of Sydney (1922). Letter from the Warden and Registrar to Norman Haire, 31 March. HC, 3.27.
University of Sydney Calendar (1914). Faculty of Medicine results, pp467, 560–61.
University of Sydney Calendar (1915). Faculty of Medicine results, pp417–18.
Victoria Barracks (1919). Military forces of the Commonwealth, 2nd Military Division, signed on behalf of Major A L Kerr, Adjutant, PRO P MQ – 'This is to certify that Dr N Zions is permitted to leave the Commonwealth, 19 August'. Sydney: Victoria Barracks.
Weeks, Jeffrey (2001). Personal communication, 26 February.
Weston, J (Canberra) (1981). Letter hand delivered to Dr Susan Fleming, Clinical Superintendent, King George V Hospital, Sydney on 16 March who forwarded it to Dr Frank Forster.

Bibliography

ABC (1944a). *The nation's forum of the air.* 'Population unlimited?' Broadcast on its National Network by the Australian Broadcasting Commission, 1, (1), 23 August.

ABC (1944b). *The nation's forum of the air.* 'The Battle for Population' Broadcast on its National Network by the Australian Broadcasting Commission, 1, (9), 29 November.

ADB (2006). Online edition, Australian National University. [Online] Available: adbonline.anu.edu.au/adbonline.htm [Accessed 19 December 2009].

Afford, Max (1974). *Mischief in the air: radio and stage plays.* St Lucia, Brisbane: University of Queensland Press.

Alexander, Peter F (1989). *William Plomer: a biography.* Oxford, New York: Oxford University Press.

Allbutt, H Arthur (1887). *The wife's handbook.* Leeds: Allbutt.

American Birth Control Conference (1921). *Birth control: what it is, how it works, what it will do.* 1922. The Proceedings of the first American Birth Control Conference, Hotel Plaza, New York, November 11, 12, 1921. New York: *The Birth Control Review.*

Arndt, HW (1987). Entry for Colin Clark in the *New Palgrave dictionary of political economy*, John Eatwell and others (Eds). London: Macmillan.

Arnold, John (Ed) (1983). *A letter from Sydney: being a long epistle from Ray Lindsay to his brother Jack relating mainly to their lives in Sydney in the nineteen-twenties*. Melbourne: Jester Press.

Asbury, Herbert (2002 [1927]). *The gangs of New York: an informal history of the underworld*. London: Arrow Books.

Atherton, Gertrude (1933). Science after fifty. *Pictorial Review*, 34: 15, 58.

—— (1932). *Adventures of a novelist*. London: Cape.

Avery, Harold (1965). Contraception through the ages. *Medical History*, 91(1): 99–100.

—— (1952). Norman Haire: a tribute. *The Journal of Sex Education*, 5(1): 2.

Ayto, John (1993). *Euphemisms*. London: Bloomsbury.

Barcan, Alan (1965). *A short history of education in New South Wales*. Sydney: Martindale Press.

Barker, Dudley (1939). Harley Street. *London Evening Standard*, 7 August, p7.

Baring-Gould, William S (1970). *The lure of the limerick*. London: Panther Books.

Baring-Gould, William S & Cecil Baring-Gould (1967). *The annotated Mother Goose. Nursery rhymes old and new, arranged and explained*. Clevelane and New York: Meridian Books.

Bashford, Alison & Strange, Carolyn (2004). Public pedagogy: sex education and mass communication in the mid-twentieth century. *Journal of the History of Sexuality*, 13 (1): 71–99.

Bauer, Bernhard (1927). *Woman and love*. Vol. 2. Translated by Eden & Cedar Paul. New York: Liveright Publishing.

Bauer, Hikie (2003). 'Not a translation but a mutilation': the limits of translation and the discipline of sexology. *The Yale Journal of Criticism*, 16(2): 381–405.

Bell, Anne Oliver (Ed) (1977). *The diary of Virginia Woolf. Vol. I: 1915–1919*. London: The Hogarth Press.

Benjamin, Harry (1969). Address. 12th annual conference of the Society for the Scientific Study of Sex, November. [Online] Available: www2.huberlin.de/sexology/GESUND/ARCHIV/REMINI.HTM [Accessed 7 June 2006].

—— (1945). Eugen Steinach: a life of research. *Scientific Monthly*, 61: 437.

—— (1944). The late Professor Steinach. *The New York Times*, 3 June, p12.

Bendiner, Elmer (1988). Brown-Sequard: scientific triumphs and fiascos. *Hospital Practice*, 23(8): 139–40.

Benn, J Miriam (1992). *The predicaments of love*. London: Pluto Press.
Bennett, Jack (Ed) (1982). *A photo album: the ABC from 1932 to 1982*. Sydney: ABC.
Billington, Michael (2001). Tynan's gift was to make criticism glamorous and sexy. *The Guardian*, 24 September.
Blacker, CP (1926). *Birth control and the state: a plea and a forecast*. London: Kegan Paul, Trench, Trubner & Co.
Bland, Caroline & Cross, Marie (Eds) (2003). *Gender and politics in the age of letter writing, 1750–2000*. Aldershot, Hants: Ashgate.
Bland, Caroline & Laura Doan (Eds) (1998). *Sexology in culture: labelling bodies and desires*. Chicago: University of Chicago Press.
Blunt, Wilfred (1983). *Married to a single life: an autobiography, 1901–1938*. London: Michael Russell.
—— (1986). *Slow on the feather: further autobiography, 1938–1959*. London: Michael Russell.
Bongiorno, Frank (2012) *The sex lives of Australians: a history*. Collingwood, Victoria: Black Inc.
Book Review Digest (1928). New York: HW Wilson Company.
Borell, Merriley (1987). Biologists and the promotion of birth control research, 1918–1938. *Journal of the History of Biology*, 20 (1), Spring: 51–87.
Bradshaw, David (1992). The eugenics movement in the 1930s and the emergence of *On the Boiler*. *Yeats Annual*, (9): 189–215.
Brandhorst, Henny (2003). From Neo-Malthusianism to sexual reform: the Dutch section of the World League for Sexual Reform. *Journal of the History of Sexuality*, 12(1): 42.
Bremmer, Robert (Ed) (1971). *Children and youth in America*. Cambridge, Mass: Harvard University Press.
Brooke, Stephen (2005). The body and socialism: Dora Russell in the 1920s. *Past & Present*, 189(1): 161.
Broun, Malcolm D (1996). Dovey, Wilfred Robert (1894–1969). *ADB*, 14, Melbourne University Press, p24.
Browne, Frances Worsley Stella (1917). Women and birth-control. In C & E Paul (Eds). *Population and birth-control* (pp243–257). New York: Critic and Guide
Brunvand, Jan Harold (1962). Further notes on sex in the classroom. *Journal of American Folklore*, 75: 62.
—— (1960). Sex in the classroom. *Journal of American Folklore*, 73: 250–251.

Buckridge, Patrick (1994). *The scandalous penton: a biography of Brian Penton*. St Lucia: University of Queensland Press.
Burman, Barbara (1995). Better and brighter clothes; the Men's Dress Reform Party, 1929–1940. *Journal of Design History*, Vol. 8, (4): 275–290.
Burke, Thomas (1925). Australians I have met. *The Triad*, 14 September, p17.
—— (1924). Profile. *The Triad*, 1 December, p15.
Burnet, FM & Clark, Ellen (1942). *Influenza: a survey of the last 50 years in the light of modern work on the virus of epidemic influenza*. (Monograph 4, Walter and Eliza Hall Institute of Research in Pathology and Medicine), Melbourne: Macmillan.
Butt, John (Ed) (1968). *The poems of Alexander Pope*. London: Methuen.
Calder-Marshall, Arthur (1959). *Sage of sex: a life of Havelock Ellis*. London: Putnam's.
Callesen, Gerd (comp.) (2001). *Socialist international: a bibliography. Publications of the social-democratic and socialist internationals, 1914–2000*. International Association of Labour History Institutions. [Online] Available: library.fes.de/pdf-files/bibliothek/01035.pdf [Accessed 19 May 2001].
Capshew, James H, Adamson, Matthew H, Buchanan, Patricia A, Murray, Narisara & Wake, Naoko (2003). Kinsey's biographers: a historiographical reconnaissance. *Journal of the History of Sexuality*, 12(3): 465–86.
Carr, Raymond (2005). Review of *DH Lawrence: the life of an outsider*. *Weekend Australian*, 14–15 May, pR12.
Champion, Ben W (1978). *The history of Newcastle Hospital, 1891–1915*. Newcastle: the Author.
Chesler, Ellen (1992). *Woman of valor: Margaret Sanger and the birth control movement in America*. New York: Simon & Schuster.
Chesser, Elizabeth Sloan (1930). The Dutch pessary. *The Lancet*, 216(5581): 377.
Churches, Kelvin (1976). Tracy-Maund memorial lecture delivered at the Royal Women's Hospital, Melbourne: '120 years of abortion in Melbourne: a social, medical and legal history'. Typescript provided by Dr Churches on 21 April 1988.
Clanchy, John (1990). Stewart, David (1883–1954). *ADB*, 12, Melbourne University Press, pp84–85.
Close, Robert (1977). *Of salt and earth: an autobiography*. Melbourne: Thomas Nelson.
—— (1945). *Love me sailor*. Melbourne: Georgian House.

Coleman, Peter (1962). *Obscenity, blasphemy, sedition: censorship in Australia.* Brisbane: Jacaranda Press.

Commonwealth of Australia (1920). *Official year book of the Commonwealth of Australia* (13). Canberra: Commonwealth Bureau of Census and Statistics.

Cook, Hera (2004). *The long sexual revolution: English women, sex, and contraception 1800–1975.* Oxford: Oxford University Press.

Cooper, James F (1928). *Technique of contraception: the principles and practice of anti-conceptional methods.* New York: Day-Nicholas.

Cooper, John (2003). *Pride versus prejudice: Jewish doctors and lawyers in England, 1890–1990.* Oxford, Portland, Ore: The Litman Library of Jewish Civilization.

Coote, Stephen (1997). *WB Yeats: a life.* London: Sceptre.

Corners, George F (1923). *Rejuvenation: how Steinach makes people young.* New York: Thomas Seltzer.

Cox, Erle (2006). *Out of the silence.* Text revised by John H Costello with permission from the estate of Erle Cox. Dimitar Guetov (Ed). First published in *The Argus* in 1919.

Craig, Alec (1963). *Suppressed books: a history of the conception of literary obscenity.* Cleveland and New York: The World Publishing Company.

—— (1962[1937]). *The banned books of England: a study of the conception of literary obscenity.* London: George Allen & Unwin.

—— (1934). *Sex and revolution.* London: George Allen & Unwin.

Croall, Jonathan (1983). *Neill of Summerhill: the permanent rebel.* London: Routledge & Kegan Paul.

Cronin, AJ (1937). *The citadel.* London: V Gollancz.

Crowlesmith, John (1949). Review of Norman Haire's *Everyday sex problems. Marriage Hygiene*, 3(4) October, p4.

Crozier, Ivan (2003). All the world's a stage: Dora Russell, Norman Haire and the 1929 London World League for Sexual Reform Congress. *Journal of the History of Sexuality*, 12(1): 16–37.

—— (2001). Becoming a sociologist: Norman Haire, the 1929 World League for Sexual Reform Congress, and organizing medical knowledge about sex in interwar England. *History of Science*, 39 Part 3(125): 299–329.

Cumpston, John Howard Lidgett (1919). *Influenza and maritime quarantine in Australia.* CofA, Quarantine Service Publication no 18. Melbourne: Government Printer.

Cumpston, John Howard Lidgett & Milton James Lewis (Eds) (1989 [1928]). *Health and disease in Australia: a history.* Canberra: AGPS Press.

Darian-Smith, Kate (1990). *On the home front: Melbourne in wartime 1939-1945.* South Melbourne: Oxford University Press.

Davidson, Graeme, Hirst, John & Macintyre, Stuart (Eds) (1998). *The Oxford companion to Australian history.* Melbourne: Oxford University Press.

Davie, Richard (1927). An Australian doctor's mission. *The Triad*, 23 May, p4.

Dawson, Lord Dawson of Penn (1922). *Love-marriage-birth control.* London: Nisbet and Co Ltd.

—— (1921). Love-marriage-birth control. *The Malthusian*, November: 87.

de Berg, Hazel (1976). 'Ruby Rich', interview. Canberra: National Library of Australia, Oral History Tape 13, 368.

de Haan, Francisca, Daskalova, Krasimira & Lotfi, Anna (Eds) (2006). *A biographical dictionary of women's movements and feminists: Central, Eastern and South Eastern Europe, 19th and 20th centuries.* Budapest and New York: Central European Press.

Dickinson, Robert L (1924). Contraception: a medical review of the situation. *American Journal of Obstetrics and Gynecology*, viii(8): 583–604, Discussion, pp654–55.

Dose, Ralf (2003). The World League for Sexual Reform: some possible approaches. *Journal of the History of Sexuality*, 12(1), January: 1–15.

—— (2005). *Magnus Hirschfeld: Deutscher – Jude – Weltbürger* [German, Jew, Citizen of the World]. Berlin: Hentric & Hentrich.

Doyle, Sir Arthur Conan (1923). *The adventure of the creeping man* was first published in *The Strand Magazine* in March and it was included in *The case book of Sherlock Holmes* in 1927.

Drysdale, BI (1922). Reports. Great Britain. In Raymond Pierpoint (Ed). *Report of the fifth International Neo-Malthusian and Birth Control Conference* (p9). London: William Heinemann Ltd.

Drysdale, CV (1922). Preface. In Raymond Pierpoint (Ed). *Report of the fifth International Neo-Malthusian and Birth Control Conference* (ppv, vii). London: William Heinemann Ltd.

Duke, Emma (1915). Infant mortality: results of a field study in Johnstown, PA. In Robert Bremmer (Ed). *Children and youth in America* (p968). Cambridge, Mass: Harvard University Press.

Dutton, Geoffrey (1986). *The innovators: the Sydney alternatives in the rise of modern art, literature and ideas*. Melbourne: The Macmillan Company of Australia.

Dutton, Ron (2003). The mystery of Li Shiu Tong. *Xtr West*, Issue 265, 16 October. [Online] Available: archives.xtra.ca/Story.aspx?s=2265328 [Accessed 7 July 2011].

Edgar, Suzanne (2006). Lionel George Logue (1880–1953). *ADB*. [Online] Available: adb.anu.edu.au/biography/logue-lionel-george-10852 [Accessed 7 July 2011].

Edsall, Nicholas C (2003). *Toward Stonewall: homosexuality and society in the modern western world*. Charlottesville: University of Virginia Press.

Edwards, Graham A & Hall, Wayne (1980). The case of William Chidley: a study of psychiatry, morality and lunacy law. *Australian and New Zealand Journal of Psychiatry*, 14(2): 133–139.

Ehrlich, Dr Paul R (1969). *The population bomb*. San Francisco: Sierra Club.

Elcano, Barrett W & Bullough, Vern (1981). Sexology: a personal guide to the serial literature. In Peter Gellatly (Ed). *Sex magazines in the library collection: a scholarly study of sex in serials and periodicals*. New York: Haworth Press, 1981.

Ellis, Albert (1952). *Sex beliefs and customs*. London: Peter Nevill.

Ellis, Henry Havelock (1939). *My life: Havelock Ellis*. London: Neville Spearman Ltd.

—— (1937). *Studies in the psychology of sex*. New York: Random House, Vol. 2, Part 2, pp232–35.

—— (1922). First Session. *Birth control: what it is how it works, what it will do*. Proceedings of the first American Birth Control Conference, 11 November 1921. New York: *The Birth Control Review*, p177.

Ellmann, Richard (1986). WB Yeats's second puberty. *Four Dubliners: Wilde, Yeats, Joyce and Beckett*. New York: George Braziller, pp38–62.

—— (1979[1948]). *Yeats: the man and the mask* (2nd edn). New York: EP Dutton.

Ensor, Jason (2009). A policy of splendid isolation: Angus & Robertson, George G Harrap and the politics of co-operation in the Australian book trade during the late 1930s. *Literature and Politics*: Third Annual Conference of the Australasian Association for Literature, Sydney University, 6 July, Politics of Literary Production session. [Online] Available: www.artsnaked.com/postscripts/?p=255 [Accessed 1 January 2010].

Eraso, Yolanda (2007). Biotypology, endrocrinology, and sterilization: the practice of eugenics in the treatment of Argentinian women during the 1930s. *Bulletin of the History of Medicine*, 81(4): 813, fn 55.

Etzioni, Amitai & Baris, Mackenzie (2005). A communitarian perspective on sex and sexuality. *International Review of Sociology*, 15(2) July: 224–26.

Fellows of the Australian Academy of Technological Sciences and Engineering, Melbourne (Eds) (2000). *Technology in Australia 1788–1988: a condensed history of Australian technological innovation and adaptation during the first two hundred years.* [Online] Available: www.austehc.unimelb.edu.au/tia/index.html.

Ferris, Paul (1993). *Sex and the British: a twentieth-century history.* London: Michael Joseph.

Fielding, Michael [pseudonym of Dr Maurice Newfield] (1928). *Parenthood: design or accident? A manual of birth control.* London: Labour Publishing Co.

Fifth Neo-Malthusian Conference (1922). *Report of the Fifth International Neo-Malthusian and Birth Control Conference.* Kingsway Hall, London, 11–14 July. Raymond Pierpoint (Ed). London: William Heinemann (Medical Books) Ltd.

Figaro (incorporated with *The Bohemian*) (1919). Melbourne: Bohemia Publishing Company, 18 October, pp7, 10 and 8 November, pp6–7.

Finneran, Richard J (Ed) (1989). *The collected poems of WB Yeats.* New York: Collier Books.

Fishbein, Morris (1927). *The new medical follies: an encyclopedia of cultism and quackery in these United States, with essays on the cult of beauty, the craze for reduction, rejuvenation, eclecticism, bread and dietary fads, physical therapy, and a forecast as to the physician of the future.* New York: Boni & Liveright.

Fisher, Patty (1976). 'Obituary. Professor VH Mottram: nutritionist who enjoyed his food.' *The Times*, 20 March, p16.

FitzGibbon, Constantine (1967). *Through the minefield: an autobiography.* London: The Bodley Head.

Flügel, Professor JC (1929). Address of welcome. WLSR: xxi. Translated from Esperanto by Kep Enderby.

Ford, Bruce (1980). *The wounded warrior and rehabilitation.* Caufield, Qld: The Alfred Healthcare Group.

Foster, RF (2003). *WB Yeats: a life. Vol. II: The arch-poet.* Oxford: Oxford University Press.

—— (1997). *WB Yeats: a life. Vol. I: The apprentice mage*. Oxford: Oxford University Press.
Fryer, Peter (1969). *British birth control ephemera 1870–1947*. Leicester: Barracuda Press.
—— (1965). *The birth controllers*. London: Secker and Warburg.
Gammage, Bill (1998). Edward 'Ned' Kelly (1855–1880). In Graeme Davidson, John Bradley Hurst & Stuart Macintyre (Eds). *The Oxford companion to Australian history* (pp362–63). Oxford: Oxford University Press.
Gathorne-Hardy, Jonathan (1998). *Alfred Kinsey: sex the measure of all things. A biography*. London: Chatto & Windus.
Gill, Brendan (1987). *Many masks: a life of Frank Lloyd Wright*. London: Putnam's.
Gilman, Sander L (1999). *Making the body beautiful: a cultural history of aesthetic surgery*. Princeton, New Jersey: Princeton University Press.
Glass, David V (1936). *The struggle for population*. Oxford: Oxford University Press.
Graham, Roy Vescya (1921). The influenza epidemic in eastern New South Wales in 1919. MD Thesis. Sydney: University of Sydney.
Grant, George (2000). *Grand illusions: the legacy of planned parenthood* (4th edn). Nashville, Tennessee: Cumberland House.
Graves, Robert & Hodge, Alan (1941). *The long weekend: a social history of Great Britain, 1918–1939*. New York: Macmillan.
Greenwood, AW (Ed) (1931). *Proceedings of the Second International Congress for Sex Research, London, 1930*. London: Oliver and Boyd.
Greer, Germaine (1984). *Sex and destiny: the politics of human fertility*. London: Secker & Warburg.
Groves, Ernest R (1929). The belated science of sex. *Social Forces*, 7(4) June: 592–95.
Griffin, Nicholas (Ed) (2001). *The selected letters of Bertrand Russell: the public years, 1914–1970*. London: Routledge.
Griffiths, Robin (Ed) (2006). *British queer cinema*. London and New York: Routledge.
Grmek, Mirko Drazen (1958). Aging and old age: basic problems and historic aspects of gerontology and geriatrics. *Monographiae Biologicae*, 5(2): 57–162.
Groopman, Jerome (2002). Hormones for men: is male menopause a question of medicine or marketing? *The New Yorker*, 29 July, pp34–38.

Grossman, Atina (1995). *Reforming sex: the German movement for birth control and abortion reform, 1920-1950*. New York, Oxford: Oxford University Press.

Grosskurth, Phyllis (1985). *Havelock Ellis: a biography*. New York: New York University Press.

Gruber, Helmut & Graves, Pamela (Eds) (1998). *Women and socialism: socialism and women: Europe between the two world wars*. New York, Oxford: Berghahn.

Haeberle, Erwin J (2004). The global future of sexology. Speech given in Berlin on 16 October. [Online] Available: www2.hu-berlin.de/sexology/GESUND/ARCHIV/BSpeech/index.htm [Accessed 7 May 2011].

—— (1983). Human rights and sexual rights: the legacy of René Guyon. *Medicine and Law*, (2): 159-172.

Haigh, Gideon (2008). *The racket: how abortion became legal in Australia*. Melbourne: Melbourne University Press.

Haire, Norman *see also* Terriss, Wykeham

—— (1952[1938]). *Sexual anomalies and perversions: physical and psychological development, diagnosis and treatment. A summary of the works of the late Professor Dr Magnus Hirschfeld*. London: Encyclopaedic Press.

—— (1951). *The encyclopaedia of sex practice* (2nd edn). London: Encyclopaedic Press.

—— (1949). National health plans (1), *Woman*, 24 January, p34.

—— (1949). National health plans (2), *Woman*, 14 February, p34.

—— (1948). *Everyday sex problems*. London: Federick Muller.

—— (1947). Havelock Ellis: adventurer in morals. *The Rationalist*, April, pp37-40.

—— (1947). Problems of euthanasia, *Woman*, 28 July, p38.

—— (1946). *Wykeham Terriss, sex talks*. Sydney: Vanguard Publications.

—— (1945). *Sex problems of to-day*. Sydney: Angus and Robertson.

—— (1945). *Birth-control methods*. Sydney: Australasian Publishing Company.

—— (1945). Wisdom of moderation. *Woman*, 14 May, p38.

—— (1943). Venereal diseases and their prevention: some recent pronouncements. *Medical Journal of Australia*, 23: 299-300.

—— (1943). Sex and the juvenile community. *New Horizons in Education*, 3(2) April: 8-14.

—— (1941). Australia's population problem. *General Practitioner*, 12: 2-6.

—— (1940). *Encyclopaedia of sexual knowledge*. New York: Eugenics Publishing Company.

—— (1936). *Birth-control methods (contraception, abortion, sterilization)*. London: George Allen & Unwin.

—— (1935). Introduction. In Magnus Hirschfeld. *Sex in human relationships* (pxii–xiii). Translated by John Rodker. London: The Bodley Head.

—— (1935). Introduction. In Anthony Ludovici. *The choice of a mate* (ppv-vi). London: The Bodley Head.

—— (1935). Magnus Hirschfeld: in memoriam. *Marriage Hygiene*, 2: 120–22.

—— (1934). Revision of the abortion laws, *Anthropos* (1), *Medical Review of Reviews*, 40, January: 47–48.

—— (1932). *Allocution du Docteur Norman Haire*, à la Séance Solennelle tenue en la Sorbonne, le 24 juin par L'Association d'Études Sexologiques, la Société Scientifique de Sexologie, la Société de Prophylaxie Criminelle, la Société d'Hygiène Mentale. Sous la Présidence de Monsieur Justin Godard, Ministre de la Sante Publique [bound with] *La Réforme Sexuelle*. Conférence faite a Paris, dans un cercle privé, le 27 juin 1932, par le Docteur Norman Haire de Londres. Co-Président de la Ligue Mondiale pour la Réform Sexuelle. CP - CP/IND/MONT/4/9. Translated by Dorothy Simons.

—— (1931). The regulation of contraception. Letter by Norman Haire. *The Eugenics Review,* 23(2): 189–90.

—— (1931). The Cromer Welfare Centre. In Margaret Sanger & Hannah M Stone (Eds). *The practice of contraception: an international symposium and survey* (pp218–19). From the Proceedings of the Seventh International Birth Control Conference, Zurich, Switzerland, September, 1930. Part 3, Clinic Reports, Section 9, England.

—— (1929). Rejuvenation. *The Realist: A New Journal of Scientific Humanism*, May: 120–29.

—— (1929). *How I run my birth control clinic*. Proceedings of the Second International Congress of the WLSR.

—— (1929). Revocable sterilization of the female. *British Medical Journal*, 2: 1134.

—— (1928). *Hymen: or, the future of marriage*. London: Kegan Paul.

—— (1928). *The comparative value of current contraceptive methods*, Proceedings of the First International Congress for Sex Research, Berlin, 10–16 October 1926. London: Cromer Welfare Centre (HC Item 7.36).

—— (1928). *Some more medical views on birth control*. New York: EP Dutton (HC Item 22).

—— (1928). World League for Sexual Reform, Copenhagen, July 1928. London: The Cromer Welfare Centre.

—— (1928). Birth control. Reviews of *The night-hoers, or the case against birth control and an alternative* by Anthony Ludovici and *Parenthood: design or accident?* by Michael Fielding. *The Saturday Review,* 5 May, pp563–65.

—— (1927). Marriage. *Practitioner* (London), 118: 227–34.

—— (1927). Quinine and chinosol suppositories. *The Lancet*, 210(5420): 143–44.

—— (1927). Quinine and chinosol suppositories. *The Lancet*, 210(5424): 360.

—— (1927). Foreword. In Anthony Mario Ludovici. *Lysistrata: or woman's future and future woman* (pp5–8). London: Kegan Paul, Trench, Trubner & Co.

—— (1924). *Rejuvenation: the work of Steinach, Voronoff, and others*. London: Allen & Unwin.

—— (1923). *Rejuvenation: Steinach's researches on the sex glands*. 'Recent developments of Steinach's work'. Publication 11, Paper 2. London: BSSSP, pp14–36. Read before the BSSSP 28 November 1921.

—— (1923). Contraceptive technique. A consideration of 1,400 cases. *Practitioner* (London), CXI: 74–90.

—— (1923). Science. Rejuvenation. Steinach's researches on the sex glands. *The Nation & The Athenaeum* (London), 33(18): 580–81.

—— (1922). Recent developments in Steinach's work. *Medical Life* (New York) XXIX: 285–307.

—— (1922). Sterilization of the unfit: a contribution to the First American Birth Control Conference. *The Birth Control Review*, VI(2): 10–11.

—— (1922). Sterilization of the unfit. *Fifth Neo-Malthusian and Birth Control Conference*. London, p236.

—— (1922). Contraceptive technique. *Fifth Neo-Malthusian and Birth Control Conference,* London, pp268–95.

—— (1922). Birth control conference in London: technique of contraception. *The Lancet*, 200(5158): 99.

—— (1922). Effect of position in the family on the health of the child. *The Lancet*, 200(5172): 835.

—— (1922). Clinic experience in contraception. *The Lancet*, 200(5164): 419 and (5167): 588.

Halford, SH (1917). Dysgenic tendencies of birth control and the feminist movement. In C & E Paul (Eds). *Population and birth-control: Symposium.* (pp225–243). New York: Critic and Guide.

Hall, Lesley A (2003). 'In great haste': the personal and political in the letters of F W Stella Browne (1880–1955), feminist socialist, sex radical. In Caroline Bland & Marie Cross (Eds). *Gender and politics in the age of letter writing, 1750–2000* (pp213–24). Aldershot, Hants: Ashgate. Quoting her letters to Havelock Ellis (BL, 1922).

—— (2000). *Sex, gender and social change in Britain since 1880*. London: Macmillan Press Ltd.

—— (1998). Feminist reconfigurations of heterosexuality in the 1920s. *Sexology in culture: labelling bodies and desires*. Cambridge: Cambridge University Press.

—— (1995). 'Disinterested enthusiasm for sexual misconduct': the British Society for the Study of Sex Psychology, 1912–47. *Journal of Contemporary History*, 30(4): 665–86.

Hall, Ruth (1977). *Passionate crusader: the life of Marie Stopes*. London: Andre Deutsch.

Hamilton, David (1986). *The monkey gland affair*. London: Chatto & Windus.

Hart-Davis, Sir Rupert (1952). *Hugh Walpole: a biography*. London: Macmillan.

Hasteltine, Nate (1963). Old birth control device stages a comeback with improvements. *The Washington Post*, 8 May, A3.

Hauck, Christina (2003). Abortion and the individual talent. *English Literary History*, 70: 228.

Henn, Thomas Rice (1965). *The lonely tower: studies of the poetry of WB Yeats*. London: Methuen.

Herman, JR (1982). Rejuvenation: Brown-Séquard to Brinkley. Monkey glands to goat glands. *New York State Journal of Medicine*, 82(12): 1731.

Hesling, Bernard (1960). The facts-of-lifeman: a memoir of Dr Norman Haire. *Nation*, 42, 23 April, pp12–14.

Hicks, Neville (1971). 'Rediscovering' the evidence of the New South Wales Birth Rate Commission. *Archives and Manuscripts*, Malvern, Victoria, 4(4): 17.

Higgins, EA (1957). *David Stewart and the WEA*. Sydney: The Workers' Educational Association of NSW.

Hilvert, John (1984). *Blue pencil warriors: censorship and propaganda in World War II*. St Lucia, Qld: University of Queensland Press.

Himes, Norman (1970[1936]). *Medical history of contraception*. New York: Schocken Books.

Himes, Norman E & Himes, Vera C (1929). Birth control for the British working classes: a study of the first thousand cases to visit an English birth control clinic. Pamphlet digitized by the British Library of Political and Economic Science. *Hospital Social Service*, XIX: 580.

Hirsch, Edwin W (1936). *The power to love: a psychic and physiologic study of regeneration*. London: The Bodley Head.

Hirschfeld, Dr Magnus (1935). *Sex in human relationships*. Translated by John Rodker with an introduction by Norman Haire. London: The Bodley Head.

Hodge, Errol (1995). *Radio wars: truth, propaganda and the struggle*. Cambridge: Cambridge University Press.

Holmes, Colin (1979). *Anti-Semitism in British society, 1876–1939*. London: Edward Arnold.

Holtby, Winifred (1928). *Eutychus, or the future of the pulpit*. To-day and to-morrow series. London: Kegan Paul, Trench, Trubner & Co.

Hone, J (1942). *WB Yeats: Man and artist*. London: Macmillan.

Horan, Ronald S (1989). *Fort Street: the school*. Sydney: Honeysett Publications.

Horsley, Keith (2007). How did the Spanish influenza come to Australia? In medicine in context: 10th Biennial Conference, Australian and New Zealand Society of the History of Medicine, 6 July. Canberra: Manning Clark Centre, ANU.

Houlbrook, Matt (2005). *Queer London: perils and pleasures in the sexual metropolis, 1918–1957*. Chicago and London: University of Chicago Press.

Hughes, Robert (2006). *Things I didn't know: a memoir*. Milsons Point, NSW: Knopf.

Huxley, Aldous (1923). *Antic hay*. New York: The Modern Library.

Huxter, Robert (1992). *Reg and Ethel*. York, UK: Sessions Book Trust.

Influenza Report (1920). *Report on the influenza epidemic in New South Wales in 1919*. Sydney: Government Printer.

Inge, William Ralph (1930). *Christian ethics and modern problems*. London: Hodder & Stoughton.

Inglis, Keith S (1983). *This is the ABC: The Australian Broadcasting Commission, 1932–1985*. Melbourne: Melbourne University Press.

Ishill, Joseph (Ed) (1929). *Havelock Ellis: in appreciation*. Berkeley Heights, New Jersey: Oriole Press.

Ives, George (1930). The taboo attitude. In Sexual Reform Congress, pp338–43. World League for Sexual Reform [WLSR] [Third] (1930). Sexual reform congress. Proceedings. London, 8–14 September 1929. London: Kegan Paul, Trench, Trubner & Co.

Jackson, A (1927). The Steinbach film: from a woman's point of view. *The Triad*, February, p32.
Jackson, Julian (1987). *The politics of depression in France, 1932–1936.* Cambridge: Cambridge University Press. Reviewed in *French History*, 1 (1), February, p145.
Jackson, Margaret (1994). *The real facts of life; feminism and the politics of sexuality, c 1850–1940.* London; Bristol, PA: Taylor & Francis.
Jacobs, Louis (1950). The Jewish attitude to artificial insemination. *The Journal of Sex Education*, 2(4): 177.
James, Clive (2007). Launching *A grand obsession: the DMS Mitchell story*, celebrating the centenary of the bequest of David Scott Mitchell, at the State Library of NSW, 20 June.
Jeffares, Norman (1998). *WB Yeats: man & poet.* New York: St Martins Press.
Jeffreys, Sheila (1997). *The spinster and her enemies: feminism and sexuality 1880–1930.* Melbourne: Spinifex.
Jewish encyclopedia (2002[1906]). [Online] Available: www.jewishencyclopedia. com/view.jsp?artid=27&letter=P&search=Plock [Accessed 5 August 2011].
Johnston, Ron (1988). Social responsibility of science: the social mirror of science. In Roy MacLeod (Ed). *The commonwealth of science: ANZAAS and the scientific enterprise in Australasia, 1888–1988* (pp308–325).
Jones, Greta (1993). Review of *Selected papers of JBS Haldane.* In Krishna R Dromraju (Ed). *Journal of the History of the Behavioral Sciences*, 29, July: 218–222.
Jones, James Howard (1997). *Alfred C Kinsey: a public/private life.* New York: Norton.
Lyons, Mark (1981). Gardiner, Albert (Jupp) (1867–1952). *ADB*. [Online] Available: adb.anu.edu.au/biography/gardiner-albert-jupp-6275 [Accessed 8 August 2011].
Kable, KJ (2006). Henry Havelock Ellis (1859–1939). *ADB*. [Online] Available: adb.anu.edu.au/biography/ellis-henry-havelock-3479 [Accessed 8 August 2011].
Keneally, Thomas (1982). *Schindler's ark.* London: Hodder and Stoughton.
Kennedy, Hubert (2003). Internet website review – *Institut für Sexualwissenschaft* (1919–1933) – [The Institute for Sexual Science]. *Journal of the History of sexuality*, 12, January: 122–126.

Kevles, Daniel (1995). *In the name of eugenics: genetics and the uses of human heredity* (2nd edn). Cambridge, Massachusetts: Harvard University Press.

Kiernan, Kathleen (1998). *Lone motherhood in twentieth-century Britain*. Oxford: Clarendon Press; New York: Oxford University Press.

Knibbs, GK (1920). The influenza epidemic of 1918–19. *Australasian Medical Congress*, 11th Session, 21–28 August, pp321–28.

Knightley, Phillip (1997). *A hack's progress*. London: Jonathan Cape.

Kolata, Gina (2000). *Flu: the story of the great influenza pandemic of 1918 and the search for the virus that caused it*. New York: Macmillan.

Knopf, S Adolphus (1921). *Aspects of birth control*. San Diego, California: The Truth Seeker Co. Inc.

Koestler, Arthur (1969). *The invisible writing: the second volume of an autobiography*. London: Hutchinson of London.

Konikow, Antoinette F (1931). *Physicians' manual of birth control*. New York: Buchholz Publishing Co.

Kuhl, Stefan (1994). *The Nazi connection: eugenics, American racism and German national socialism*. New York, Oxford: Oxford University Press.

Kunitz, Stanley & Howard Haycraft (1966). *Twentieth century authors: a biographical dictionary of modern literature*. New York: H W Wilson.

Lambert, JW & Ratcliffe, Michael (1987). *The Bodley Head 1887–1987*. London: The Bodley Head.

Lancaster, Paul AL (2006). Sir Norman McAlister Gregg (1902–1966). *ADB*. [Online] Available: adb.anu.edu.au/biography/gregg-sir-norman-mcalister-10362 [Accessed 8 August 2011].

Landy, Marcia & Fischer, Lucy (Eds) (2004). *Stars: the film reader*. New York: Routledge.

Lawson, Valerie (2000). Norton, Ezra (1897–1967). *ADB*, 15, Melbourne University Press, pp495–497.

Ledbetter, Rosanna (1976). *A history of the Malthusian League, 1877–1892*. Columbus, Ohio: Ohio State University Press.

Lehfeldt, Hans (1981). Norman Haire (1892–1952). *Reports of the Magnus Hirschfeld Society*, (15): 18–22. Translated from the German by Dorothy Simons.

LeVay, Simon (1996). *Queer science: the use and abuse of research into homosexuality*. Boston, Massachussets: MIT Press.

Leslie, Anita (1972). *Edwardians in love*. London: Hutchinson of London.

Lewis, Jane & Brookes, Barbara (1983). A reassessment of the work of the Peckham Health Centre, 1926–1951. *The Milbank Memorial Fund Quarterly*, 61(2): 307–50.

Lewis, Jeremy (2004). *Rupert Hart-Davis: man of letters* by Philip Ziegler, a pompous publisher from the old school. *The Independent*, 25 May. [Online] Available: www.independent.co.uk/arts-entertainment/books/reviews/rupert-hartdavis-man-of-letters-by-philip-ziegler-756663.html [Accessed 22 October 2012].

Lewis, John (Ed) (1997). *Reminiscences of the Royal: Royal Newcastle Hospital: celebrating 180 years of health and healing.* Newcastle: Royal Newcastle Hospital Heritage Committee.

Lewis, Roy (1974). How accurate were the visions of the twenties prophets? *The Times*, 26 August, p6.

Licht, Hans (1932). *Sexual life in ancient Greece.* London: Routledge.

Lindsay, Jack (1960). *The roaring twenties: literary life in New South Wales in the years 1921–1926.* London: The Bodley Head.

Lindsey, Judge Ben (1920). Horses' rights for women. In Ben Barr Lindsey & Harvey Jerrold O'Higgins (Eds). *The Doughboy's religion and other aspects of our day* (p65). London: Harper and Brothers.

Litvinoff, Barnet (1969). *A peculiar people: world Jewry today.* London: Weidenfeld & Nicholson.

Lock, Stephen, (1983). 'Oh that I were young again': Yeats and the Steinach operation. *British Medical Journal*, 287, 24–31 December: 1965–66.

Lockie, Ruby (1936). A problem in ethics. *Eugenics Review*, 28(July): 161.

Loftin, Craig M (2007). Unacceptable mannerisms: gender anxieties, homosexual activism and swish in the United States, 1945–1965. *Journal of Social History*, 40(3), Spring: 577–596.

Lomask, Milton (1987). *The biographer's craft.* New York: Perennial Library, Harper and Row.

Loudon, Dr Irvine (1992). *Death in childbirth: an international study of material care and maternal mortality 1800–1950.* Oxford: Clarendon Press.

Lowenstein, Andrew Freud (1993). *Loathsome Jews and engulfing women: metaphors of projection in the works of Wyndham Lewis, Charles Williams and Graham Green.* New York: New York University.

Ludovici, Anthony M (2010). Anthony M Ludovici webpage. [Online] Available: www.anthonymludovici.com/ [Accessed 8 August 2011].

—— (1935). *The choice of a mate* [The international library of sexology and psychology]. With an introduction by Norman Haire. London: The Bodley Head.

—— (1928). *The night-hoers, or the case against birth control and an alternative.* London: Herbert Jenkins Ltd.

—— (1927[1925]). *Lysistrata: or woman's future and future woman* [To-day and To-morrow] (2nd edn). Foreword by Norman Haire. London: Kegan Paul, Trench, Trubner & Co.

Lyons, Dame Enid (1972). *Among the carrion crows.* Adelaide: Rigby.

McLaren, Angus (2007). Smoke and mirrors; Willy Clarkson and the role of disguises in inter-war England. *Journal of Social History*, 40(3): 606.

—— (1995). *Twentieth-century sexuality: a history.* Oxford: Blackwell.

—— (1990). *A history of contraception: from antiquity to the present day.* London: Basil Blackwell.

—— (1977). Abortion in England, 1890–1914. *Victorian Studies*, 20(4): 379–400.

Macnicol, John (1989). Eugenics and the campaign for voluntary sterilization in Britain between the wars. *Social History of Medicine*, 2(2), August: 147–169.

MacNiven, Ian S & Moore, Harry T (Eds) (1981). *Literary lifelines: the Richard Aldington–Lawrence Durrell correspondence.* New York: Viking Press.

McPhee, Peter (1999). *'Pansy': a life of Roy Douglas Wright.* Melbourne: Melbourne University Press.

Maddox, Brenda (1999). *George's ghosts: a new life of WB Yeats.* London: Picador.

Mannin, Ethel (1971). *Young in the twenties: a chapter of autobiography.* London: Hutchinson.

—— (1939). *Privileged spectator.* London: Hutchinson.

—— (1930). *Confessions and impressions.* London: Hutchinson.

Marr, David (1992). *Patrick White: a life.* Sydney: Vintage Books.

Marsden, Susan (2005). *The Royal: a castle grand, a purpose noble. The Royal Newcastle Hospital 1817–2005.* Newcastle: Hunter New England Area Health Service.

Marshall, Jane (1998). *Jock Marshall: one armed warrior.* [Online] Available: www.asap.unimelb.edu.au/bsparcs/exhib/marshall/marshall.htm [Accessed 15 May 2006].

Maude, Alymer (1924). *The authorised life of Marie C Stopes.* London: Williams & Norgate.

Masters, REL (1962). *Forbidden sexual behavior and morality: an objective re-examination of perverse sex cultures in different cultures.* New York: The Julian Press, Inc.

McClure, D (1920). The modern elixir of life. Experiments in the rejuvenation of aged animals by the grafting of special organs. *Scientific American Monthly*, 2, November: 203.

Medical directory for Australia (1935). Sydney: EG Knox.

Mitchell Bruce (2006). Alexander James Kilgour (1861–1944). *ADB.* [Online] Available: adb.anu.edu.au/biography/kilgour-alexander-james-6954 [Accessed 8 August 2011].

Mitchell, Bruce & Rutledge, Martha (2006). George Mackaness (1882–1968). *ADB.* [Online] Available: adb.anu.edu.au/biography/mackaness-george-7376 [Accessed 8 August 2011].

Moffat, Wendy (2010). *EM Forster: a new life.* London: Bloomsbury.

Moggridge, Donald Edward (1992). *Maynard Keynes: an economist's biography.* London and New York: Routledge.

Molnar, George (1952). And when will we get the money? [Cartoon]. *The Daily Telegraph*, 3 December.

Monk, Ray (2001). *Bertrand Russell: the ghost of madness, 1921–1970.* London: Vintage.

Montagu, Ivor (1970). *The youngest son: autobiographical sketches.* London: Lawrence and Wishart.

—— (1967). *With Eisenstein in Hollywood: a chapter of autobiography.* New York: International Publishers.

Moonan, Wendy (2008). What the British saw when they looked at China. *The New York Times*, 5 September, pE28.

Moore, Nicole (2002). Obscene and over here: national sex and the *Love Me Sailor* obscenity case. *Australian Literary Studies*, 20(4): 316–29.

—— (1975). Secrets of the censors; obscenity in the archives, speech given at the National Archives of Australia, 2 May. [Online] Available: www.naa.gov.au/about_us/nicolemoore.html [Accessed 10 June 2009].

Moran, Jean (1986). Australian scientists and the cold war. *Martin*, pp11–30.

—— (1983). Scientists in the political and public arena: a social-intellectual history of the Australian Association of Scientific Workers, 1939–1949. M Phil thesis, Griffith University.

Mudd, Emily (1998). [Obituary for] a pioneer in marriage and family counselling. *Almanac*, 44, (33), 12 May. [Online] Available: www.upenn.edu/almanac/v44/n33/deaths.html [Accessed 1 January 2010].

Munster, George (1983). Only shadowy clues left by a reviled prophet of sexual liberation. The Good Weekend. *Sydney Morning Herald*, 24 September, p38.

Neill, AS (1945). *Hearts not heads in the school*. London: Herbert Jenkins.

Newsholme, Arthur (1926). Broadcasting birth control. *The Times* (London), 18 November, p15.

Nottingham, Chris (1999). *The pursuit of serenity: Havelock Ellis and the new politics*. Amsterdam: Amsterdam University Press.

O'Faolain, Sean (1953). Love among the Irish: a Catholic blames celibacy and censorship. *Life*, 16 March, p152.

Orwell, George (2004[1941]). The lion and the unicorn: socialism and the English genius. *George Orwell Essays*, pp138–188. London: Penguin.

—— (2004[1946]). Why I write. *George Orwell Essays*, pp1–7. London: Penguin.

Osborne, Graeme (1979). Bennett, Henry Gilbert (1877–1959). *ADB*, 7, Melbourne University Press, pp268–269.

Passmore, John (1997). *Memoirs of a semi-detached Australian*. Melbourne: Melbourne University Press.

Paul, Eden (1923). Steinach's rejuvenation experiments. Publication no 11, Paper 1. *Rejuvenation: Steinach's researches on the sex glands*. London: British Society for the Study of Sex Psychology, pp1–13.

Peel, John (Secretary of the Galton Institute) (1994). Is it a boy? Problems of sex determination. *The Galton Institute Newsletter*, 12. [Online] Available: www.galtoninstitute.org.uk/Newsletters/GINL9403/is_it_a_boy.htm [Accessed 8 August 2011].

Peel, John (1964). Contraception and the medical profession. *Population Studies*, 18(2): 133–45.

Penchaszadeh, Victor B (1996). Review of *The Nazi connection: eugenics, American racism and German national socialism*, by Stefan Kuhl. *Journal of Public Health Policy*, 17 (1), pp115–117.

Perez, Manuel L (1940). Paper given at the 4th Argentine Congress of Obstetrics and Gynecology (cited by Yolanda Esaro, 2009).

Peters, George (2001). Colin Clark (1905–89) economist and agricultural economist (Oxford: International Development Centre, University of Oxford). QEH Working Paper – QEHWPS69, April, pp9–10.

Piddington, AB (1921). *The next step: a family basis income*. Melbourne: Macmillan.
Ploetz, Alfred (1912). Neo-Malthusianism and race hygiene. *Problems in Eugenics*. First International Eugenics Congress, London, pp183–89. [Online] Available: www.archive.org/stream/problemsineugeni02inte/problemsineugeni02inte_djvu.txt [Accessed 8 August 2011].
Plomer, William (1958). *Mrs Fernandez and Dr Pood. At home: memoirs*. London: Jonathan Cape.
—— (1932). *The case is altered*. London: Published by Leonard and Virginia Woolf at The Hogarth Press.
Porritt, Annie G (1922). Propaganda and general section, publicity in the birth control movement. In Raymond Pierpoint & New Generation League (Eds). *Report of the fifth International Neo-Malthusian and Birth Control Conference, Kingsway Hall, London, July 11th to 14th, 1922* (p305). London: William Heinemann Medical Books.
Porter, Roy & Lesley Hall (1995). *The facts of life: the creation of sexual knowledge in Britain, 1650–1950*. New Haven: Yale University Press.
Pruitt, Virginia D (1982). Yeats, the mask, and the poetry of old Age. *Journal of Geriatric Psychiatry*, 15(1): 99–112.
Pruitt, Virginia D & Pruitt, Raymond D (1989). Yeats and the Steinbach operation: a further analysis. Finneran (1989).
Pullan, Robert (1984). *Guilty secrets: free speech in Australia*. North Ryde, NSW: Methuen.
Pyke, Margaret (1939). The Abortion Report. Correspondence, *British Medical Journal* 2: 5 August, 308.
Radi, Heather (2006). Millicent Fanny Preston Stanley (1883–1955). *ADB*. [Online] Available: adb.anu.edu.au/biography/preston-stanley-millicent-fanny-8107 [Accessed 8 August 2011].
Raitt, Suzanne (2004). Early British psychoanalysis and the Medico-Psychological Clinic. *History Workshop Journal*, (58): 7.
Randall, EG (1930). The individual aspects of prostitution among the English middle class. World League for Sexual Reform [Third]. (1929, 254–67).
Reis, Elizabeth (Ed) (2001). *American sexual histories*. Malden, Massachusetts, Oxford: Blackwell.
Report on the Influenza Epidemic in New South Wales in 1919 (1920). Sydney: Government Printer.

Reports of the Advisory Committee for Military Hospitals and Convalescent Homes, New South Wales (1918). Upon the Administration of No. 4 Australian General (Military) Hospital, Randwick, NSW. The Parliament of the Commonwealth of Australia, Paper (92) – F.9097. Melbourne: Albert J Mullett, Government Printer to the State of Victoria, 6 June.

Riordan, Jim (2008). The Hon Ivor Montagu (1904–1984): founding father of table tennis. *Sport in History*, 28(3) September, pp512–530.

Roberts, Michael (Ed) (1933). *New country: prose and poetry by the authors of New Signatures*. London: Leonard and Virginia Woolf's Hogarth Press.

Roland, Betty (1990). *The devious being*. Sydney: Angus & Robertson.

Rose, June (1992). *Marie Stopes and the sexual revolution*. London: Faber and Faber.

Rout, Ettie A (1922). *Safe marriage: a return to sanity*. London: William Heinemann (Medical Books) Ltd.

—— (1922). Clinical experience in contraception. *The Lancet*, 200(5167): 588–89.

Rowbotham, Sheila (2008). *Edward Carpenter: a life of liberty and love*. London, New York: Verso.

Royal Commission on the Decline of the Birth-Rate and on the Mortality of Infants in New South Wales (1904). Vol. 1. Report, together with copies of commissions, diagrams, statistical evidence, and statistical exhibits, etc.; Vol. 2. Minutes, evidence, exhibits, index. Sydney: Government Printer.

Rubinstein, Helge (Ed) (1990). *The Oxford dictionary of marriage*. Oxford: Oxford University Press.

Rubinstein, WD (1996). *A history of the Jews in the English-speaking world: Great Britain*. London: St Martins Press.

Ruck, Berta (1935). *A story teller tells the truth: reminiscences and notes*. London: Hutchinson.

—— (1929). *The unkissed bride*. New York: Dodd, Mead & Co.

Russell, Dora (1977). *The tamarisk tree. Vol. 1: My quest for liberty and love*. London: Virago.

Rutgers, Johannes (1924). *The sexual life and its biological significance*. Translated by Norman Haire. Dresden: RE Giesecke. (HC. 26).

—— (1923). *Eugenics and birth control*. Translated by Clifford Courdray. Dresden, Germany: RA Giesecke.

Rutland, Suzanne D (2005). *The Jews in Australia*. Port Melbourne, Vic: Cambridge University Press.

Ryan, Edna (1989). Notes from the past. *WEL Informed*, (189), May: 33–34.
Saddlemyer, Ann (2002). *Becoming George: the life of Mrs WB Yeats*. Oxford: Oxford University Press.
Sagarin, Edward (1975). *Structure and ideology in an association of deviants*. New York: Arno Press.
Sanger, Alexander C (1995). In his grandmother's footsteps. *The New York Times*, p1.
Sanger, Margaret (1970). *Margaret Sanger: an autobiography*. New York: Maxwell Reprint Co.
—— (Ed) (1934). *Biological and medical aspects of contraception*. Washington: National Committee on Federal Legislation for Birth Control, Inc. (HC, Item 25).
—— (1925). One week's activity in England. *Birth Control Review*, 1925: 219–20.
—— (1921). Impressions of the Amsterdam Conference. *The Birth Control Review*, V(11): 11.
—— (1920). *Woman and the new race*. New York: Bretano's.
—— (1917). *The case for birth control: a supplementary brief and statement of facts*. New York: Modern Art Print Co.
Sanger, Margaret & Stone, Hannah M (Eds) (1931). The practice of contraception: an international symposium and survey. Proceedings of the Seventh International Birth Control Conference, Zurich, Switzerland, September, 1930. London: Bailliere, Tindall and Cox.
Scammell, Michael (2009*). Koestler: the literary and political odyssey of a twentieth-century skeptic*. New York: Random House.
Schmidt, Peter (1930). Six hundred rejuvenation operations: a nine years' survey. In Norman Haire (Ed). *WLSR: proceedings of the Third Congress* (pp574–81). London: Kegan Paul, Trench, Trubner & Co.
Schultheiss, D, J Deni & U Jonas (1997). Rejuvenation in the early 20th century. *Andrologia*, 29(6): 353.
Seidelman, William E (1999). Medicine and murder in the Third Reich. *Dimensions: A Journal of Holocaust Studies*, 13, (1). [Online] Available: www.jewishvirtuallibrary.org/jsource/Holocaust/medmurder.html [Accessed 2 June 2006].
Senar, Canon Howard (1983). *Little Gaddesden and Ashridge*. Cheshire, UK: Phillimore & Co.

Sengoopta, Chandak (1993). Rejuvenation and the prolongation of life: science or quackery? *Perspectives in Biology and Medicine*, 37(1): 55-66.

—— (2006). Glands and rejuvenation: sex and life in the twenties (and beyond). *The Galton Institute Newsletter*, (59): 9.

—— (2000). The modern ovary: construction, meanings, uses. *History of Science*, 38(Pt 4) (122): 425-88.

—— (2006). *The most secret quintessence of life: sex, glands and hormones, 1850-1950*. Chicago and London: The University of Chicago Press.

Serle, Geoffrey (1993). *Sir John Medley: a memoir*. Melbourne: Melbourne University Press.

Shanks, Edward (1927). Reviews marriages: comments about Haire's *Hymen* and Sanger's *Happiness in marriage*. *The Saturday Review*. 1 October, 430.

Shepherd, John (2004). A Life on the left. George Lansbury (1859-1940): a case study in recent Labour biography. *Labour History*, 87, November. [Online] Available: www.historycooperative.org/journals/lab/87/shepherd.html [Accessed 7 January 2010].

Siedlecky, Stefania & Wyndham, Diana (1990). *Populate and perish: Australian women's fight for birth control*. North Sydney: Allen & Unwin.

Simmer, Hans (1970). On the history of hormonal contraception. 1. Ludwig Haberlandt (1885-1932) and his concept of 'hormonal sterilisation'. *Contraception*, 1(1): 3-27.

Simms, Madeleine (1975). Marie Stopes memorial lecture 1975. The compulsory pregnancy lobby: then and now. *Journal of the Royal College of General Practitioners*, 25: 712.

Simpson, Jean (1998). *A history of Nettleden Lodge*. A copy is filed in the Dacorum Heritage Trust, The Museum Store, Berkhampstead, Herts.

Sinclair, Alison (2003). The World League for Sexual Reform in Spain: founding, infighting, and the role of Hildegart Rodriguez. *Journal of the History of Sexuality*, 12(1): 98-108.

Skinner, Graeme (1991). Music's pale rider: a great void filled, he then left town: profile of Paul Lowin, benefactor of the Paul Lowin Prize for Composition. *Sydney Morning Herald*, 30 July [Online] Abaliable: newsstore.smh.com.au/apps/viewDocument.ac?docID=news910729_0003_0775 [Accessed 8 June 2012].

Slee, John (2002). Shand, John Wentworth (1897-1959). *ADB*, 16, Melbourne University Press, pp216-217.

Smith, Babette (2008). *Australia's birthstain: the startling legacy of the convict era*. Crows Nest, NSW: Allen & Unwin.

Socialist Review: A Monthly Review of Modern Thought (Independent Labour Party. Great Britain) (1933). New Series 3, 5: 56.

Soloway, Richard Allen (1995). The 'perfect contraceptive': eugenics and birth control research in Britain and America in the interwar years. *Journal of Contemporary History*, 30(4), October: 637–664.

—— (1982). *Birth control and the population question in England, 1870–1930*. Chapel Hill, North Carolina: University of North Carolina Press.

Southern, George William Robert (1934). *Making morality modern*. Mosman, NSW: Southern.

Spar, Debora L (2006). *The baby business: elite eggs, designer genes, and the thriving commerce of conception*. Boston, Massachusetts: Harvard Business School Press.

Steketee, Mike (2008). Illegimate [sic] claim in Enid Lyons's closet. *The Australian*, 7 June. [Online] Available: www.theaustralian.com.au/news/illegimate-claim-in-enid-lyonss-closet/story-e6frg6ox-1111116564749 [Accessed 14 January 2011].

Steinach, Eugen (1940). *Sex and life: forty years of biological and medical experiments*. New York: Viking Press.

—— (1920). Rejuvenation by experimental revitalization of the ageing puberty gland. *Archiv Fur Entwicklungsmech*, 46: 553.

Stephensen, PR (1935). *The foundations of culture in Australia: an essay towards national self-respect*. The Percy Stephensen Collection. Part 2, Section 34: 'Export of Genius'. First published in *Australian Mercury*. [Online] Available: home.alphalink.com.au/~radnat/stephensen/prs5.html [Accessed 2 May 2010].

Still, John (1937). Population in Australia. *The Eugenics Review*, 28–29, April 1937–January 1938: 286.

Stivens, Dal (1970) *A horse of air*. Ringwood, Vic: Penguin.

Stone, Hannah (1937). Birth control wins. *The Nation*, 144(3), 16 January, pp70–71.

Stone, Hannah M and Stone, Abraham, A (1935) *A Marriage manual. A practical guide-book to sex and marriage*. New York: Simon and Schuster.

Stopes, Marie (1952[1923]). *Contraception (birth control): it's theory and practice. A manual for the medical and legal professions* (5th edn). London: John Bale, Sons & Danielsson Ltd.
—— (1941[1918]). *Married love: a new contribution to the solution of sex difficulties* (25th edn). London: Putman.
—— (1922). A new gospel to all peoples: a revelation of god uniting physiology and the religions of man. First delivered to the Bishops in session at Lambeth. London: Arthur L Humphreys.
—— (1922). Clinic experience in contraception. *The Lancet*, 200(5163): 539 and 200(5166): 357–58.
Suitters, Beryl (1973). *Be brave and angry: chronicles of the International Planned Parenthood Federation*. London: The International Planned Parenthood Federation.
Sutherland, Halliday Gibson (1922). *Birth control, a statement of Christian doctrine against the Neo-Malthusians*. New York: P J Kennedy and Son.
Sutherland, Halliday Gibson (1922). Birth control: a statement. *Literary Review* (NY), 14 November, pp107.
Sutherland, Halliday Gibson (1944). *Control of life*. London: Burns, Oates and Washbourne.
Sweetman, David (1990). *Van Gogh: his life and art*. New York: Crown.
Swenson, Kristine (2003). The menopausal vampire: Arabella Kenealy and the boundaries of true womanhood. *Women's Writing*, 10(1): 27–46.
Symonds, John (1989). *The king of the shadow realm*. London: Duckworth.
Talbot, Margaret (2000). The placebo prescription. *New York Times*, (6), 9 January, p34.
Tamagne, Florence (2004). *A history of homosexuality in Europe: Berlin, London, Paris, 1919-1939* (2 Vols). New York: Algora.
Terriss, Wykeham (Norman Haire) (1950). Intelligence is lower. *Woman*, 26 June, p22.
—— (1949). National health plans. *Woman*, 24 January, p34.
—— (1949). National health plans. *Woman*, 14 February, p34.
—— (1949). Should she marry him? *Woman*, 17 October, p8.
—— (1949). Working of health scheme. *Woman*, 21 November, p28.
—— (1947). Ignorance and suicides. *Woman*, 21 July, p38.
—— (1946). Think of the child. *Woman*, 29 April, p38.
—— (1946). These men need treatment. *Woman*, 19 August, p39.

—— (1945). Wisdom of moderation. *Woman,* 14 May, p38.
—— (1944). Abortion: those good old days. *Woman,* 15 May, p9.
—— (1944). Hospital or home birth? *Woman,* 27 November, p12.
—— (1943). Babies from test tubes. *Woman,* 21 June, p8.
—— (1943). The terror by night. Woman, 22 November, p9.
The history of the University of Oxford (1994). *Vol. 8. The twentieth century.* Edited by Brian Harrison. Oxford: Clarendon Press; New York; Oxford University Press.
Thiery, M (1997). Pioneers of the intrauterine device. *The European Journal of Contraception and Reproductive Health Care,* 2(1), March, pp15–33.
Thomas, Alan (1980). *Broadcast and be damned: the ABC's first two decades.* Melbourne: Melbourne University Press.
Thompson, Charles Willis (1925). Little hope remains for men. [Reviews of Ludovici's *Lysistrata* and Dora Russell's *Hypatia*]. *The New York Times.* 9 August, ppBR 1.
Tolerton, Jane (1992). *Ettie: a life of Ettie Rout.* Auckland, New Zealand: Penguin.
Tregenza, John (1965). *Australian little magazines 1923-1954: their role in forming and reflecting literary trends.* Adelaide: Libraries Board of SA.
Trimmer, Eric J (1967). *Rejuvenation: the history of an idea.* London: Hale.
Tuchman, Barbara (1978). *A distant mirror: the calamitous 14th century.* New York: Knopf.
Turtle, Alison M (1987). History and philosophy of science at the University of Sydney: a case of non-innovation. *Historical Records of Australian Science,* 7 (1), December: 27–37.
van de Velde, Theodoor H (1931[1929]). *Fertility and sterility in marriage: their voluntary promotion and limitation.* Translated by FW Stella Browne. New York: Covici Friede Medical Books.
—— (1930[1926]). *Ideal marriage: its physiology and technique.* Translated by FW Stella Browne. New York: Random House.
van Poppel, Frans & Hugo Röling (2003). Physicians and fertility control in the Netherlands. *Journal of Interdisciplinary History,* xxxiv(2): 163, 168.
Vercoe, RH (1922). The effect of position in the family on the health of the child. *The Lancet,* 200(5171): 758–59.
Vickery, Edward Louis (2003). Telling Australia's story to the world: the department of information 1939-1950. Canberra: Australian National University, PhD Thesis, August.

Viner, Katharine (2002). Look back in awe. *The Guardian*, 26 January. [Online] Available: www.guardian.co.uk/books/2002/jan/26/referenceandlanguages. artsandhumanities/print [Accessed 1 January 2010].

Voronoff, Dr Serge (1925). Can old age be deferred? *Scientific American*, (133): 227.

Wade, William A (1954). *The letters of WB Yeats*. London: Hart-Davis.

Ward, John M (1988). Nicholas, Harold Sprent (1877–1953). *ADB*, 11, Melbourne University Press, pp21.

Waters, Chris (1998). Havelock Ellis, Sigmund Freud and the state: discourses of homosexual identity in interwar Britain. In Lucy Bland & Laura Doan (Eds). *Sexology in culture: labelling bodies and desires* (pp174–76). Chicago: University of Chicago Press.

Waynberg, J (2009). '1908–2008: un siècle de sexologie et toujours pas de légitimité?' (1908–2008: a century of sexology and still no legitimacy?), *Sexologies*, 18(1), January–March: 19–21.

Weeks, Jeffrey (1977). *Coming out: homosexual politics in Britain, from the nineteenth century to the present*. London: Quartet Books.

Welby, William (1945). *Naked and unashamed: nudism from six points of view*. London: Thorsons. (HC, Item 24).

Wells, HG (1927). The way the world is going. Man becomes a different animal: delusions about human fixity. *Los Angeles Times*, 9 January, ppB.

West, Nigel (2002). 'Venona': the British dimension, *Intelligence and National Security*, 17, (1), March, pp117–134.

Who's Who in Australia (Imprint varies) (1933/34). Melbourne: *The Herald*: 1935–1988. Melbourne: Herald and Weekly Times.

Willett, Graham (1997). The darkest decade: homophobia in 1950s Australia. *Australian Historical Studies*, (109): 129.

Wills, W David (1964). *Homer Lane: a biography*. London: Allen & Unwin.

Wilson, Bee (2001). Queen-size appetite. Food. *New Statesman*, 12: 48–49.

Winspear, Rosalind (2004). A college benefactor: Frank Forster – obstetrician, gynaecologist, medical historian and bibliophile. *Australian and New Zealand Journal of Obstetrics and Gynaecology*, 44, pp4

Wolfe, Beran (1934). *How to be happy though human*. London: Routledge.

Wolff, Charlotte (1986). *Magnus Hirschfeld: a portrait of a pioneer in sexology*. London: Quartet Books.

Wood, Clive & Beryl Suitters (1970). *The fight for acceptance: a history of contraception*. Aylesbury, Buckinghamshire: Medical and Technical Publishing Co Ltd.

World League for Sexual Reform, Third [WLSR] (1930). *Sexual reform congress. Proceedings*. London, 8–14 September 1929. London: Kegan Paul, Trench, Trubner & Co.

——, Second [WLSR] (1929). *Sexual Reform Congress. Proceedings*. Copenhagen 1–5 July 1928. Copenhagen/Leipzig: Levin & Munksgaard. Haire Collection. (10).

Wright, Helena (1947). *Sex fulfillment in married women*. London: William & Norgate.

Wyndham, Diana (2003). *Eugenics in Australia: striving for national fitness*. London: Galton Institute.

—— (2000). Misdiagnosis or miscarriage of justice? Dr Norman Haire and the 1919 influenza epidemic at Newcastle Hospital. *Health and History*, 2(1): 3–26.

—— (1996). Striving for national fitness. Eugenics in Australia. PhD thesis, University of Sydney.

Zimmermann, Susan (2006). Countess Apponyi. In Francisca de Haan, Krasimira Daskalova & Anna Loutfi (Eds). *A biographical dictionary of women's movements and feminists: Central, Eastern and South Eastern Europe, 19th and 20th centuries* (pp25–26). Budapest; New York: Central European Press.

Zweiniger-Bargielowski, Ina (2006). Building a British superman: physical culture in interwar Britain. *Journal of Contemporary History*, 4(4): 595–610.

Index

The abbreviation NH = Norman Haire.

A

Aarons, Solomon Jervois 73
ABC population debate 343–359
abortifacients 225
  antiseptic paste 211
  Beecham's Pills 25
  RU 486 385
abortion 16, 19, 25, 96, 151, 158, 164, 174, 179, 183, 189, 203, 207, 209, 211–214, 285, 307, 314, 337, 339, 341, 359, 365, 367, 376–377, 385, 390, 401
  laws and reform 211–214, 217, 223, 275, 291, 380, 384
  septic abortion 85–86, 100, 275
Adler, Alfred 259
Afford, Max 309
Albrecht, Berty 202–203, 213, 215–216
Aldington, Richard 285, 292
Allen & Unwin 94, 97, 126, 234–239, 378, 395
American Birth Control League 83, 127, 169
American Conference on Birth Control (Washington) 230
American Eugenics Society 243
American Gynecological Society 169
Angus & Robertson 126, 316, 327

Animal Defence and Anti-Vivisection Society 163
anthropology 172, 177, 213, 369, 414
anti-Semitism 67–68, 70–71, 112–113, 116, 227–228, 230, 274, 290, 299
Archbishop of Canterbury 75, 159, 381–382
artificial insemination (AI) 73–75, 91, 155, 372, 381–382, 391, 417. *See also* IVF
Asche, Oscar 37–38
atheism 235, 420
Atherton, Gertrude 92–93
Auden, WH 112, 122, 226, 256
Australasian Publishing Co 126
Australia
  expatriates in Britain 275–276
  sense of cultural inferiority 275
Australian Association of Scientific Workers (AASW) 313–317
Australian Broadcasting Commission (ABC) 343–345, 384, 397
  The army wants to know 334
  The battle for population 358
  The nation's forum of the air 343–345, 355
Avery, Harold 103, 296, 400–401

B

Ballarat Eisteddfod 40–41
Ball, William Macmahon 344–347, 352–353, 355–358
Barrett, Lady Florence Elizabeth 159
Barr, Sir James 157–158
Bateson, William 182
Bauer, Bernhard A 132–133
BBC 93, 130, 215, 329, 343, 388
Bean, CEW 334
Benjamin, Harry 91–92, 119, 307, 391–392, 400
Bennett, Arnold 70, 78, 167, 173
Bennett, H Scott 159
Besant, Annie 83, 192, 325
bestiality 141, 293, 332
birth control clinics 15, 76, 77, 78, 191, 217, 295, 397, 399, 407. *See also* Malthusian League: birth control clinic; Stopes, Marie: birth control clinic; Cromer Welfare and Sunlight Centre
Birth Control International Information Centre 207
Birth Control Investigation Committee 207
birth control movement 16–19, 71, 82–83, 86, 94, 179, 190, 209–210, 225, 290, 365, 368, 397, 415. *See also* sex reform movement
birthrates 15–16, 128, 323, 345–346, 356, 358–359, 385
'birth rationing'. *See* population debate

Blacker, CP 157, 243–245
Bloch, Iwan 227, 375
Blunt, Sir Anthony 167
Blunt, Wilfred 74, 165
The Bodley Head press 219, 221, 234, 289, 292
Bohun, GR 327, 331, 333
Bölsche, Wilhelm 209
Bonney, EG 344
Boothby, Sir Robert 225, 297
Bourne, Aleck 158, 384, 385
Bradlaugh, Charles 83, 192
British Empire Exhibition 122
British Medical Association (BMA) 157, 296, 315, 328, 335, 345–346
British Museum 239, 362, 405
British Social Hygiene Association 369
British Society for the Study of Sex Psychology (BSSSP) 69, 77, 82, 90, 93, 113, 114, 116, 118, 122, 178, 209, 294, 398, 419, 421
Brooklyn Gynecological Society 128
Browne, Frances Stella 72, 113–115, 161, 171, 174–175, 190, 210, 212–213, 409–410
Browning, Robert 195
'Burr, Jane' (Rosalind Mae Guggenheim) 71
Butler, Samuel 141–142

C

Calwell, Arthur 327, 331–333, 344–345, 354–355, 368

INDEX

Cardus, Sir Neville 281
Carlyle, Thomas 259–260
Carpenter, Edward 77, 178, 182
Carr-Saunders, Alexander 173
Catholic Action 331
Catholic Chemists' Guild 327
celibacy 254–255
censorship 82, 179, 186, 189–190, 227, 230–232, 236, 239, 286–290, 292, 295, 322, 340, 344, 349, 351, 358, 364, 391, 415. *See also* World War II: wartime censorship
  laws 288
Chance, Janet 171, 213
Charles, Enid 207, 227
chastity 143, 223, 241, 284
Chidley, William 232
childbirth 15, 125, 348–350
  dangers of 45, 279–280
circumcision 194, 238
Clark, Colin 345, 348, 351–353, 355–359
Close, Robert 63
Cohen, Norman (relative of NH) 16
Cold War 389
Coleman, Peter 131, 322, 413
Cole, P Tennyson 276–277, 285
communism 93, 115, 135, 182–183, 183–184, 209, 212, 232, 274, 310, 317, 385
Communist Party 300–301
Conan Doyle, Arthur 91
conservatism 130, 274, 293, 315
contraception 17, 95, 163–164, 213, 216, 241, 307, 341, 351–352, 354, 357

and women's rights 408
benefits of 120, 161, 210
difficulties in giving contraceptive advice 45, 103, 142, 159, 258, 397
difficulties in obtaining contraceptive advice 16, 399
history of 157, 226–227
laws regarding 314
published works on 265, 286, 424
safety and reliability of 15, 86, 99, 109, 208, 284
selling 417, 425
use of contraception as normal 142, 387
contraceptives 203, 353, 390
  abstinence 351
  cervical cap 99
  chemical douches 286
  Chinosol suppositories 146
  coitus interruptus 109, 208
  condoms 109, 208, 289, 314, 331, 333, 382–384, 395
  contraceptive jelly 128
  diaphragm 95
  douching 110
  female sheath 409
  gold-pin pessary 84–86, 99–100, 146
  Gräfenberg ring 187, 207–208, 218, 225, 417
  Haire pessary 95, 101
  hormonal contraceptives 115
  intrauterine devices 84, 207
  Japanese pessary 287
  lactic acid jelly 187
  Mensinga pessary 84, 103, 109, 145–146

the Pill 16, 115
quinine 208
rubber pessary 95, 128, 187
'safe period' 109–110, 239
spermicidal paste 103, 286
Cornelius, Stella 258
'Corners, George F(our)' (George Sylvester Viereck) 118–119, 288
Cox, Erle 91
Cox, Oswald 297
Craig, Alec 224, 239–240, 362
Crew, FAE 158, 160, 176, 204
Cromer Welfare and Sunlight Centre 147–151, 148, 191, 208, 265
Cronin, AJ 340
Crowley, Aleister 214–215, 293
Crozier, Ivan 38, 68, 151, 409–411, 423
Cumpston, JHL 54, 57, 333–334
Curtin, John 343–344, 346
Cust, Harry 74

D

da Costa, Sybil 'Sybil Starr' 269
Daniels, Elizabeth 146
Dare, Lionel 199, 338, 403
Dawson, Bertrand Edward (Lord Dawson of Penn) 80, 83, 94, 96, 104, 157, 192, 227
Departmental Commission on Sterilisation (UK) 243
depression (financial) 193, 217, 222, 408
depression (medical) 252, 262, 281, 398
de Sade, Marquis 216

de Walden, Baroness Howard 153
Dickinson, RL 127, 161, 169–170, 286–287, 374
Dick, Sir William Reid 281
diet (healthy food) 123, 125, 131, 179, 232, 258–259, 279, 305, 329–330, 341, 378, 416
disability 46, 141, 421
divorce 98, 143, 175, 179, 187, 191, 199, 316, 341, 361–362, 408, 424
Dose, Ralf 110–111, 202, 204, 209, 238, 261, 267–268, 375, 420, 424
Dovey, Justice Wilfred 335–336
Doyle, Martin 55, 60, 62
dress reform movement 187–188, 205–206, 209
Drysdale, Alice Vickery 72, 83, 86
Drysdale, Bessie 71, 78–79, 80, 84, 120
Drysdale, Charles Robert 83, 96
Drysdale, Charles Vickery 78–79, 80–81, 84, 95, 104, 120, 128, 187, 401
Duncan, WGK 356

E

ectogenesis 408–409
Eder, MD 'David' 157, 158, 196, 198, 200, 222, 244, 281–283
Ellis, Albert 395
Ellis, Havelock 18, 34, 35, 71, 97, 99, 104, 137–138, 155–156, 191, 221–222, 227–232, 235, 238, 259, 276–277, 281–285, 362, 375, 410, 417–418.

See also World League for Sexual Reform (WLSR): International Congress of the World League for Sexual Reform (Third, 1929, London)
correspondence with NH 127–128, 133, 241–242, 268, 405
disagreements with NH 114, 145–146, 369–372
ethics of birth control 94
involvement with the BSSSP 76–78, 112–117, 209
patronage of NH 68–69
Sexual inversion 167
Studies in the psychology of sex 33, 283
Ellmann, Richard 248, 252–253, 255, 257
Ernst, Morris 287–288
eugenics 76, 84, 94, 104, 109, 142–143, 152, 157, 184–186, 204, 279, 308, 316, 418. *See also* sterilisation
Eugenics Society (UK) 77, 157, 178, 239, 241–245, 249, 250, 365, 373, 415, 416
Evans, CBS 221
Evans, Ernestine 191
Evatt, HV 332–333

F

FA Davis Company 137
family planning. *See* birth control movement
Family Planning Association of New South Wales (FPA) 15, 148
Family Planning Association (UK) 83, 178, 207, 384
fascism 202, 232
Federation of Progressive Societies 225
Federation of Socialist Doctors 209
female suffrage 159, 190
feminism 15, 18, 71–72, 76, 115–116, 132, 170, 178, 193, 213, 217, 241, 269, 323, 356, 384
Ferris, Paul 235–236
'Fielding, William J' (Maurice Newfield) 235
Fink, Averil 381
Fink, Lotte 311, 362, 381, 417
Fisher, Sir Warren 297
Fitton, Dame Doris 309
Flügel, Ingeborg 187, 368
Flügel, Jack 180, 187–189, 368
Forel, August 179, 184, 227
Forster, EM 167, 423
Forster, Frank 7, 68, 107, 279–280, 300, 327, 404–406, 419
free love 115, 176, 189
Freemasons 62, 336, 378
Freud, Sigmund 11, 18, 70, 77, 90, 187, 219, 227, 371, 375
Friedjung, Josef K 205

G

Galton Institute 415. *See also* Eugenics Society (UK)
Geddes, Patrick 179
General Medical Council 81, 162, 221
Gernsback, Hugo 391
Gielgud, Sir John 349

Giese, Karl 204, 208, 211, 224, 228–229, 266–268, 405
Gillett, Henry 206
glands, transplantation of 87–88, 90, 155, 163, 252
Goddard, Charles R 158
Gogarty, Oliver 250–252
Golders Green Ethical Society 123
Gräfenberg, Ernst 204, 306, 393–394
Grant, George 70
Greer, Germaine 132, 359
Gruner, Elioth 200
Guyon, René 223–224, 231, 295, 375
Gynaecological Congress (1931, Frankfurt) 207
gynaecology 73–76, 85–86, 123, 127, 148, 152, 157, 371, 397, 400, 407

H

Haire, Norman (né Zions)
  as a captain in the Australian Army Medical Corps (AAMC) 45–46
  as a gourmet and gourmand 131, 164, 223, 258, 310, 378, 401, 408
  as a humanist 10, 359, 397, 417
  as a lover of Asian art 67, 153–155, 271–272
  as a lover of theatre 36, 131, 164, 199, 249, 310, 330, 391, 393, 399
  as a medical student 36–39, 43–46
  as an actor 31, 36–41, 44, 63, 203, 308–310, 316, 322, 337, 397, 399, 411
  as an editor of *The Journal of Sex Education* (*JSE*) 295, 375, 386, 399, 400–401
  as a rationalist 274, 358, 397, 399, 414–415, 420
  as a school student 27, 27–29, 28, 28–36, 195
  as 'Dr Wykeham Terriss' in *Woman*. See *Woman*: articles written by NH as 'Dr Wykeham Terriss'
  as Medical Superintendant, Newcastle Hospital 49–65, 68, 397
  attracting the attention of the security services 18, 32, 297, 300–301, 304, 313, 327, 332, 334, 397
  attractive voice of 10, 41–42, 153, 249, 308, 334, 349–350, 397
  bequest to the University of Sydney 402–406
  birth of 15, 23
  censorship of 327, 331, 333–334, 338, 340, 413, 421
  changes his name 15
  charity work of 111–112, 191, 380–382, 397, 410–411, 417
  childhood of 24–28, 35, 425
  conference papers given by 86, 94–96, 99, 105, 111, 120, 127, 204–205, 217
  death of 395, 400–402, 407–408, 423

death of father 69
death of mother 176–177
direct style of approach of 285, 293–295, 328–329, 345, 355, 400
family background of 16, 21, 68, 129, 138, 304–305, 389
financial situation of 151, 268, 276, 297, 306, 370, 376, 379, 393, 395, 398, 414–415, 417
homosexuality of 129, 131, 199, 215, 311, 397, 399
illness and health of 61–63, 208, 214–215, 225, 229, 265, 272, 275, 279, 281–283, 288, 296–298, 299, 305–306, 314, 317, 329–330, 358, 377–378, 391–393, 397–404
images of 166, 187–188, 204–205, 218, 220
lectures and speeches by 18, 29, 116–117, 122, 126–128, 130, 134, 233, 397
legal troubles of 335–338
library of 362–364, 402–406
medical practices of 18, 72–74, 102, 129, 152–153, 299, 305–306, 327, 361, 376, 397, 410, 414, 426
musical tastes of 41–42
partner of. *See* van de Hagt, Willem
physical appearance of 28, 44–45, 129, 131, 195, 305, 372, 378, 399, 407, 414–415
publications by. *See* publications by NH

publications edited by. *See* publications edited by NH
radio broadcasts by 328, 334, 343
rejuvenation procedures by 105, 107–108, 117, 151, 244–245
residences of NH 18, 23–25, 68, 152–156, 233, 249, 270–271, 273–276, 282, 285, 295, 300, 303–304, 310, 376, 402
return to Australia 299–321
ships travelled on by 67, 230, 233, 299, 361
Halford, SH 114
Hall, Radcliffe 167–168, 386
Hammond, Canon Thomas 357
Hampstead General Hospital (London) 68, 72
Hare, Bert (né Zions) (brother of NH) 17, 217, 307
Hare, Sir John 68
Harmsworth, Alfred 222
Hawthorne, Janie 158
Herzer, Manfred 420
Hesling, Bernard 111, 131, 312, 322, 349
Higgins, EM 317–322
Hill, Arthur 'Bung' 75, 275
Himes, Norman 18, 77, 133, 164, 192, 239–240, 367
contraceptive advice 286
correspondence with NH 145–146, 149–150, 221
criticism of the work of NH 109, 169
disagreement with NH 365, 372–374

Medical history of contraception 103, 226, 287
visit to Nettleden Lodge 295
Himes, Vera 77, 192
Hirschfeld, Magnus 108, 132–133, 143, 146, 198, 201–205, 208, 210–211, 217–219, 228, 236, 265–268, 375, 405. *See also* Institute for Sexual Research (*Institut für Sexualwissenschaft*); International Congress for Sex Research (First, 1926, Berlin)
    disagreement with Albert Moll 176
    establishment of WLSR 163, 165, 167–168
    homosexuality of 18, 224–225, 417–418
Holiday, Billie 329
Hollinworth, May 308, 337
Holtby, Winifred 143
homosexuality 112, 113, 116, 122, 142, 165, 165–166, 171, 175, 177, 183, 196, 202, 209, 223–224, 270, 274, 291–293, 336, 373, 377, 383, 386–391, 393, 417–424. *See also* lesbianism
    laws regarding 217, 223, 389–391, 421
    persecution of homosexuals 202
Horan, Ronald 29, 36
Horder, Lord Thomas 156–157, 226, 365–366
Houlbrook, Matt 291–292
Housman, Laurence 173, 189
How-Martyn, Edith 72, 299, 308, 376

Hoyer, Niels 222
Humbert, Eugène 178
Hunter, John 74
Huxley, Aldous 92, 173, 184, 284, 409
Huxley, Julian 176–178, 231–232, 244
hygiene 81, 104, 163, 286, 318, 328, 365
    in hospitals 45, 49–52

I

impotence 75, 248, 249, 253, 254–255, 259, 260, 261–262, 341
incest 141, 143, 223
infertility 74, 75, 321, 341, 368
influenza pandemic 53–61, 397. *See also* quarantine
    The Influenza Report 53–54, 64
    McAlister, Frederick 56–59
Inge, Dean William 142–143
Institute for Sexual Research (*Institut für Sexualwissenschaft*) 108, 111, 171, 211, 214, 227, 261, 266. *See also* Hirschfeld, Magnus
Institute for Sexual Science 171
Institute of Family Relations 76
International Birth Control Conference, (Sixth, 1925, New York) 127
International Birth Control Conference (Seventh, 1930, Zurich) 204–205, 219, 245
International Congress for Sex Research (First, 1926,

Berlin) 77–79, 90, 130, 133, 169, 171, 181–183, 190
International Congress for Sex Research (Second, 1930, London) 203
International Eugenics Congress (First, 1912, London) 102
International Federation of Socialist Doctors 208
International Medical Group for the Investigation of Contraception 206
International Meeting for Sexual Reform on a Sexological Basis (1921) 171
International Planned Parenthood Federation 375
Isherwood, Christopher 419–420, 423
Ives, George 115, 189, 377, 418
IVF 409. *See also* artificial insemination (AI)

J

Jacobs, Aletta 158
James, Henry 35
James, William 125
Jeffreys, Sheila 178
Jerdan, Ernest 193–202, 268, 283, 395, 407
Jerdan, Rachael 194–199
Jorgensen, Christine née George 222

K

Kapp, Edmond X 164–165
Kenna, Florence 331–332

Keynes, John Maynard 108, 112, 144, 172
Kilgour, AJ 28–31
Kinsey, Alfred 18, 26, 295, 375, 382, 390–391
Kirkby, Elisabeth 415
Kisch, EH 227
Knowlton, Charles 83
Koestler, Arthur 237, 394–395
Kollontai, Alexandra 189
Kortum, LA 59, 61–62
Krafft-Ebing, Richard 132, 227, 367

L

Lafitte-Cyon, Françoise 181–185, 276–277, 281, 362, 369–373
Lambert Pharmacal Company 145
Lambeth Conference 80, 352
Lampel, Peter Martin 201–202
Lanchester, Elsa 166
Lane, Allen 221
Lane, John 219, 234, 282
Lane, Sir William Arbuthnot 70, 94, 96, 99, 157–158, 160, 222
Lansbury, George 136
Laski, Frida 130, 171
Laski, Harold 130, 172
Latukefu, Ruth 209, 311, 311–312, 381
League of Catholic Women 331
League of Nation Life 120
Leask, Eric 33
Lehfeldt, Hans 187, 407
lesbianism 167, 178, 217, 386. *See also* homosexuality
Leunbach, JH 185, 205, 211
Lewis, Joseph 235

Lewis, Roy 408
Lindsay, Jack 194, 201
Lindsey, Judge Ben 73, 375
Lockie, Ruby 198, 203, 282
London Jewish Medical Society 227, 268
Lowin, Paul 310
Ludovici, Anthony M 117–118, 123–124, 162
Lutyens, Sir Edwin 281
Lyons, Dame Enid 346–349, 352–353, 356–357, 415

M

Mackaness, George 29
Magnus Hirschfeld Society 420
Malinowski, Bronislaw 172, 177–178, 231
Malthusianism 115
Malthusian League 76–77, 81–86, 94, 105, 115, 148, 192, 224, 351, 402. See also New Generation League
 birth control clinic 81–82, 84
 The Malthusian 401
 Walworth Clinic 208
Mannin, Ethel 155, 187, 197–199, 221, 247, 249–255, 271, 293, 299, 370, 411, 414–416
marriage 115, 179, 184, 213, 339, 341. See also trial marriage
Marshall, Alan John 'Jock' 361–362
masturbation 32, 109, 141, 143, 240, 248, 293, 339, 341, 373, 388, 391, 424
McLaren, Angus 26, 259, 416, 421
medical ethics 81, 86, 94, 115, 119, 125, 132, 143–144, 184, 190, 217, 223, 328, 339, 340, 351, 355
mental illness 45, 201
Menzies, Robert 349
miscarriage 211, 212
Moll, Albert 171, 176, 181, 203–204. See also Hirschfeld, Magnus: disagreement with Albert Moll
Mond, Alfred (Baron Melchett) 96
monogamy 125
Monson, Jan 306
Montagu, Ivor 173, 182, 189
 Bluebottles 39, 165–166
mortality
 infant 15–16, 25, 102–103, 212
 maternal 15–16, 323
motherhood 115, 159, 348–350, 356
Mottram, VH 180–181
Munster, George 29, 413–414, 417
Murray, Gilbert 170

N

National Archives of Australia 300
National Birth Control Association 207
National Birth-Rate Commission 134
National Council for Combating Venereal Disease 395
National Health and Medical Research Council 315, 333
National Health Service (NHS) 377
National Library of Australia (NLA) 363

National Security Act and
   regulations 301, 312,
   331–332, 383
Natusch, Guy 330, 340
Neo-Malthusian Conference (1922)
   86, 94
Neo-Malthusian League 119, 121
New Education Fellowship 318,
   411
Newfield, Maurice 162
New Generation League 149, 174.
   See also Malthusian League
Newton, Ivor 278, 281
Nicholas, Harold 357
Nightingale, Florence 128,
   388–389
No. 4 Military Hospital (Randwick)
   45, 49, 54
Nordau, Max 276
Norman Haire Fellowship 16
North Kensington Women's
   Welfare Clinic 192

O

obscenity. *See also* censorship
   charges of 64, 98, 235, 237, 325,
   327
   laws 287, 289
   trials 78, 221, 386
obstetrics 73, 152
O'Connor, Armand Stiles 'Paddy'
   251–252, 380
Olfield, Josiah 329
Order of the Golden Dawn 248
orgasm 238, 293, 409, 420
Orwell, George 193
O'Sullivan, Chris 312

P

Paul, Eden 90, 93, 117, 118, 122
Pearce, GF 45–46
Peckham Health Centre 134
Peel, Sir John 157
Piddington, Marion Louisa 76–77
Pillay, AP 365–367, 370–371,
   373–374, 376
placebo effect 92, 257–258
Planned Parenthood Federation
   390
Plomer, William 269–270, 407
Poland 16, 21–22
polyandry 408
polygamy 125, 141, 143, 187, 272
Pope Pius XII 186–187, 274, 359,
   369, 391
population debate 307, 341, 356,
   361, 366, 368, 397
pornography 236
pregnancy 341, 376, 381
pre-marital sex 142–143, 330
Preston-Stanley, Millicent 73
Preterm (abortion clinic, Sydney)
   385
Priestley, JB 173
Promethean Society 229–230
pronatalism 146
prostitution 132, 143, 179, 203,
   216, 245, 341, 391
'Pry, Paul' (Thomas Burke) 129,
   131, 275–276, 291–292
psychiatry 260, 390
psychoanalysis 69, 77, 196, 198,
   200
psychology 77, 201, 259, 323
psychosocial medicine 212

puberty 32, 341, 383, 391, 413, 424
publications by NH
  Birth-control methods 110, 283, 287, 289, 316–317, 334, 395, 401
  The comparative value of current contraceptive methods 409
  Everyday sex problems 185, 236, 384, 412
  The future of marriage 283
  Hymen 137–143, 167, 279, 286, 408
  Manual of contraceptive technique for medical practitioners and students 97
  Marriage hygiene 267
  Methods and technique of prevention of contraception 290
  Rejuvenation 107, 117, 126–127
  'Sex and the juvenile community' 333
  Sex problems of today 317, 320, 325
  Sex talks 107, 327, 424
  Some more medical views 25, 157, 160–161
  Through a doctor's spectacles 44
publications edited by NH
  The encyclopaedia of sex practice 240, 262
  The encyclopaedia of sexual knowledge 235, 237–240, 284–287, 416
  The encyclopaedia of sexual knowledge Volume II 240
  'The international library of sexology and psychology' series 93, 117, 219, 221, 289

Medical views on birth control 157

Q

quarantine 53–57. See *also* influenza pandemic
Queen Victoria 15, 131

R

Racial Hygiene Association 316
radio 362, 387
  as an effective method of communication 339
Reddie, Cecil 178
Reich, Annie 219
rejuvenation 87–92, 119, 163, 184, 241, 248, 252–255, 260–262, 417. See *also* vasectomy
  Benda, Carl 90
  Benjamin, Harry 91
  Blum, Victor 92
  Brown-Séquard, Charles-Édouard 87
  Cavazzi, Franscisco 146
  Lichtenstern, Robert 92
  Schmidt, Peter 92
  Testogan 261
  Yohimbine 261
religious opposition to birth control 84, 100, 109, 120–121, 135–136, 142, 157, 158, 160–161, 186, 206, 223, 230–231, 242–243, 321, 327, 329, 331–332, 334, 339, 346, 352–355, 357–358, 367, 373, 379, 381, 391, 398, 411–412, 415
rickets 149

Riddell, Elizabeth 323, 325–326, 329–330, 413, 415
Rodriguez, Hildegart 228–229
Roland, Betty 300, 309–310, 378
Roman Catholic Federation for Large Families 120
Ross, Marjorie 369–371
Rout, Ettie 99–100
Royal Hospital for Women (Paddington) 44
Royal Institute of Public Health 128
Ruben-Wolf, Martha 189
Rublee, Juliet 128, 191
Ruck, Berta 271–272, 398
Russell, Dora 18, 125, 130, 177, 198, 212, 213, 225, 230, 270, 279, 404–405, 409. *See also* World League for Sexual Reform (WLSR): International Congress of the World League for Sexual Reform (Third, 1929, London)
  financial situation of 276
  marketing for the WLSR 114–115, 180, 184
  pregnancy 202–203
  treasurer of the WLSR 179
Russell, Lord Bertrand 98, 142, 170, 186, 189, 193–195, 233, 249, 305, 375
Rutgers, Johannes 'Jan' 119–122

S

Saffron Hill Welfare Maternity Centre 100
Sanger, Margaret 18, 26, 97–98, 133, 137, 143, 148, 164, 191, 204, 222, 227–228, 230–231, 290, 368–369, 382. *See also* International Birth Control Conference (Seventh, 1930, Zurich); World League for Sexual Reform (WLSR): International Congress of the World League for Sexual Reform (Third, 1929, London)
  Birth Control International Centre 224
  correspondence with NH 80–83, 365, 376, 390, 402
  Critic and guide 82, 190
  disagreements with Marie Stopes 78–79
  disagreements with NH 114–116
  funding of the Malthusian League 94
  invitation to visit Nettleden Lodge 270, 282
  opinion on access to contraceptives 120–127
  opinions on eugenics 104, 308
  opposition to laws regarding contraceptives 287
  perception of 70–71
Savill, Gloria (niece of NH) 17–18, 408
Scharlieb, Dame Mary 163
Schmidt, Peter 206
sectarianism 353, 357
Semmler, Clement 351
sex advice 323, 339. *See also Woman*

sex aids 289, 387
sex change 239
sex determination 416–417
sex education 32, 108, 128,
    145–146, 185–186, 200, 223,
    230, 258, 286, 289, 295, 307,
    314–316, 320–321, 323,
    330–332, 338, 341, 345–346,
    373, 375, 398–400, 411. *See
    also* sex advice; *Woman*
Sex Education Society (SES)
    300–301, 375–377, 379, 391,
    398, 400, 404, 421
sexology 105, 108, 132, 190, 224,
    238, 305–306, 375, 388,
    391–392, 397, 400
sex reform movement 410. *See
    also* World League for
    Sexual Reform (WLSR);
    birth control movement
sexual anxieties 35, 36, 245, 248,
    278
sexual morality 142, 398
Shand, Justice John 335–336
Shaw, Sir George Bernard 44, 70,
    76, 167, 186, 189, 232, 274,
    275, 322, 337, 349, 395
Shenfield, Gillian (relative of NH)
    7, 17, 68, 129, 261
Shrank, Ettie (relative of NH) 16
Siedlecky, Stefania 15, 17, 312
Sieff, Israel 179
Smith, Hamblin 158
socialism 136–137, 164, 208, 209,
    213
Society for Constructive Birth
    Control and Racial Progress
    84, 87

Society for the Prevention of
    Venereal Disease 395
Society for the Provision of Birth
    Control Clinics 151, 208
Society for the Scientific Study of
    Sexuality 391
Southern, George 231–232
Sprott, WJH 'Sebastian' 107–108,
    141, 144, 153, 173
statistics, imortance of 204–205
Steinach, Eugen 87, 88–91, 93, 108,
    119, 152, 252, 257, 262, 400.
    See also rejuvenation
Stein, Gertrude 193
Stekel, Wilhelm 238
Stephensen, Percy 'Inky' 275–276
sterilisation 94–95, 97, 104, 116,
    143, 145, 152, 179, 185–186,
    241, 244, 250, 284–286, 290,
    307, 366, 368, 376–377,
    390, 401. *See also* eugenics;
    rejuvenation
  laws 242–244
  methods of 117
  Nazi sterilisation program 243
sterility 96, 236, 254, 307
Stewart, David 'Dave' 317–319
Stone, Abraham 217, 285, 288
Stone, Hannah 127, 158, 217,
    287–288
Stopes, Marie 18, 71, 97–100,
    111–112, 134, 158, 187, 196,
    244, 382
  birth control clinic 77, 80, 84,
    148, 192
  Committee of Research into
    Contraceptives 86
  Contraception 210, 290

disagreements with NH 103–104, 116, 177, 191, 209–210, 233–234, 402
Married love 26, 139
A new gospel to all peoples 100
public advocation of birth control 83–86
representation of 26
Stopes v. Sutherland 84, 146
Wise parenthood 100
Storer, Robert 234–235
Strachey, Lytton 173
Street, Jessie 205, 348, 353, 356–357
suicide 33, 151, 183, 193, 196, 196–200, 267–269, 323, 329, 395, 418
Sumner, Sir John 77
Supervia, Conchita 278–281, 395
Sutherland, Halliday 84, 102, 110–111, 120, 158, 163, 176
Sydney University Dramatic Society (SUDS) 17, 41, 195, 308, 322

T

taboos 418
'Tao Li' (Li Shiu Tong) 224, 266–267
transvestitism 112, 224, 367
trial marriage 316, 408
Tynan, Kenneth 215

U

Ulrichs, Karl 132
United Associations of Women 320

United Nations 368
University of Sydney 16, 39, 41, 44, 193, 242, 279, 311, 313, 318–320, 424
urolagnia 369

V

Vachet, Pierre 205–208, 210–215
van de Hagt, Willem 112, 228, 297, 371, 402, 422–425
van de Velde, Theodoor 237, 259
van Gogh, Vincent 19, 398
van Wein, Mona 310, 349
vasectomy 88–89, 107, 241
venereal disease (VD) 16, 72, 99, 156, 179, 226, 272, 314–315, 317, 319–320, 323, 325, 328, 330–331, 333, 340–341, 345, 358, 382–383
Vercoe, Richard H 102–103
Viner, Katharine 409
Voge, Cecil 230
Voronoff, Serge 88, 93, 163, 252

W

Walpole, Hugh 173, 184, 297
Walworth Women's Welfare Centre 192, 399, 401
Watt, Chris 123
Weatherhead, Leslie 315
Weisskopf, Josef 218
Wells, HG 76, 117, 165, 179, 183, 229, 232, 285
White, Patrick 193
Whitlam, Gough 17
Whitlam, Margaret 17, 308, 335
Wigmore Hall 18, 114, 172–173, 190, 281

Wilde, Oscar 115, 421
Wilmot, Chester 334
Windeyer, Justice WC 325
Woman 17, 322, 323, 325–326, 329–331, 337, 340–342, 358, 361, 377–378, 398, 401, 411–413, 415, 424
  articles written by NH as 'Dr Wykeham Terriss' 323, 325–327, 334, 336, 341, 399, 413, 415
Women's Christian Temperance Union 318, 331, 358
Woolf, Leonard 167, 269
Woolf, Virginia 113, 167, 254, 269
Workers' Birth Control Group 130, 171
Workers' Educational Association (WEA) 317–319, 411
World League for Sexual Reform (WLSR) 215, 233, 266, 282, 395, 404
  association with socialism 209, 228
  committment to education 242
  decline of 218–219, 265, 320, 375
  founding of 163, 165, 168, 170
  International Congress of the World League for Sexual Reform (First, 1921, London) 168, 293–294
  International Congress of the World League for Sexual Reform (Third, 1929, London) 114, 169–191, 170–173, 179, 181–183, 187–188, 191, 194–195, 203, 234, 244, 397, 400, 409–410
  International Congress of the World League for Sexual Reform (Fourth, 1930, Vienna) 202–203, 206–207, 219
  International Congress of the World League for Sexual Reform (Fifth, 1932, Brno) 121, 193–194, 205, 212, 218, 220
  Le problème sexuel 203
  membership of 204, 212–213
  SEXUS 208, 287
  work towards law reform 424
World Population Congress (1927, Geneva) 219
World War I 41, 44, 53, 107, 172, 424
World War II 32, 225, 227, 287, 288, 290, 295–297, 308, 375, 380, 385
wartime censorship 397. See also censorship
wartime security 300–302, 304, 312–313, 333–334, 343
Worrall, Ralph 75
Wright, Helena 208, 419–420
'Wykeham Terriss'. See *Woman*: articles written by NH as 'Dr Wykeham Terriss'
Wyndham, Diana 110

Y

Yeats, WB 107, 245–246, 248, 249, 250–256, 260–262

Z

Zajac, Louis Levy (grandfather of NH) 21
Zajac, Simon (uncle of NH) 21
Zajac, Solomon (uncle of NH) 21
Zions, Clara (mother of NH) 23–25, 140
Zions, Henry (né Zajac) (father of NH) 21–24, 26

www.ingramcontent.com/pod-product-compliance
Lightning Source LLC
Chambersburg PA
CBHW071958150426
43194CB00008B/920